Talar Osteochondral Defects

C. Niek van Dijk • John G. Kennedy
Editors

Talar Osteochondral Defects

Diagnosis, Planning, Treatment, and Rehabilitation

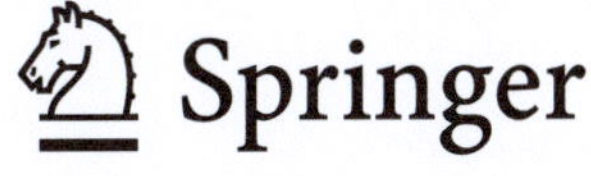

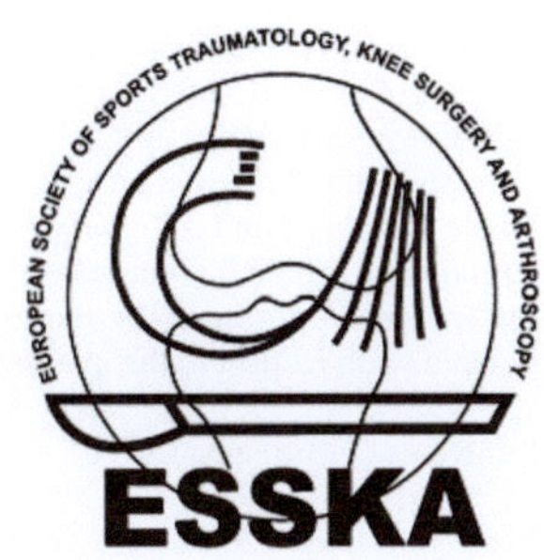

Editors
C. Niek van Dijk, MD, PhD
Department of Orthopaedic Surgery
and Traumatology
Academic Medical Center
University of Amsterdam
Amsterdam
The Netherlands

John G. Kennedy, MD, MCh,
FRCS (Orth)
Department of Orthopaedic Surgery
Hospital for Special Surgery
New York, NY
USA

Project coordinators
Arthur J. Kievit, MD, PhD Fellow
Department of Orthopaedic Surgery
Orthopaedic Research Centre Amsterdam
Academic Medical Center
University of Amsterdam
Amsterdam
The Netherlands

Christopher D. Murawski, BS
Department of Orthopaedic Surgery
Hospital for Special Surgery
New York, NY
USA

ESSKA ASBL
Centre Médical
Fondation Norbert Metz
76, rue d'Eich
1460 Luxembourg
Luxembourg

ISBN 978-3-662-51462-7   ISBN 978-3-642-45097-6   (eBook)
DOI 10.1007/978-3-642-45097-6
Springer Heidelberg New York Dordrecht London

Springer is part of Springer Science+Business Media (www.springer.com)

Preface

This book on Talar Osteochondral Defects is the first publication of ESSKA-AFAS. The book is a compilation of opinion from world experts assembled at the first International Congress on Cartilage Repair of the Ankle ESSKA-AFAS Dublin 2012.

ESSKA is the European Society of Sports Traumatology, Knee Surgery and Arthroscopy and AFAS is one of its specialised sections – Ankle and Foot Association.

ESSKA-AFAS is the European forum for sports-related ankle and foot pathology (and the use of arthroscopy). It brings together all the leading lights and, having formed such a pool of expertise, it promotes their endeavours. It ensures that discoveries and new techniques are promptly disseminated; it nurtures an environment for research; and it enforces strict professional standards.

By doing all this, it can ensure that its patients – those with sports-related ankle and foot injuries – receive the very best treatment that is available.

We hope there will be many more such contributions from ESSKA-AFAS. If you are interested in the activities of ESSKA and its specialised sections and committees, please consult the website on www.esska.org where you will find membership details.

We acknowledge Arthur J. Kievit, as the book's co-ordinator, and Christopher D. Murawski for his assistance.

Amsterdam, The Netherlands   C. Niek van Dijk
New York, USA   John G. Kennedy

Contents

1 Diagnosis of Chondral Injury After Supination Trauma 1
Wataru Miyamoto, Masato Takao, and Hajo Thermann

2 Arthroscopy After Ankle Fracture 9
James W. Stone, Jin Woo Lee, Hang Seob Yoon,
and Woo Jin Choi

3 Diagnosis of Osteochondral Lesions by MRI 21
Thomas M. Link, Patrick Vavken, and Victor Valderrabano

**4 Diagnosis of Osteochondral Defects of the Talus
by Computerized Tomography (CT) and Single-Photon
Emission Computed Tomography (SPECT-CT)** 31
Mies A. Korteweg, Martin Wiewiorski, Geert J. Streekstra,
Klaus Strobel, Victor Valderrabano, and Mario Maas

5 Diagnosis of Osteochondral Defects by Arthroscopy 43
David E. Oji, David A. McCall, Lew C. Schon,
and Richard D. Ferkel

6 Preoperative Planning for Osteochondral Defects 51
Inge C.M. van Eekeren, Arthur J. Kievit,
and C. Niek van Dijk

7 Surgical Approach to Lateral OLT 55
Mark E. Easley and Samuel B. Adams Jr.

8 Approach to Osteochondral Lesions of the Medial Talus 67
Keir A. Ross, Niall A. Smyth, and John G. Kennedy

9 Approach to Osteochondral Lesions of the Tibial Plafond . . . 75
Steven M. Raikin

10 Meta-analysis on Therapy 83
Maartje Zengerink and C. Niek van Dijk

11 Outcome Scores 95
Inger N. Sierevelt, Christiaan J.A. van Bergen,
Karin Grävare Silbernagel, Daniel Haverkamp,
and Jón Karlsson

12 Follow-up Imaging for Osteochondral Lesions of the Ankle 105
Keir A. Ross, Niall A. Smyth, Francesca Vannini, and John G. Kennedy

13 Return to Sports 113
Inge C.M. van Eekeren and C. Niek van Dijk

14 Rehabilitation After Bone Marrow Stimulation 119
Inge C.M. van Eekeren, Kyriacos I. Eleftheriou, Christiaan J.A. van Bergen, and James D.F. Calder

15 Rehabilitation After Replacement Procedures (i.e., OATS, Allograft) 129
Ágnes Berta, László Hangody, and Mark E. Easley

16 Rehabilitation After Cartilage Reconstruction 135
Tomasz T. Antkowiak, Richard D. Ferkel, Martin R. Sullivan, Christopher D. Kreulen, Eric Giza, and Scott R. Whitlow

17 Talar Dome Resurfacing with the HemiCap Prosthesis 145
Mikel L. Reilingh and C. Niek van Dijk

Index 151

Contributors

Samuel B. Adams, Jr., MD Department of Orthopaedic Surgery, Duke University Medical Center, Durham, NC, USA

Tomasz T. Antkowiak, MD, MS Department of Orthopaedic Surgery, Southern California Orthopedic Institute, University of California, Los Angeles, Van Nuys, CA, USA

Ágnes Berta, MD, MSc, MRes Department of Orthopaedics and Traumatology, Uzsoki Hospital, Budapest, Hungary

Department of Traumatology, Semmelweis University, Budapest, Hungary

James D.F. Calder, MD, FRCS (Tr&Orth), FFSEM Department of Trauma and Orthopaedics, Chelsea and Westminster Hospital, The Fortius Clinic, London, UK

Woo Jin Choi, MD, PhD Department of Orthopaedic Surgery, Yonsei University College of Medicine, Seoul, South Korea

Mark E. Easley, MD Department of Orthopaedic Surgery, Duke University Medical Center, Durham, NC, USA

Kyriacos I. Eleftheriou, MBBS, MD, FRCS (Tr&Orth) Department of Trauma and Orthopaedics, Hippocrateon Private Hospital, Nicosia, Cyprus

Richard D. Ferkel, MD Department of Orthopaedic Surgery, University of California Los Angeles, Los Angeles, CA, USA

Southern California Orthopedic Institute, Van Nuys, CA, USA

Eric Giza, MD Department of Orthopaedics, Foot and Ankle Surgery, University of California, Sacramento, CA, USA

László Hangody, MD, PhD, DSc Department of Orthopaedics and Traumatology, Uzsoki Hospital, Budapest, Hungary

Department of Traumatology, Semmelweis University, Budapest, Hungary

Daniel Haverkamp, MD, PhD Department of Orthopaedic Surgery, Slotervaart Hospital, Amsterdam, The Netherlands

Jón Karlsson, MD, PhD Department of Orthopaedics, Sahlgrenska University Hospital, Gothenburg University, Gothenburg, Sweden

John G. Kennedy, MD, MCh, FRCS (Orth) Department of Orthopaedic Surgery, Hospital for Special Surgery, New York, NY, USA

Arthur J. Kievit, MD, PhD Department of Orthopaedic Surgery, Orthopaedic Research Centre Amsterdam, Academic Medical Center, University of Amsterdam, Amsterdam, The Netherlands

Mies A. Korteweg, MD, PhD Department of Radiology, Academic Medical Center, University of Amsterdam, Amsterdam, The Netherlands

Christopher D. Kreulen, MD, MS Department of Orthopaedic Surgery, SutterAuburn Orthopaedics, Sutter Medical Group, Auburn, CA, USA

Jin Woo Lee, MD, PhD Department of Orthopaedic Surgery, Yonsei University College of Medicine, Seoul, South Korea

Thomas M. Link, MD, PhD Department of Radiology and Biomedical Imaging, University of California, San Francisco, CA, USA

Mario Maas, MD, PhD Department of Radiology, Academic Medical Center Amsterdam, University of Amsterdam, Amsterdam, The Netherlands

David A. McCall, MD Department of Orthopaedic Surgery, Southern California Orthopedic Institute, University of California, Los Angeles/Van Nuys, CA, USA

Wataru Miyamoto, MD, PhD Department of Orthopaedic Surgery, Teikyo University School of Medicine, Tokyo, Japan

Christopher D. Murawski, BS Department of Orthopaedic Surgery, Hospital for Special Surgery, New York, NY, USA

David E. Oji, MD Division of Foot and Ankle, Department of Orthopaedics, Medstar Union Memorial Hospital, Baltimore, MD, USA

Steven M. Raikin, MD Department of Orthopaedic Surgery, Rothman Institute, Jefferson Medical College, Thomas Jefferson University Hospital, Philadelphia, PA, USA

Mikel L. Reilingh, MD, PhD Department of Orthopaedic Surgery, Orthopaedic Research Centre Amsterdam, Academic Medical Center, University of Amsterdam, Amsterdam, The Netherlands

Keir A. Ross, BS Department of Orthopaedic Surgery, Hospital for Special Surgery, New York, NY, USA

Lew C. Schon, MD Department of Orthopaedics, Medstar Union Memorial Hospital, Baltimore/Washington, DC, USA

Division of Foot and Ankle, Johns Hopkins School of Medicine and Georgetown School of Medicine, Johns Hopkins University, Baltimore/Washington, DC, USA

Inger N. Sierevelt, PT, MSc Department of Orthopaedic Surgery, Orthopaedic Research Centre Amsterdam, Academic Medical Center, University of Amsterdam, Amsterdam, The Netherlands

Karin Grävare Silbernagel, PT, ATC, PhD Department of Physical Therapy, Samson College of Health Sciences, University of the Sciences in Philadelphia, Philadelphia, PA, USA

Niall A. Smyth, MD Department of Orthopaedic Surgery, Hospital for Special Surgery, New York, NY, USA

James W. Stone, MD Department of Orthopaedic Surgery, Medical College of Wisconsin, Milwaukee, WI, USA

Geert J. Streekstra, PhD Department of Radiology, Academic Medical Center, University of Amsterdam, Amsterdam, The Netherlands

Klaus Strobel, MD, PhD LA Nuklearmedizin/Radiologie, Luzerner Kantonsspital, Luzern, Switzerland

Martin Sullivan, MBBS(Hons), FRACS, FAOrthA Department of Orthopaedic Surgery, St Vincent's Clinic, Sydney, NSW, Australia

Masato Takao, MD, DMSc Department of Orthopaedic Surgery, Teikyo University School of Medicine, Tokyo, Japan

Hajo Thermann, MD, PhD ATOS Clinic, Center for Hip, Knee and Foot Surgery, Sport Surgery, Heidelberg, Germany

Victor Valderrabano, MD, PhD Orthopaedic Department, University Hospital of Basel, Basel, Switzerland

Christiaan J. A. van Bergen, MD, PhD Orthopaedic Research Centre Amsterdam, Department of Orthopaedic Surgery, Academic Medical Center, University of Amsterdam, Amsterdam, The Netherlands

C. Niek van Dijk, MD, PhD Department of Orthopaedic Surgery and Traumatology, Academic Medical Center, University of Amsterdam, Amsterdam, The Netherlands

Inge C.M. van Eekeren, MD, PhD Orthopaedic Research Centre Amsterdam, Department of Orthopaedic Surgery, Academic Medical Center, University of Amsterdam, Amsterdam, The Netherlands

Francesca Vannini, MD, PhD First Clinic of Orthopaedics and Traumatology, Rizzoli Orthopaedic Institute, University of Bologna, Bologna, Italy

Patrick Vavken, MD Orthopaedic Department, University Hospital of Basel, Basel, Switzerland

Scott R. Whitlow, MD Department of Orthopaedics, University of California, Sacramento, CA, USA

Martin Wiewiorski, MD Orthopaedic Department,
University Hospital of Basel, Basel, Switzerland

Hang Seob Yoon, MD Department of Orthopaedic Surgery,
Seoul Wooridul Hospital, Seoul, South Korea

Maartje Zengerink, MD, PhD Department of Orthopaedic Surgery,
Orthopaedic Research Centre Amsterdam, Academic Medical Center,
University of Amsterdam, Amsterdam, The Netherlands

Introduction

We are proud to present you the first ESSKA-AFAS production on the subject of talar osteochondral defects (OCD).

Current areas of interest in the field of talar OCDs are improvements in accurate diagnosis, sound pre-operative planning, optimal treatment and procedure specific rehabilitation protocols. This book will address these topics with special emphasis on diagnosis and rehabilitation. The technical difficulties on these subjects are discussed and the guidelines are based on the currently best available evidence.

Adequate treatment is important since the majority of these lesions occur in young and active individuals.

As physical examination is insufficient for diagnosing an OCD, surgeons are dependent on additional imaging. Imaging modalities used are standard radiography, computed tomography (CT), magnetic resonance imaging (MRI) and positron emission tomography–computed tomography (PET-CT). For each different surgical method specific imaging techniques can aid the surgeon in planning the procedure.

The choice of treatment is mostly guided by the localization and size of the lesion. Different treatment options can be considered. Options include both arthroscopic and open approaches, with additional osteotomies or ligament turndowns for better access to lesions. Current treatment options include bone marrow stimulation (BMS), fixation, retrograde drilling and autologous chondrocyte implantation (ACI). Larger lesions can be treated with autologous osteochondral transfer (OATS), osteochondral allograft, or HemiCap. Orthobiologics are playing an expanding role in all procedures. Also, corrective osteotomy has to be considered.

There are still clear challenges in optimizing rehabilitation following treatment of ankle OCDs. Advancements have been made with fast track rehabilitation protocols. This book will provide an overview of the direct post-operative treatment and rehabilitation protocols for all the different treatment options.

The content of this book has been written by a team of experts in the field of foot and ankle surgery. Their review and opinions are based on the best currently available evidence. It is filled with the ins and outs of diagnosis, planning, treatment and rehabilitation of talar OCDs and will provide the reader with an up-to-date handbook in approaching a patient with a talar OCD.

Amsterdam, The Netherlands
New York, USA
C. Niek van Dijk
John G. Kennedy

Diagnosis of Chondral Injury After Supination Trauma

Wataru Miyamoto, Masato Takao, and Hajo Thermann

Take-Home Message
- *CT scan and MRI have a similar accuracy for detection of a talar OCD; CT scan is preferred for preoperative planning.*
- *New imaging techniques include SPECT-CT scan and dGEMRIC.*
- *Arthroscopic examination is the definitive method for assessment.*

1.1 Introduction

Ankle injuries caused by forced supination are the most common injuries affecting the foot and ankle. Recent investigation revealed that an osteochondral lesion (OCL) of the ankle is an increasingly common injury following the common ankle sprain [22]. Berndt and Harty reported on possible mechanisms for the occurrence of OCL on the talar dome after supinating ankle trauma. They reported two predilection sites, the lateral and medial side [3]. According to their report, an ankle positioned in inversion and dorsiflexion predisposes for an OCL on the lateral side, while medial lesions occur mostly with the ankle positioned in inversion and plantar flexion [3]. They also reported that 57 % of OCL to the talar dome were located medially and 43 % laterally [3].

Clinical symptoms and physical examination are the bases for correct diagnosis of an OCL in the ankle. However, because clinical findings can be nonspecific, diagnostic imaging is routinely performed if an OCL is suspected. Routine X-rays have long been the first choice for diagnostic imaging, but due to lack of detail on aspect and location, there is usually a necessity for further imaging such as computed tomography (CT) or magnetic resonance imaging (MRI) [17]. Recent advances of MRI in detecting injury of articular cartilage are remarkable; there are several established classification systems for OCL of the talus based on MRI findings [11, 15, 21]. Despite these advances, CT remains the imaging of choice for talar OCL. Imaging is effective not only for diagnosis of OCL but also for deciding on treatment options.

1.2 History

The classic history preceding an OCL is supination or pronation trauma. Furthermore, hindfoot valgus and "flatfoot type" can be predisposing factors for injury. A combination of complaints of persistent pain, hematoma, and swelling over a

W. Miyamoto, MD, PhD (✉) • M. Takao, MD, DMSc
Department of Orthopaedic Surgery, Teikyo
University School of Medicine, Tokyo, Japan
e-mail: miyamotokumakura@yahoo.co.jp;
mtakao@med.teikyo-u.ac.jp

H. Thermann, MD, PhD
ATOS Clinic, Center for Hip, Knee and Foot Surgery,
Sport Surgery, Heidelberg, Germany
e-mail: hajo.thermann@atos.de

C.N. van Dijk, J.G. Kennedy (eds.), *Talar Osteochondral Defects*,
DOI 10.1007/978-3-642-45097-6_1, © ESSKA 2014

period of 3–4 weeks following an ankle sprain is suspect for an osteochondral or chondral lesion of the talus.

1.3   Clinical Evaluation

In the acute phase, it can be difficult to clinically diagnose an OCL of the ankle due to severe pain resulting from the primary supination trauma. If there are remaining symptoms following treatment of acute supination trauma such as dull deep ankle pain, swelling, restriction of range of motion, locking, or crepitus, surgeons should suspect an OCL. As mentioned above, the two predilection sites are the lateral and medial talar dome. OCL on the medial side tends to be located more posterior while OCL on the lateral side tends to be located more anterior [3]. Therefore, palpation for tenderness should be performed with the ankle in full plantar flexion if a medial lesion is suspected, but mild plantar flexion can be sufficient if a lateral lesion is suspected.

Sharp deep pain located at the medial or lateral joint space longer than 1 or 2 weeks after trauma is clinically suspect for more than just ligament injury. That is why, and even more so in athletes, there is an indication for a further imaging using CT or MRI.

1.4   Radiological Examination

As mentioned above, routine diagnostic imaging, such as radiography assisted by CT and/or MRI, is necessary for the correct diagnosis of an OCL because there is no specific definitive clinical finding.

1.4.1   Radiography (Fig. 1.1a-2)

If an OCL of the ankle is suspected, anteroposterior radiographs with additional lateral and mortise views are the first choice for radiological examination [17]. Berndt and Harty established a 4-stage classification system of OCL of the ankle by evaluating the severity of the lesion through plain radiographs. The four stages are I, a small compression fracture; II, an incomplete avulsion fracture; III, a complete avulsion of a fragment without displacement; and IV, a displaced fragment. This system remains the basis of other classification systems in radiological investigations [3]. However, up to 50 % of OCL of the ankle is missed if only plain radiography is indicated as diagnostic imaging [13]. Because of the lack of detailed information on the articular cartilage and subchondral bone, plain radiography alone is insufficient for diagnosing an ankle OCL.

1.4.2   CT (Fig. 1.1a-1, 3, b-1, 2)

CT produces detailed information on the size, shape, and extent of displacement of the bony injury. It is especially effective for the evaluation of subchondral (cystic) lesions [7]. Because of its effectiveness, a CT-based classification system was established. The stages of this system are I, a cystic lesion in the talar dome with an intact roof; IIA, a cystic lesion with communication to the talar dome surface; IIB, an open articular surface lesion with an overlaying non-displaced fragment; III, a non-displaced lesion with lucency; and IV, a displaced fragment [8]. A common reported disadvantage of CT compared to MRI is the insufficient ability to evaluate the articular cartilage [17]. To overcome this disadvantage, CT techniques which contain a CT arthrography and helical technology with multiplanar reconstructions have been advanced recently. A study on the comparison of MR arthrography and CT arthrography for the evaluation of cartilage lesions in the ankle joint revealed that CT arthrography was superior to MR arthrography with regard to interobserver variability and detecting articular cartilage lesions [20]. It has also been reported that the diagnostic value of MRI did not prove to be better than high-resolution multidetector helical CT for the detection or exclusion of an OCL of the ankle [23]. Furthermore, single-photon emission computed tomography (SPECT)-CT, a combination of a 3-dimensional scintigraphy bone scan and CT, was introduced as a new tool in the

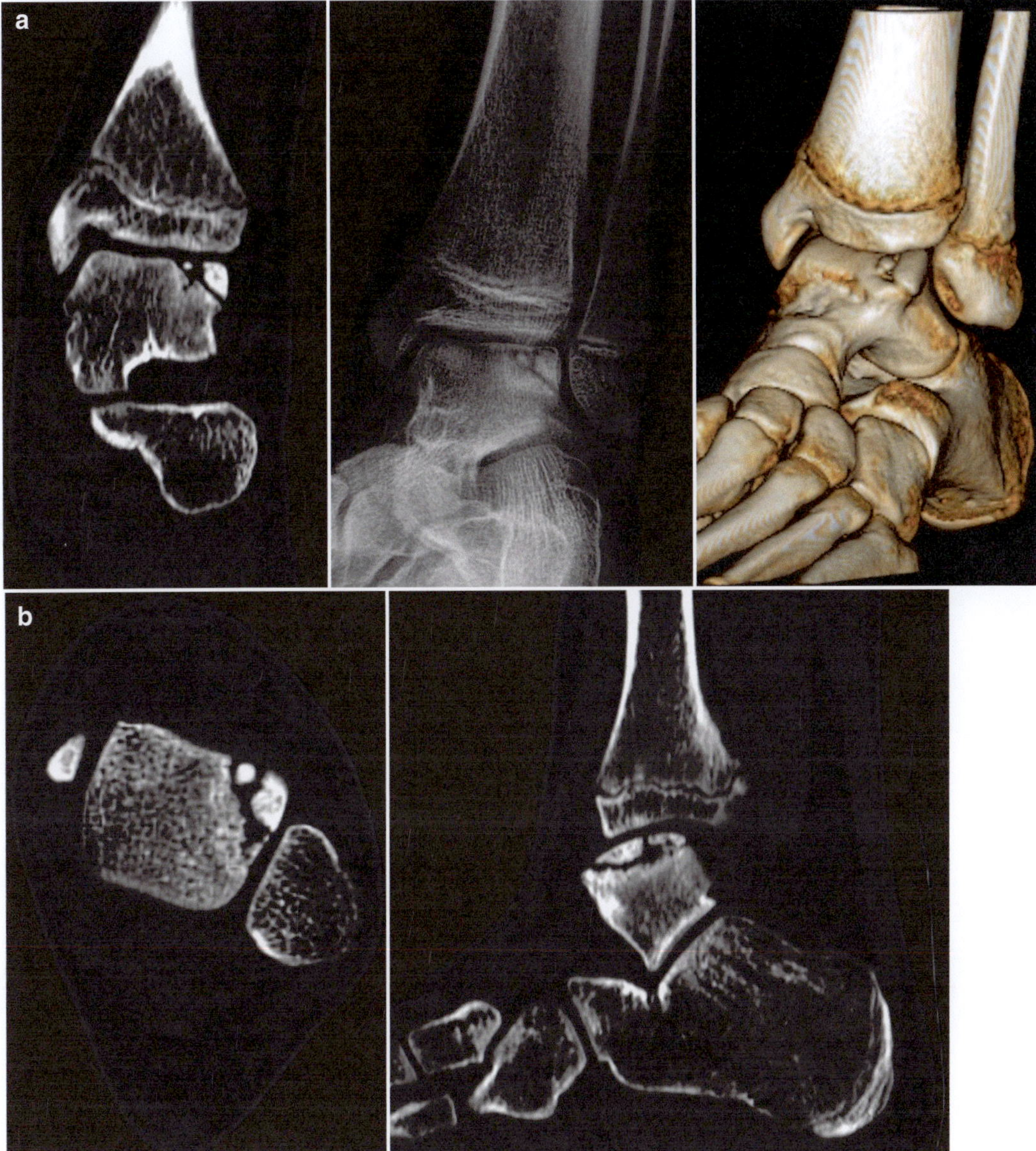

Fig. 1.1 (**a–b**) Osteochondral fracture diagnosed one year after trauma by radiograms and CT scan. (**a**) Coronal view; anteroposterior X-ray; 3D reconstruction. (**b**) Transversal and sagittal view

orthopedic field recently [12, 14]. SPECT-CT detects scintigraphic osteoblastic activity in the area of interest in combination with the anatomic resolution of a CT scan. The effectiveness of SPECT-CT to diagnose OCL of the ankle has been proven in previous literature [12, 14]. SPECT-CT has been compared to MRI for imaging interpretation and decision making in OCL of the ankle [12]. Ankle OCL was evaluated by MRI, SPECT-CT, or a combination of both. SPECT-CT provided additional information and influenced decision making, and it was recommended in this study to perform both MRI and SPECT-CT for diagnostic evaluation in OCL [12]. Another study on the usefulness of SPECT-CT reported that the advantage was an ability to identify the active lesion, especially in multifocal disease or revision surgeries [14].

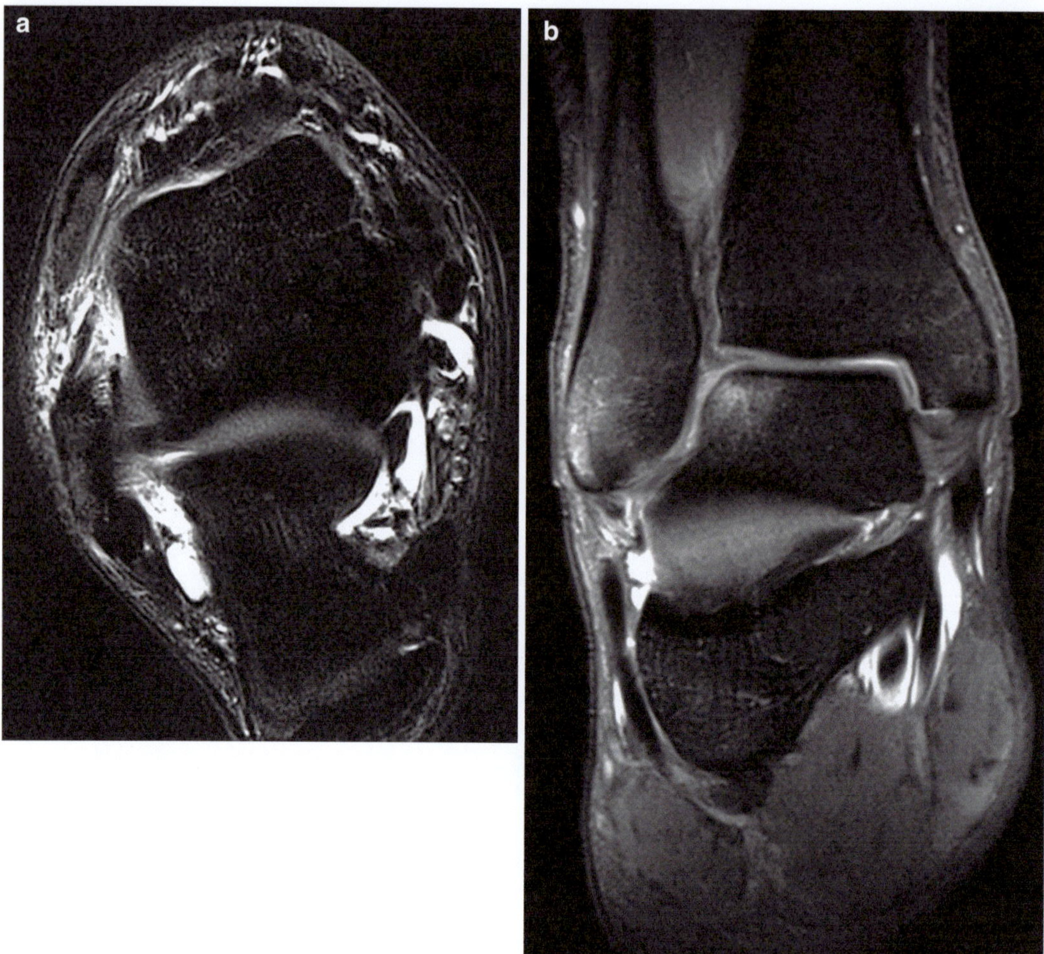

Fig. 1.2 (**a–b**) Professional soccer player with an ankle sprain. MRI revealed FTA rupture and medial talar dome edema

1.4.3 MRI (Figs. 1.2a, b and 1.3a)

MRI has been reported by some as a noninvasive diagnostic imaging of choice for OCL of the ankle [6, 19]. It visualizes the surface of articular cartilage and subchondral bone by means of multiplanar evaluation. There are several classification systems using MRI [11, 15, 21]. One classification system for MRI was based on Berndt and Harty's 4-stage radiographic classification [11]. Another classification system for MRI was based on arthroscopic findings [15]. T2-weighted MRI provides extra information on articular cartilage status and the subchondral bone. A high-intensity area between a fragment and its attachment to the talar dome can indicate instability of the fragment [4].

Three Tesla (T) MRI has also been applied as a diagnostic tool with the expectation of improved visualization of multiple organ systems. The usefulness of such high-resolution imaging is mostly for the diagnosis of OCL in an ankle with thin cartilage [1, 24]. The imaging quality and ability of 3 T MRI to assess cartilage, ligament, and tendon pathology have been tested in fresh human cadaver specimens and compared to 1.5 T MRI. In this study, the imaging quality was found to be significantly higher ($P < 0.05$) at 3 T than at 1.5 T [1]. Furthermore, they emphasized the usefulness of 3 T MRI in assessing cartilage pathology. However, because signal patterns in the talus can exaggerate the severity of the bone injury due to its high

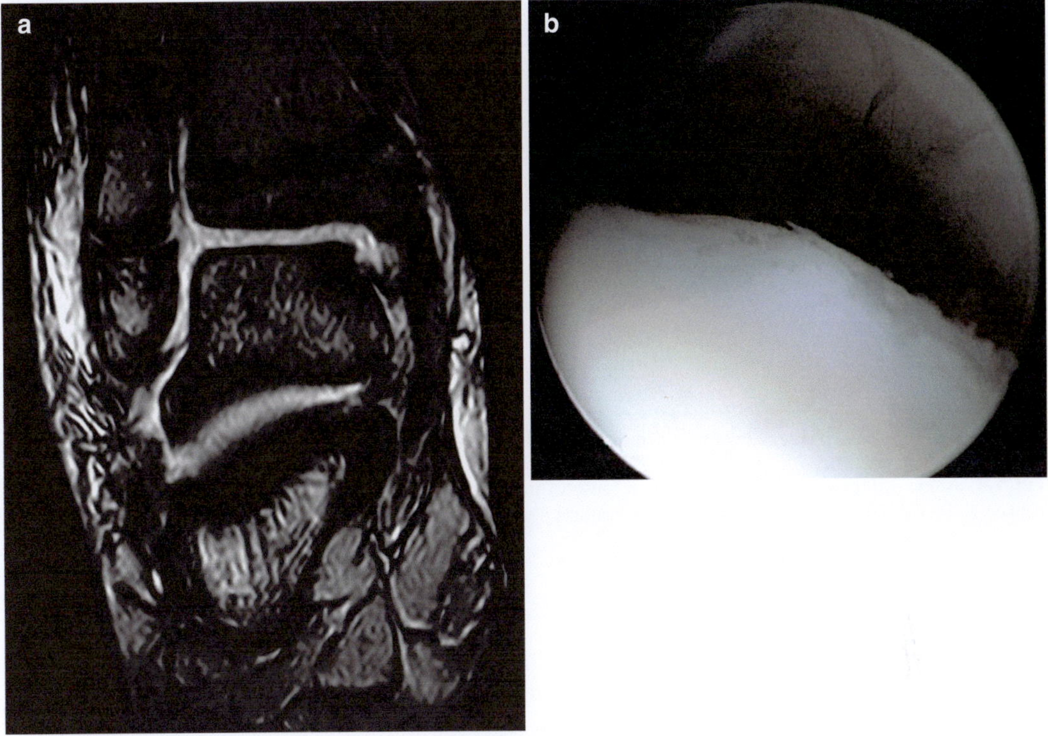

Fig. 1.3 (**a–b**) Small chondral flake medial talus after supination trauma. (**a**) MRI. (**b**) Ankle arthroscopy

sensitivity, the decision making of treatment should be decided through a combination of imaging evaluations [7, 17].

Although MRI is useful for detecting articular cartilage injury with morphological abnormality, it cannot detect degenerative cartilage without morphological change. Recently, new techniques which can quantify the structural and composition change of degenerative articular cartilage have been developed and its application to detect OCL in the ankle is expected [2, 16]. Delayed gadolinium-enhanced magnetic resonance imaging of cartilage (dGEMRIC) technique is considered to be specific for assessing the concentration of glycosaminoglycan (GAG) in cartilage which generally reduces in accordance to degeneration of the cartilage [2]. In this technique, negatively charged gadolinium diethylenetriamine pentaacetic acid (Gd-DTPA^{2-}) is injected intravenously which distributes inversely to the concentration of negatively charged GAG and alters T1 depending on the amount of GAG [2]. The effectiveness of dGEMRIC has been reported for

assessing the thin cartilage layer of the ankle. The technique was used for evaluation of cartilage following matrix-associated autologous chondrocyte implantation [5]. Furthermore, T2 mapping permits evaluation of changes in collagen arrangement and water content in the articular cartilage [16]. Normal articular cartilage contains a close and regular arrangement of collagen with fixed water content. However, as degeneration of the articular cartilage advances, the collagen arrangement becomes irregular and the amount of water content increases, and such changes make T2 intenser than that of normal articular cartilage [16]. This is useful for detection of early-stage degenerative change of articular cartilage and quantitative evaluation of cartilage degeneration [16]. As a clinical evaluation method for OCL of the ankle, T2 mapping has already been used to evaluate cartilage after autologous chondrocyte implantation for OCL of the ankle [10]. Further studies which apply these new techniques for diagnosis of OCL of the ankle are to be expected.

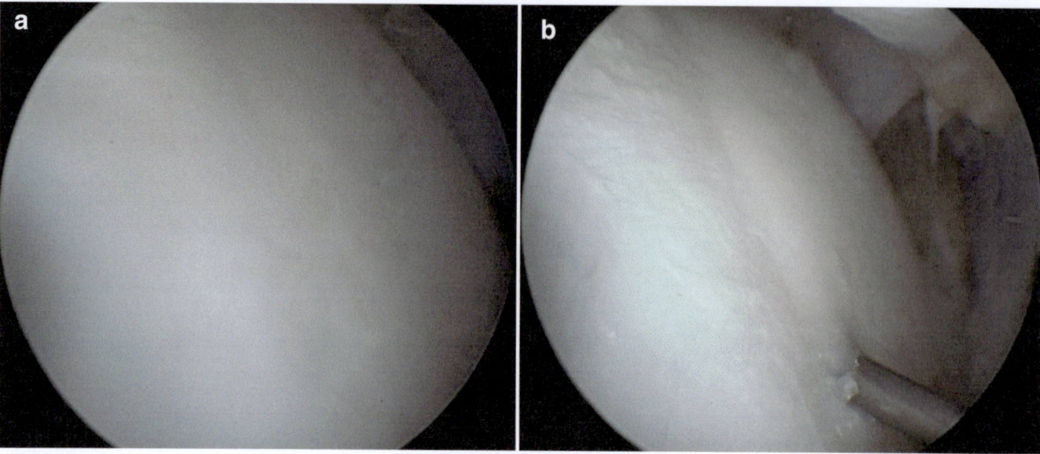

Fig. 1.4 Ankle arthroscopy after 14 months because of pain on exercising: (**a**) Stable cartilage coverage tested by a probe. (**b**) PRP (ACP) injection to enhance subchondral healing response

1.5 Arthroscopic Examination (Figs. 1.3b and 1.4a, b)

Arthroscopy is the most effective diagnostic and staging tool because of direct visualization of articular cartilage injury [18]. Even if cartilage damage cannot easily be confirmed through direct visualization, arthroscopy enables the surgeon to diagnose such lesions by probing the articular surface and feeling for softening and/or fissures. Probing makes it possible to not only diagnose OCL but also to evaluate the extent of the lesion and instability of the fragment. The prospective study by van Dijk and coworkers demonstrated a higher accuracy for arthroscopy in the detection of a talar OCD when compared to MRI and CT scan [23]. Significant correlations between arthroscopic stage and clinical outcome have been reported where no correlation has been found for plain radiographs, computed tomography, or magnetic resonance imaging staging [9]. Generally, arthroscopic diagnosis is combined by surgical intervention such as excision of the fragment, debridement, microfracture, and AMIC procedure.

remains first choice as it is easy and inexpensive, despite reports mentioning its limited value. Further imaging such as CT and/or MRI is necessary for suspected patients. CT is effective especially for cases with subchondral cystic lesions because of its ability to depict the subchondral character of the OCL. Moreover, CT scan is preferred for preoperative planning. Some studies have reported advancement of CT by helical technology with multiplanar reconstructions and SPECT-CT. MRI has been reported as a popular diagnostic tool for OCL of the ankle because it can assess articular cartilage. New uses of MRI are being developed, and recent techniques (dGEMRIC, T2 mapping) make it possible to evaluate degenerative change of articular cartilage quantitatively. However, there is no evidence to support a gold standard for imaging with respect to the diagnosis of ankle OCL. Evaluation using a combination of CT and MRI may be necessary in some cases. Arthroscopic examination is invasive, but it provides the best assessment for the extent of the lesion and (in)stability of the fragment.

> **Conclusion**
> Although clinical findings are important to diagnose an OCL of the ankle, it always needs to be supported by imaging. Radiography

Conflict of Interests The author has no current conflict of interests with the products presented.

References

1. Barr C, Bauer JS, Malfair D, Ma B, Henning TD, Steinbach L, Link TM. MR imaging of the ankle at 3 Tesla and 1.5 Tesla: protocol optimization and application to cartilage, ligament and tendon pathology in cadaver specimens. Eur Radiol. 2007;17:1518–28.
2. Bashir A, Gray ML, Hartke J, Burstein D. Nondestructive imaging of human cartilage glycosaminoglycan concentration by MRI. Magn Reson Med. 1999;41:857–65.
3. Berndt AL, Harty M. Transchondral fractures (osteochondritis dissecans) of the talus. J Bone Joint Surg Am. 1959;41:988–1020.
4. De Smet AA, Fisher DR, Burnstein MI, Graf BK, Lange RH. Value of MR imaging in staging osteochondral lesions of the talus (osteochondritis dissecans): results in 14 patients. Am J Radiol. 1990;154: 555–8.
5. Domayer SE, Trattnig S, Stelzeneder D, Hirschfeld C, Quirbach S, Dorotka R, Nehrer S, Pinker K, Chan J, Mamisch TC, Dominkus M, Welsch GH. Delayed gadolinium-enhanced MRI of cartilage in the ankle at 3 T: feasibility and preliminary results after matrix-associated autologous chondrocyte implantation. J Magn Reson Imaging. 2010;31:732–9.
6. Dunfee WR, Dalinka MK, Kneeland JB. Imaging of athletic injuries to the ankle and foot. Radiol Clin North Am. 2002;40:289–312.
7. Easley ME, Latt LD, Santangelo JR, Merian-Genast M, Nunley II JA. Osteochondral lesions of the talus. J Am Acad Orthop Surg. 2010;18:616–29.
8. Ferkel RD, Sgaglione NA, Del Pizzo W. Arthroscopic treatment of osteochondral lesions of the talus: technique and results. Orthop Trans. 1990;14:172–3.
9. Ferkel RD, Zanotti RM, Komenda GA, Sgaglione NA, Cheng MS, Applegate GR, Dopirak RM. Arthroscopic treatment of chronic osteochondral lesions of the talus: long-term results. Am J Sports Med. 2008;36:1750–62.
10. Giannini S, Battaglia M, Buda R, Cavallo M, Ruffilli A, Vannini F. Surgical treatment of osteochondral lesions of the talus by open-field autologous chondrocyte implantation: a 10-year follow-up clinical and magnetic resonance imaging T2-mapping evaluation. Am J Sports Med. 2009;37 Suppl 1:112S–8.
11. Hepple S, Winson IG, Glew D. Osteochondral lesions of the talus: a revised classification. Foot Ankle Int. 1999;20:789–93.
12. Leumann A, Valderrabano V, Plaass C, Rasch H, Studler U, Hintermann B, Pagenstert GI. A novel imaging method for osteochondral lesions of the talus- comparison of SPECT-CT with MRI. Am J Sports Med. 2011;39:1095–101.
13. Loomer R, Fischer C, Llpyd-Smith R, Sisler J, Cooner T. Osteochondral lesions of the talus. Am J Sports Med. 1993;21:13–9.
14. Meftah M, Katchis SD, Scharf SC, Mintz DN, Klein DA, Weiner LS. SPECT/CT in the management of osteochondral lesions of the talus. Foot Ankle Int. 2011;32:233–8.
15. Mintz DN, Tashjian GS, Connell DA, Deland JT, O'Malley M, Potter HG. Osteochondral lesions of the talus: a new magnetic resonance grading system with arthroscopic correlation. Arthroscopy. 2003;19: 353–9.
16. Nieminen MT, Rieppo J, Töyräs J, Hakumäki JM, Silvennoinen J, Hyttinen MM, Helminen HJ, Jurvelin JS. T2 relaxation reveals spatial collagen architecture in articular cartilage: a comparative quantitative MRI and polarized light microscopic study. Magn Reson Med. 2001;46:487–93.
17. O'Loughlin PF, Heyworth BE, Kennedy JG. Current concepts in the diagnosis and treatment of osteochondral lesions of the ankle. Am J Sports Med. 2010;38:392–404.
18. Pritsch M, Horoshovski H, Farine I. Arthroscopic treatment of osteochondral lesions of the talus. J Bone Joint Surg Am. 1986;68:862–5.
19. Sanders RK, Crim JR. Osteochondral injuries. Semin Ultrasound CT MR. 2001;22:352–70.
20. Schmid MR, Pfirrmann CWA, Hodler J, Vienne P, Zanetti M. Cartilage lesions in the ankle joint: comparison of MR arthrography and CT arthrography. Skeletal Radiol. 2003;32:259–65.
21. Taranow WS, Bisignani GA, Towers JD, Conti SF. Retrograde drilling of osteochondral lesions of the medial talar dome. Foot Ankle Int. 1999;20:474–80.
22. Van Buecken K, Barrack RL, Alexander AH, Ertl JP. Arthroscopic treatment of transchondral talar dome fractures. Am J Sports Med. 1989;17:350–6.
23. Verhagen RAW, Maas M, Dijkgraaf MGW, Tol JL, Krips R, van Dijk CN. Prospective study on diagnostic strategies in osteochondral lesions of the talus: is MRI superior to helical CT? J Bone Joint Surg Br. 2005;87:41–6.
24. Welsch GH, Mamisch TC, Weber M, Horger W, Bohndorf K, Trattnig S. High-resolution morphological and biochemical imaging of articular cartilage of the ankle joint at 3.0 T using a new dedicated phased array coil: in vivo reproducibility study. Skeletal Radiol. 2008;37:519–26.

Arthroscopy After Ankle Fracture

James W. Stone, Jin Woo Lee, Hang Seob Yoon, and Woo Jin Choi

Take-Home Message

- *There is a general agreement that there is a high incidence of intra-articular lesions associated with ankle fractures.*
- *In acute ankle injury, some of these conditions may be missed, resulting in chronic ankle pain.*
- *Although the available data do not conclusively support the use of arthroscopy, it has become an important adjunct to the management of ankle fractures to prevent chronic complaints.*

J.W. Stone, MD (✉)
Department of Orthopedic Surgery,
Medical College of Wisconsin,
Milwaukee, Wisconsin, USA

Department of Orthopedic Surgery,
3111 W. Rawson Ave., Suite 200,
Franklin, WI 53132, USA
e-mail: jamesstonemd@gmail.com

J.W. Lee, MD, PhD • W.J. Choi, MD, PhD
Department of Orthopaedic Surgery,
Yonsei University College of Medicine, Seoul, South Korea
e-mail: ljwos@yuhs.ac; choiwj@yuhs.ac

H.S. Yoon, MD
Department of Orthopaedic Surgery,
Seoul Wooridul Hospital, Seoul, South Korea
e-mail: hsyoon79@yuhs.ac

2.1 Introduction

Ankle fractures are some of the most common lower extremity injuries. In treating these fractures, emphasis has been placed on strict adherence to the principles of anatomical restoration of the ankle joint and mortise with rigid fixation and early movement in order to achieve improved functional outcomes [2, 11, 31]. However, some studies of ankle fractures have shown poor clinical results, including chronic pain, arthrofibrosis, recurrent swelling, and perceived instability despite anatomical restoration of the ankle joint and mortise following fractures [4, 8]. Some patients develop posttraumatic degenerative arthritis despite apparent anatomic restoration of the joint surfaces as evaluated by postoperative radiographs. Although the reasons for this remain unclear, many have postulated that occult articular cartilage injury or imprecise restoration of the articular cartilage surface may be responsible for gradual joint degeneration [1, 6, 10, 14, 15, 20, 21, 23].

Our understanding of arthroscopic anatomy improved in the latter half of the twentieth century. Refinements in equipment and technique have allowed many procedures for ankle surgery formerly performed using open exposures to be effectively performed using minimally invasive arthroscopic techniques. The main indications for ankle arthroscopy include treatment of soft tissue impingement lesions, anterior bony impingement, degenerative arthritis, and osteochondral lesions of the talus [27]. Ankle arthroscopy has been recommended in the definitive treatment of

C.N. van Dijk, J.G. Kennedy (eds.), *Talar Osteochondral Defects*,
DOI 10.1007/978-3-642-45097-6_2, © ESSKA 2014

ankle fractures to confirm and manage associated intra-articular injuries in order to reduce the incidence of chronic complaints following fixation of severe ankle fractures [1, 10, 14, 15, 20, 21].

The incidence of intra-articular injuries following ankle fractures and their optimal treatment remain unclear despite multiple clinical investigations. This chapter reviews the incidence of intra-articular lesions at the time of acute ankle fracture to determine the scope of the clinical problem. Concomitant treatments for these articular injuries at the time of the operation for the ankle fracture are discussed to outline the current evidence for the optimal approach to this clinical problem.

2.2 Incidence of Articular Cartilage Injury at the Time of Ankle Fracture

There is a wide variability in the reported incidence of articular cartilage injury at the time of ankle fracture. Our ability to assess and compare studies on this topic is impaired because of variability of inclusion criteria, nonuniform classification schemes, lack of control groups, inconsistent length of follow-up, and variable evaluation criteria utilized in these studies. Grouped together, these studies suggest that the incidence of articular cartilage injury in acute ankle fracture is between 17 and 79.2 % [1, 6, 13–15, 20].

In 1991, Lantz and co-workers [13] retrospectively reviewed the intraoperative findings of 63 inspections for operatively reduced malleolar fractures. They found "cartilaginous injury" on the talar dome in 31 patients. There was only one full-thickness articular cartilage injury with exposure of the subchondral bone, with the others constituting partial-thickness articular cartilage injuries of varying depth. However, the fact that this study utilized direct visualization of the dome of the talus via arthrotomy rather than performing arthroscopy may have resulted in less complete visualization of the talar surface.

In 2000, Hintermann and co-workers [10] prospectively studied 288 consecutive patients who underwent surgical treatment for acute fractures of the ankle. Articular cartilage lesions were noted at arthroscopic evaluation in 79.2 % of ankles, more often on the talus (69.4 %) than on the distal tibia (45.8 %), fibula (45.1 %), or medial malleolus (41.3 %). This incidence of articular defects (79.2 %) is higher than that generally quoted in the literature, and the authors attributed this difference to the inclusion of "any articular cartilage injury" including those on the talus, distal tibia, fibula, and medial malleolus. The frequency and severity of the cartilage lesions were also demonstrated to increase with increasing severity of ankle fracture from type B to type C when the fractures were categorized according to the AO-Danis-Weber classification [19]. They stressed that arthroscopy is useful in identifying associated intra-articular lesions in acute fractures of the ankle.

In 2002, Loren and Ferkel [15] reported a retrospective review of 48 consecutive patients with acute unstable fractures of the ankle who underwent ankle arthroscopy followed by open reduction and internal fixation. Traumatic articular surface lesions, including chondral defects and osteochondral lesions measuring greater than 5 mm in diameter, were identified in 30 of the 48 ankles (63 %). Eleven lesions were localized to the tibia and 19 noted on the talus. Similar to the Hintermann study, they found an increased incidence of traumatic articular cartilage injuries with increasing injury severity from Danis-Weber B injuries (41.7 %) to Danis-Weber C injuries (72.7 %).

More recently, Leontaritis and co-workers [14] analyzed the correlation between severity of an acute ankle fracture and number of arthroscopically detected intra-articular chondral lesions. The severity of the fracture was found to be associated with an increased number of chondral lesions.

Associated lesions of articular cartilage remain a diagnostic challenge in acute ankle fracture. Given the lack of evidence-based literature, it is not possible to definitively recommend the use of arthroscopy for the management of ankle fractures. Although there is ample evidence documenting a high incidence of articular cartilage injuries in ankle fractures requiring open reduction and internal fixation along with the ability of arthroscopic techniques to diagnose and treat these lesions, there is not definitive evidence that arthroscopic treatment of these lesions affects the clinical results in the short or long term.

Glazebrook and coauthors reviewed 92 studies of ankle arthroscopy published as of August 2008 [9]. Each article was assigned a level of evidence I–IV based on the type of study using the criteria of Wright and coauthors [30]. A level of grade of recommendation was then determined for each procedure ranging from A (good evidence), B (fair evidence), and C (poor-quality evidence) to I (insufficient or conflicting evidence not allowing a recommendation for or against intervention) [29]. There were two level I studies and two level IV studies of ankle arthroscopy in the treatment of acute ankle fractures included in their review. They suggested an "I" grade of recommendation (insufficient evidence to recommend for or against intervention) for arthroscopy for acute ankle fractures based upon their review.

2.3 Treatment of Articular Cartilage Injury at the Time of Operative Treatment of Ankle Fracture

The indications for nonoperative and operative treatment of osteochondral lesions of the talus are controversial due to conflicting reports regarding efficacy. The concept that osteochondral lesions are best treated surgically dates back to at least the publication of study by Berndt and Harty in 1959 [5]. In their review of the literature and using their own clinical evidence, poor results were seen in a high proportion of patients treated nonoperatively. In contrast, good results were obtained in 84 % of patients treated surgically. Another study also showed that outcome was less satisfactory in ankle fractures when there was a talar dome lesion identified at the time of original treatment [13].

Options for operative treatment of acute osteochondral fractures include internal fixation of separated lesions which demonstrate uninjured articular cartilage with sufficient subchondral bone to support fixation or fragment excision followed by stimulation of the base using curettage, abrasion, or microfracture. These procedures may be performed either by open arthrotomy of the ankle joint or by arthroscopy performed prior to definitive fixation of the ankle fracture.

Arthroscopy has evolved into a safe and effective technique for debridement, curettage, and drilling of osteochondral lesions of the talus. Arthroscopy is a good adjunct to fracture management in patients with acute osteochondral injury associated with an ankle fracture requiring reduction and fixation. Although clinical outcomes of arthroscopic treatment for chronic osteochondral lesions have been well reported, a paucity of literature exists regarding the outcome of arthroscopic treatment of acute osteochondral fractures.

In a prospective randomized controlled trial of 19 patients with ankle fractures, Thordarson and co-workers [25] compared open reduction and internal fixation with and without arthroscopy. Although eight of nine patients in the arthroscopy group had articular damage to the talar dome, no difference in outcome was noted between the two groups at a mean of 21 months follow-up.

In a large prospective study of 153 patients with ankle fractures, Boraiah and co-workers [6] performed ankle arthroscopy followed by open reduction and internal fixation and reported similar results. Although they found 26 (17 %) associated osteochondral lesions on the talar dome, no interventions were performed on these lesions when detected. No significant difference in the functional outcome was noted between patients with and those without osteochondral lesions among various fracture patterns.

In a recent study by Aktas and co-workers [1], the authors performed arthroscopic debridement and drilling of acute cartilage lesions when required in acute ankle fractures. No significant difference in functional outcomes was noted between patients with or without osteochondral lesions among various fracture patterns. They concluded that an arthroscopic or open inspection of the talar dome should be routinely considered in the surgical repair of ankle fractures.

Although previous studies of osteochondral lesions contain occasional reports of internal fixation, no large studies are available on which to base definite recommendations. The best candidate for internal fixation is a young patient with an acute large osteochondral fracture. The larger the piece of attached subchondral bone and the healthier the articular cartilage, the greater the likelihood that internal fixation will be successful. These acute osteochondral lesions of the talar dome which may be suitable for open reduction and internal fixation are almost always located on the anterolateral talar surface. The medial lesions tend to be more chronic in nature with poor-quality articular cartilage and bone and are usually most appropriately treated by debridement and stimulation of the bony base. Both open and arthroscopic methods have been used for internal fixation of acute osteochondral fractures in acute ankle fractures. Options for internal fixation of osteochondral fracture include screws, Kirschner wires, and bioabsorbable pins. One of the potential difficulties inherent in fixation with screws is that lesions located posteriorly on the talar dome are challenging to approach using open techniques. It can be difficult to insert the screws. In addition, screws used for fixation may require a second surgery for removal after healing. Fixation with Kirschner wires is less secure than screw fixation, and compression across the fragment cannot be achieved. However, Kirschner wires have the advantage that they can be placed percutaneously into the nonarticular portion of the talus while the joint is monitored arthroscopically.

Methods of internal fixation involving the use of bioabsorbable pins have been studied recently. Advantages over metallic fixation include gradual stress transfer to bone during the resorption process and no need for subsequent removal of the devices [12]. Unfortunately, significant complications from biodegradable fixation methods have been reported in other joints [3, 7], but there is inadequate evidence to establish whether this is also a problem in the treatment of osteochondral lesions of the talus.

There is no evidence regarding the effectiveness of arthroscopic treatment in articular cartilage injuries associated with ankle fractures. Without extended clinical follow-up, it is not possible to determine if early arthroscopic intervention will minimize poor outcomes following ankle fractures. In the future, a large prospective randomized study with long-term follow-up care may provide more conclusive results.

2.4 Role of Arthroscopy in Residual Pain After Ankle Fracture

The goal of treatment of ankle fractures is to obtain an anatomic reduction of the articular surfaces and to hold that position until bony union is achieved, using internal fixation if necessary. Malunion of the articular surfaces is the most important factor contributing to poor long-term outcome following an ankle fracture [18]. Other factors include the presence of various intra-articular abnormalities including associated chondral and osteochondral defects of the articular surfaces. Complaints may be caused by bony spurs, irritation from internal fixation hardware, and soft tissue impingement [24, 26]. Complaints may also be generalized and caused by synovitis or posttraumatic arthritis. However, the etiology of residual pain after ankle fractures and the optimal treatment remain unresolved. Only small case series exist in the English-language literature regarding arthroscopic treatment for residual pain after ankle fractures [16, 24, 26, 28]. Van Dijk and co-workers [28] reported good or excellent results for arthroscopic treatment of residual complaints following ankle fracture in 76 % of patients if complaints could be attributed clinically to anterior bony or soft tissue impingement. If complaints were more diffuse and the definitive diagnosis was not clear before arthroscopy, 43 % of patients reported good or excellent results.

Thomas and co-workers [24] retrospectively reviewed 50 patients who had ankle arthroscopy to evaluate residual pain after an ankle fracture. They found synovitis in 46 ankles and arthrofibrosis in 20 ankles. Chondral lesions of the talus or tibia were present in 45 (90 %) patients. However, they did not analyze the various treatment modalities of the postfracture complaints, nor did they analyze the clinical outcome of arthroscopic treatment.

Utsugi and co-workers [26] performed arthroscopy at the time of hardware removal in 33 consecutive patients who had undergone open reduction and internal fixation for ankle fractures. Articular cartilage damage was noted in 33 % and arthrofibrosis in 73 % of patients. Arthroscopic debridement of fibrous tissue led to improved joint function in 89 % of patients with functional deterioration after an ankle fracture.

These results suggest that ankle arthroscopy may be of value in identifying and managing chronic pain caused by various intra-articular lesions after ankle fracture.

2.5 Role of Arthroscopy in Diagnosis of Syndesmotic Injury

Injuries to the distal tibiofibular syndesmosis frequently accompany rotational ankle fractures. Syndesmotic disruption is typically associated with fibular fractures above the level of the distal syndesmotic ligament [15, 17]. Because syndesmotic instability may lead to chronic ankle pain [6], surgeons must always be aware of this possibility.

The diagnosis of unstable syndesmotic injuries related to acute ankle fracture is based on preoperative radiographs, intraoperative stress testing, and sometimes intraoperative fluoroscopy. Assessment for syndesmotic injury can be augmented with arthroscopic visualization of the syndesmosis while applying rotational stress to the ankle.

Arthroscopy has been shown to demonstrate greater sensitivity in diagnosing syndesmosis injury compared with anteroposterior and mortise radiography [22]. Moreover, patients with unstable syndesmotic injuries are at high risk of associated articular cartilage injury of the talar dome, which can be managed at the time of arthroscopic evaluation of the ankle fracture [15].

In a study of 105 patients with ankle fractures who underwent surgical fixation along with arthroscopic evaluation, Ono and co-workers [20] reported arthroscopic evidence of ligament injury in 54 patients (51.4 %), among whom sole injury to the anterior tibiofibular ligament was most common.

Hintermann and co-workers [10] reported that ligaments around the ankle could not always be identified by arthroscopy, and there were significant differences among those. The anterior tibiofibular ligament was the most commonly seen ligament. The frequency of damage to this ligament was correlated with the severity of the ankle fracture.

Currently, arthroscopy can be indicated for the evaluation of syndesmotic injury. A problem remains in the definition of instability. As some syndesmotic laxity is normal, how much displacement is pathologic and how do we measure this displacement? Although the use of arthroscopy in ankle fractures is increasing, the effectiveness of arthroscopic treatment for syndesmotic injury has yet to be determined.

2.6 Arthroscopic Procedure

Ankle arthroscopy performed in the setting of an acute ankle fracture presents some special considerations when compared to routine ankle arthroscopy. The ankle is usually swollen, and it may be more difficult to locate the anatomic landmarks which determine good portal placement. In addition, careful fluid management is necessary since soft tissue injury to the joint capsule may allow extravasation of fluid to a greater degree than standard arthroscopy.

The patient is placed supine on the operating table with the ipsilateral hip and knee flexed and supported by a well-padded leg holder. A tourniquet is placed on the thigh but only inflated as necessary to control bleeding. A commercially available noninvasive joint distraction device is applied to the ankle. Routine anteromedial, anterolateral, and posterolateral portals are created using a "nick and spread" technique to minimize the risk of injury to superficial neurovascular structures. The location for each portal is determined by first passing an 18 gauge hypodermic needle across the joint to be certain that the position optimizes the ease of passage of instruments across the joint. The anteromedial portal is placed first, immediately adjacent to the medial margin of the tibialis anterior tendon. The 2.7 mm diameter arthroscope is introduced and the location for the posterolateral portal is determined using an 18 gauge needle.

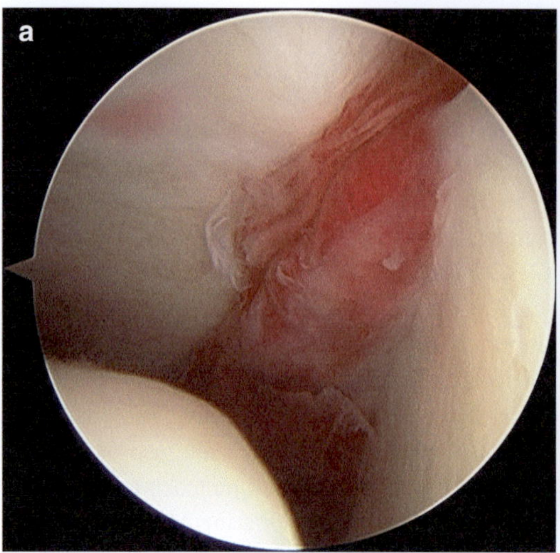
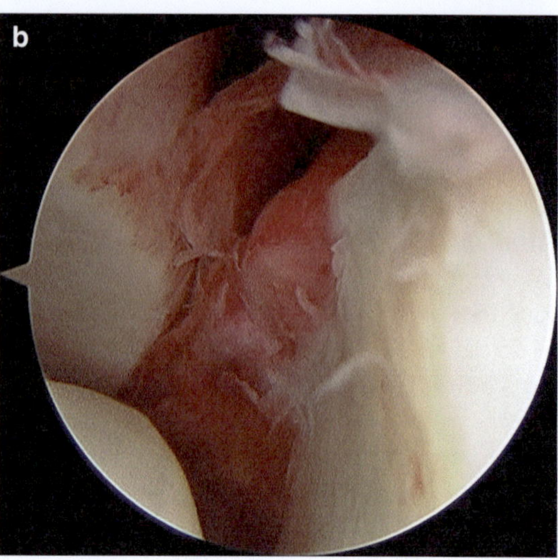

Fig. 2.1 (**a**) Arthroscopic view of distal tibiofibular joint in a left ankle with medial mortise widening on preoperative radiographs. (**b**) Widening of the syndesmosis is demonstrated when external rotation force is applied to the ankle confirming injury to the syndesmosis and the need to stabilize the distal tibiofibular joint, in this case with syndesmosis screw placement

A separate inflow cannula is placed into the posterolateral portal to act as a dedicated inflow portal. The anterolateral portal is placed in a similar fashion just lateral to the peroneus tertius tendon.

The inflow is attached to an arthroscopic fluid pump with the pump pressure set low, approximately 20–25 mmHg, and the flow rate also set on low, approximately 0.5 l/min. The arthroscope is removed from the anteromedial cannula and the joint is irrigated out thoroughly to remove blood, clots, and debris. The inflow pressure and flow rates are adjusted to achieve adequate irrigation at the lowest settings possible to minimize the risk of fluid extravasation. It is very important to monitor the leg intraoperatively on a frequent basis to be certain that there is no excessive swelling.

The arthroscope is reintroduced into the cannula and further debridement of clots and blood may be performed using a shaver. Once good visualization is achieved, the joint is examined in a systematic manner using a probe to examine all of the articular cartilage surfaces for possible chondral or osteochondral injury. Small chondral or osteochondral fragments are removed using a loose body forceps or the shaver (Fig. 2.1).

If an acute osteochondral fragment is noted, the surgeon must decide whether internal fixation or debridement is the appropriate treatment. In general, anterolateral acute osteochondral lesions of the talus have the highest likelihood of having sufficient size and quality of bone to justify internal fixation. If this type of lesion is encountered, internal fixation can be performed arthroscopically or via a small anterolateral arthrotomy approach. If it is elected to debride an osteochondral lesion, then the major fragments are removed using loose body forceps, and the articular cartilage at the periphery is debrided back to well-attached cartilage with perpendicular margins. The base then is stimulated by curettage, abrasion, or microfracture.

If the procedure is being performed for a Maisonneuve injury, it is important to assess the medial gutter for tearing of the deltoid ligament and possible impingement of torn deltoid fibers that could impair anatomic reduction. Torn fibers should be debrided using a shaver, and the ability to anatomically reduce the medial disruption can be assessed arthroscopically.

If there is a suspected syndesmosis injury, then it is important to carefully assess the distal tibiofibular joint arthroscopically. Abnormal motion at the tibiofibular joint can be detected by observing the joint as an external rotation force is

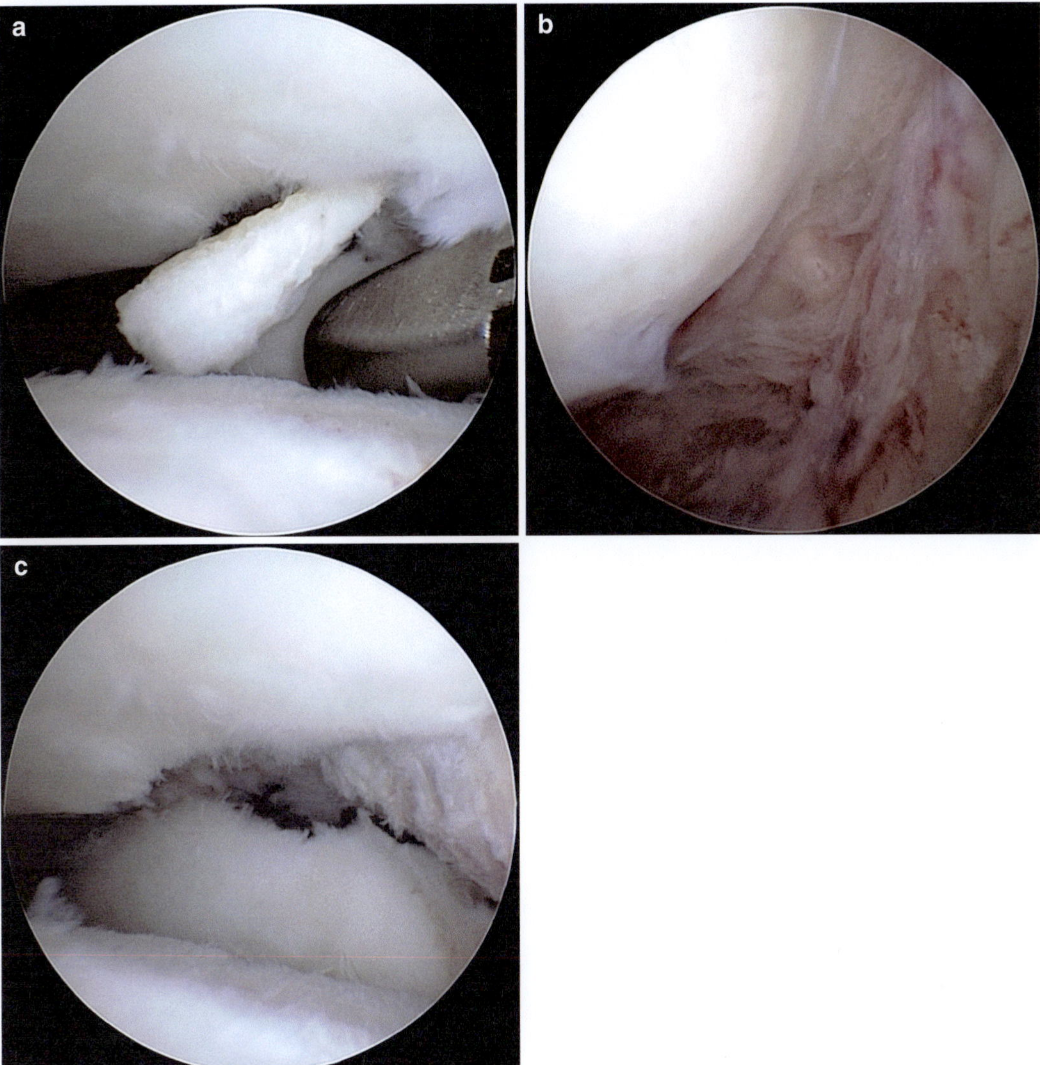

Fig. 2.2 (**a**) This patient presented for treatment of a distal fibula fracture accompanied by widening of the medial mortise which had been neglected for 6 weeks. Initial arthroscopic evaluation of this left ankle demonstrated a loose osteochondral fragment which was removed using a loose body forceps. (**b**) Arthroscopic view of the medial gutter with the medial malleolus on the left and the deltoid below after debridement of clot and debris from the medial gutter. (**c**) Arthroscopic view of lateral malleolus fracture at the level of the joint after debridement of clot and debris. Fixation of the lateral malleolus was then performed using a plate and screws along with a syndesmosis screw to stabilize the distal tibiofibular joint

applied to the ankle joint which will usually cause the joint to visibly spread and then reduce into anatomic position as an internal rotation force is applied (Fig. 2.2).

When arthroscopy is performed in conjunction with internal fixation of an intra-articular fracture of the tibia, such as a medial malleolar fracture or tibial plafond fracture, the fluoroscope is useful as the fracture is temporarily fixed with smooth Kirschner wires. The articular cartilage is anatomically reduced using arthroscopic guidance and major fragments are held with the Kirschner wires. After confirming good position, fixation is performed using cannulated screws.

This type of minimally invasive arthroscopic-assisted internal fixation is particularly useful

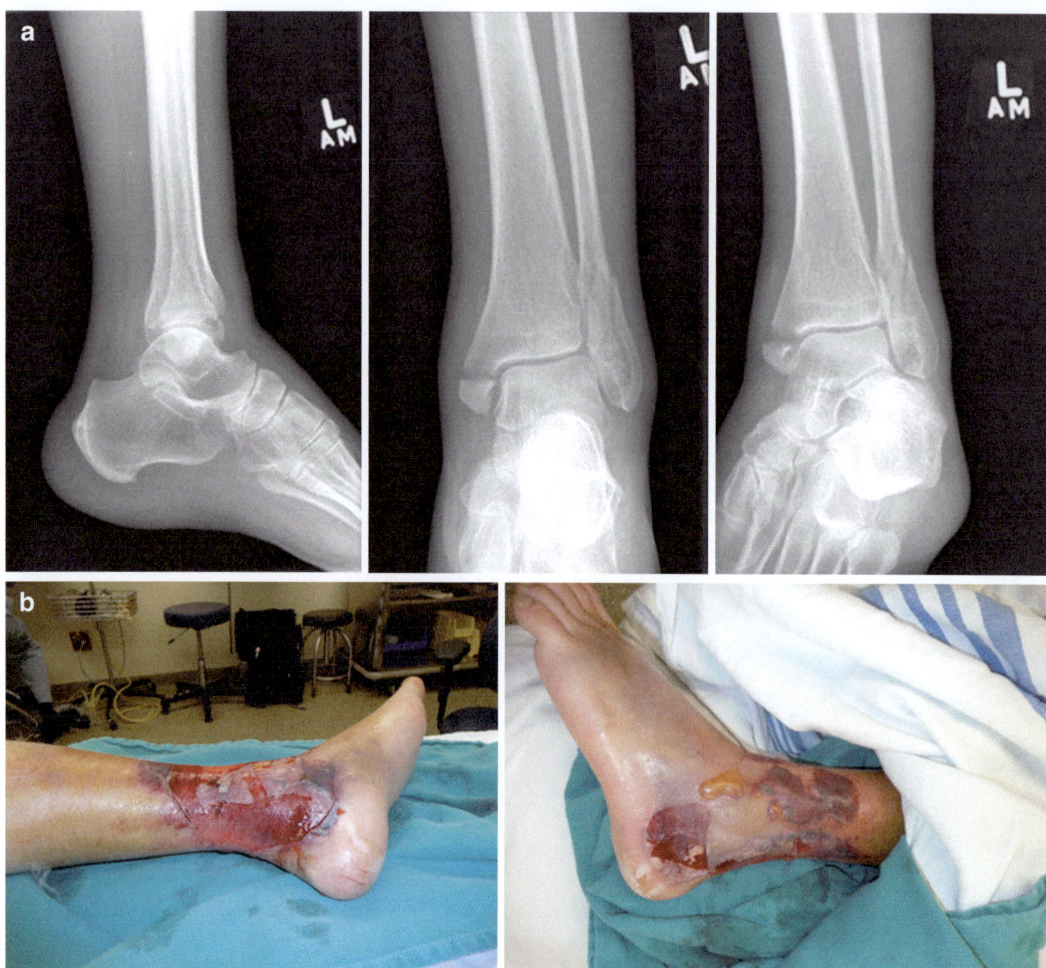

Fig. 2.3 A 65-year-old obese, diabetic female sustained a bimalleolar ankle fracture with significant soft tissue injury. (**a**) Anteroposterior, lateral, and mortise radiographs show the bimalleolar ankle fracture with displacement of the medial malleolar fragment along with slight shortening and rotation of the fibular fracture. (**b**) Photographs of the patient's leg document the severity of soft tissue injury which includes severe swelling with fracture blisters. The treating physician felt that the combination of the soft tissue injury and underlying medical factors including diabetes increased the likelihood of postoperative complications including infection and wound healing and therefore opted to utilize a minimally invasive arthroscopic-assisted approach in treating this patient. (**c**) Intraoperative photograph documenting injury to the syndesmosis. Fibula at right, tibia at upper left, and talus at lower left in this left ankle. (**d**) Intraoperative photograph showing injury to the posterior tibiofibular ligament. (**e**) Intraoperative photograph showing the displaced medial malleolar fracture. (**f**) Intraoperative photograph documenting accurate reduction of the medial malleolar fracture. Provisional fixation was then obtained using smooth K-wires under fluoroscopic guidance, and then screws were utilized to achieve final fixation. (**g–h**) Radiographs show final fixation which includes screw fixation of the medial malleolus, percutaneous intramedullary fixation of the lateral malleolus, and screw stabilization of the syndesmosis. The fractures healed uneventfully, and there were no wound healing complications (This case was contributed by Dr. Alastair Younger, Vancouver, BC, Canada)

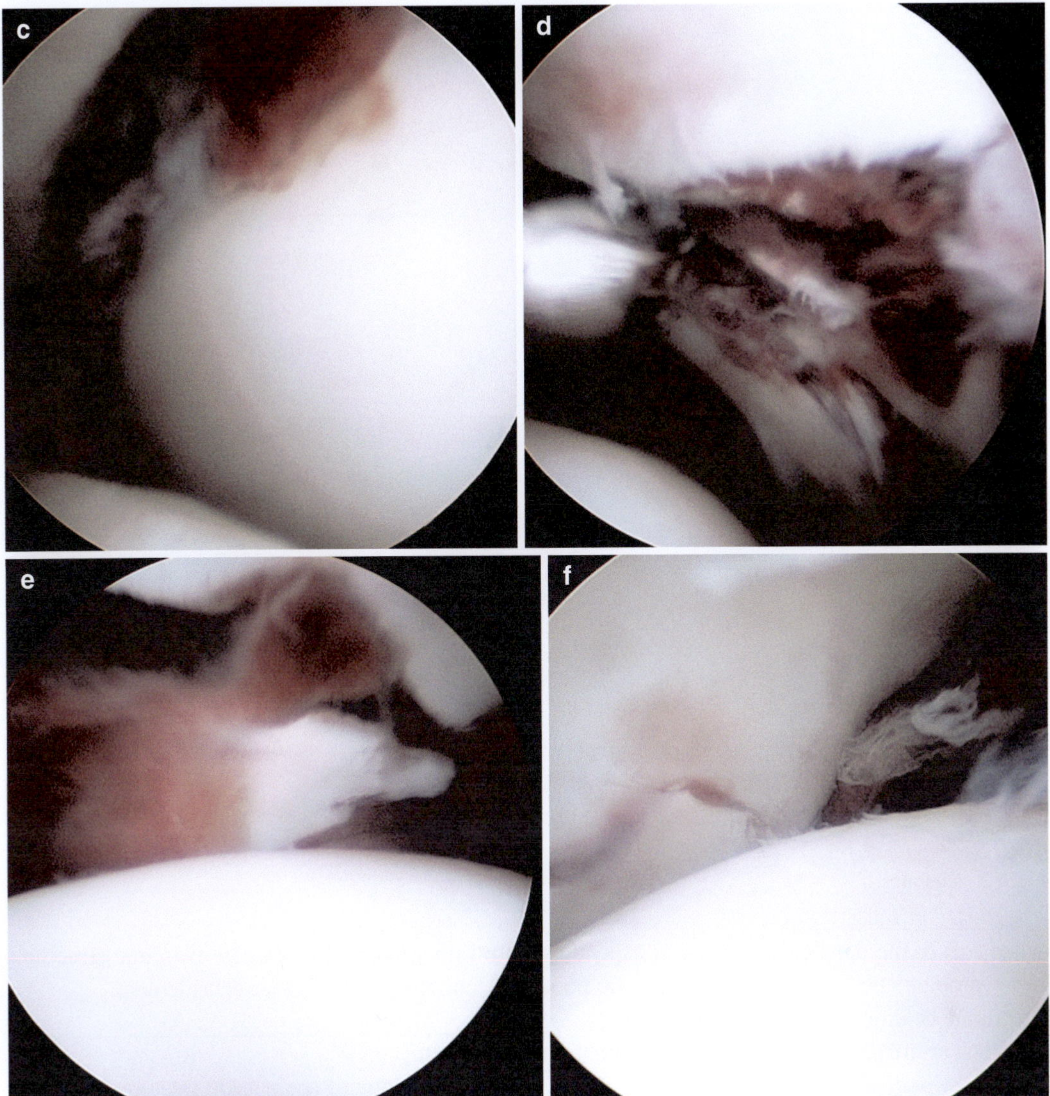

Fig. 2.3 (continued)

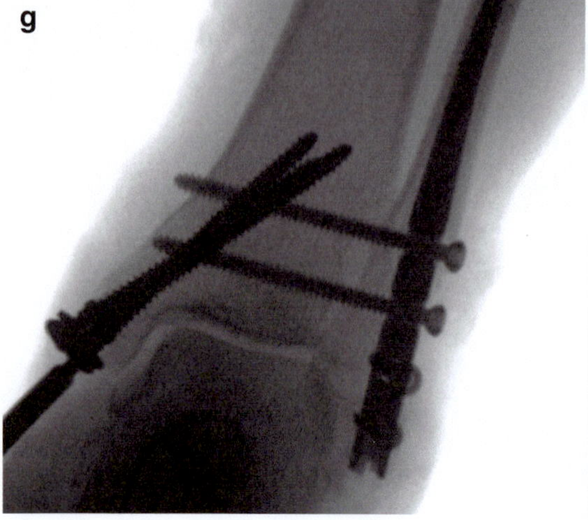

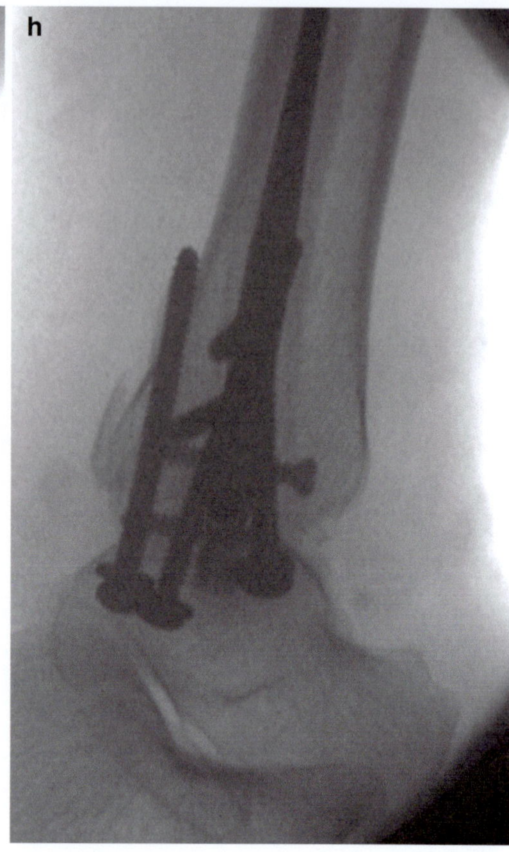

Fig. 2.3 (continued)

when soft tissue damage makes open exposures more problematic, because of the risk of poor soft tissue healing and infection (Fig. 2.3).

When arthroscopy is performed for evaluation of chronic pain after ankle fracture, either in the case of a fracture treated nonoperatively or a fracture treated with open reduction and internal fixation, the procedure is performed in a similar fashion. It is however easier because soft tissue injuries including swelling, possible fracture blisters, and acute injury to the muscle, tendon, or capsule are absent. The same setup with noninvasive distraction and use of a three-portal technique is recommended. In cases where significant adhesions cause painful limitation of range of motion, initial visualization may be difficult. Careful insertion of the arthroscope and shaver will allow initial debridement with creation of a working space. This minimizes the potential for injury to the articular surfaces or inadvertent penetration of the anterior capsule with the potential

for injury to the anterior neurovascular structures or tendons during further debridement.

Conclusions

Arthroscopy of acute ankle fractures is gaining acceptance as a valuable tool for identifying and treating pathology. Identification of intraarticular pathology may allow a more accurate prognosis regarding the outcome of ankle fractures. Arthroscopic examination at the time of open reduction and internal fixation allows the diagnosis and treatment of otherwise unrecognized intra-articular pathology, which may decrease early postoperative complications and improve long-term outcomes. With many potential benefits and minimally increased risks, arthroscopy of acute ankle fractures should be seriously considered in operative cases.

Conflict of Interests The author has no current conflict of interests with the products presented.

References

1. Aktas S, Kocaoglu B, Gereli A, Nalbantodlu U, Guven O. Incidence of chondral lesions of talar dome in ankle fracture types. Foot Ankle Int. 2008;29(3):287–92. PubMed PMID: 18348824. Epub 2008/03/20. eng.

2. Ali MS, McLaren CA, Rouholamin E, O'Connor BT. Ankle fractures in the elderly: nonoperative or operative treatment. J Orthop Trauma. 1987;1(4):275–80. PubMed PMID: 3146619. Epub 1987/01/01. eng.

3. Barfod G, Svendsen RN. Synovitis of the knee after intraarticular fracture fixation with Biofix. Report of two cases. Acta Orthop Scand. 1992;63(6):680–1. PubMed PMID: 1471523. Epub 1992/12/01. eng.

4. Beris AE, Kabbani KT, Xenakis TA, Mitsionis G, Soucacos PK, Soucacos PN. Surgical treatment of malleolar fractures. A review of 144 patients. Clin Orthop Relat Res. 1997;(341):90–8. PubMed PMID: 9269160. Epub 1997/08/01. eng.

5. Berndt AL, Harty M. Transchondral fractures (osteochondritis dissecans) of the talus. J Bone Joint Surg Am. 1959;41-A:988–1020. PubMed PMID: 13849029. Epub 1959/09/01. eng.

6. Boraiah S, Paul O, Parker RJ, Miller AN, Hentel KD, Lorich DG. Osteochondral lesions of talus associated with ankle fractures. Foot Ankle Int. 2009;30(6):481–5. PubMed PMID: 19486623. Epub 2009/06/03. eng.

7. Cahill BR. Osteochondritis dissecans of the knee: treatment of juvenile and adult forms. J Am Acad Orthop Surg. 1995;3(4):237–47. PubMed PMID: 10795030. Epub 1995/07/01. Eng.

8. Day GA, Swanson CE, Hulcombe BG. Operative treatment of ankle fractures: a minimum ten-year follow-up. Foot Ankle Int. 2001;22(2):102–6. PubMed PMID: 11249218. Epub 2001/03/16. eng.

9. Glazebrook MA, Ganapathy V, Bridge MA, Stone JW, Allard JP. Evidence-based indications for ankle arthroscopy. Arthroscopy. 2009;25(12):1478–90. PubMed PMID: 19962076.

10. Hintermann B, Regazzoni P, Lampert C, Stutz G, Gachter A. Arthroscopic findings in acute fractures of the ankle. J Bone Joint Surg Br. 2000;82(3):345–51. PubMed PMID: 10813167. Epub 2000/05/17. eng.

11. Hughes JL, Weber H, Willenegger H, Kuner EH. Evaluation of ankle fractures: non-operative and operative treatment. Clin Orthop Relat Res. 1979;(138):111–9. PubMed PMID: 445892. Epub 1979/01/01. eng.

12. Jani MM, Parker RD. Internal fixation devices for the treatment of unstable osteochondritis dissecans and chondral lesions. Oper Tech Sports Med. 2004;12(3):170–5. PubMed PMID: WOS:000226020600004. English.

13. Lantz BA, McAndrew M, Scioli M, Fitzrandolph RL. The effect of concomitant chondral injuries accompanying operatively reduced malleolar fractures. J Orthop Trauma. 1991;5(2):125–8. PubMed PMID: 1861185. Epub 1991/01/01. eng.

14. Leontaritis N, Hinojosa L, Panchbhavi VK. Arthroscopically detected intra-articular lesions associated with acute ankle fractures. J Bone Joint Surg Am. 2009;91(2):333–9. PubMed PMID: 19181977. Epub 2009/02/03. eng.

15. Loren GJ, Ferkel RD. Arthroscopic assessment of occult intra-articular injury in acute ankle fractures. Arthroscopy. 2002;18(4):412–21. PubMed PMID: 11951201. Epub 2002/04/16. eng.

16. Lui TH, Chan WK, Chan KB. The arthroscopic management of frozen ankle. Arthroscopy. 2006;22(3):283–6. PubMed PMID: 16517312. Epub 2006/03/07. eng.

17. Lui TH, Ip K, Chow HT. Comparison of radiologic and arthroscopic diagnoses of distal tibiofibular syndesmosis disruption in acute ankle fracture. Arthroscopy. 2005;21(11):1370. PubMed PMID: 16325090. Epub 2005/12/06. eng.

18. Milner SA, Davis TR, Muir KR, Greenwood DC, Doherty M. Long-term outcome after tibial shaft fracture: is malunion important? J Bone Joint Surg Am. 2002;84-A(6):971–80. PubMed PMID: 12063331. Epub 2002/06/14. eng.

19. Müller ME, Perren SM, Allgöwer M, Arbeitsgemeinschaft für O. Manual of internal fixation: techniques recommended by the AO-ASIF Group. 3rd ed. Berlin/New York: Springer; 1991.

20. Ono A, Nishikawa S, Nagao A, Irie T, Sasaki M, Kouno T. Arthroscopically assisted treatment of ankle fractures: arthroscopic findings and surgical outcomes. Arthroscopy. 2004;20(6):627–31. PubMed.

21. Stufkens SA, Knupp M, Horisberger M, Lampert C, Hintermann B. Cartilage lesions and the development of osteoarthritis after internal fixation of ankle fractures: a prospective study. J Bone Joint Surg Am. 2010;92(2):279–86. PubMed PMID: 20124053. Epub 2010/02/04. eng.

22. Takao M, Ochi M, Naito K, Iwata A, Kawasaki K, Tobita M, et al. Arthroscopic diagnosis of tibiofibular syndesmosis disruption. Arthroscopy. 2001;17(8):836–43. PubMed PMID: 11600981. Epub 2001/10/16. eng.

23. Takao M, Ochi M, Uchio Y, Naito K, Kono T, Oae K. Osteochondral lesions of the talar dome associated with trauma. Arthroscopy. 2003;19(10):1061–7. PubMed PMID: 14673447. Epub 2003/12/16. eng.

24. Thomas B, Yeo JM, Slater GL. Chronic pain after ankle fracture: an arthroscopic assessment case series. Foot Ankle Int. 2005;26(12):1012–6. PubMed PMID: 16390631. Epub 2006/01/05. eng.

25. Thordarson DB, Bains R, Shepherd LE. The role of ankle arthroscopy on the surgical management of ankle fractures. Foot Ankle Int. 2001;22(2):123–5. PubMed PMID: 11249221. Epub 2001/03/16. eng.

26. Utsugi K, Sakai H, Hiraoka H, Yashiki M, Mogi H. Intra-articular fibrous tissue formation following ankle fracture: the significance of arthroscopic debridement of fibrous tissue. Arthroscopy. 2007;23(1):89–93. PubMed PMID: 17210432. Epub 2007/01/11. eng.

27. van Dijk CN, Scholte D. Arthroscopy of the ankle joint. Arthroscopy. 1997;13(1):90–6. PubMed PMID: 9043610. Epub 1997/02/01. eng.

28. van Dijk CN, Verhagen RA, Tol JL. Arthroscopy for problems after ankle fracture. J Bone Joint Surg Br. 1997;79(2):280–4. PubMed PMID: 9119857. Epub 1997/03/01. eng.
29. Wright JG, Einhorn TA, Heckman JD. Grades of recommendation. J Bone Joint Surg Am. 2005;87(9):1909–10. PubMed PMID: 16140803.
30. Wright JG, Swiontkowski MF, Heckman JD. Introducing levels of evidence to the journal. J Bone Joint Surg Am. 2003;85-A(1):1–3. PubMed PMID: 12533564.
31. Yde J, Kristensen KD. Ankle fractures: supination-eversion fractures of stage IV. Primary and late results of operative and non-operative treatment. Acta Orthop Scand. 1980;51(6):981–90. PubMed PMID: 6782823. Epub 1980/12/01. eng.

Diagnosis of Osteochondral Lesions by MRI

3

Thomas M. Link, Patrick Vavken, and Victor Valderrabano

> **Take-Home Points**
> - *While numerous imaging modalities exist and are valid and valuable diagnostic modalities, MRI has the unparalleled benefit of showing cartilage and soft tissues directly.*
> - *Especially for early stages and pediatric patients, MRI offers a valuable diagnostic tool that allows assessing the subchondral bone without exposure to radiation.*

3.1 Introduction

MRI is the best available clinical imaging technique that can provide direct visualization of the ankle cartilage; it is also superior to all other imaging techniques in directly depicting the bone marrow, ligaments, and tendons. MRI is therefore an excellent imaging technique to diagnose and monitor osteochondral lesions and osteochondritis dissecans (OCD). MRI of the ankle, however, is technically challenging as the joint cartilage is thin and high spatial resolution and adequate signal-to-noise ratios (SNR) are required. With recent improvements in MRI hardware, coil design, and sequences, imaging of the cartilage has been substantially improved; improvements include high field scanners that operate at 3 T and provide superior spatial resolution and SNR, new multichannel coils that allow parallel imaging and provide higher SNR, and thin section and high-resolution sequences that provide better visualization of cartilage defects.

It should be noted, however, that MRI also has pertinent disadvantages, which include the inability of standard clinical sequences to directly demonstrate bone architecture and stability. Also assessing the viability of osteochondral lesions with MRI and their stability is limited. Studies comparing CT and MRI for detection of a symptomatic OCD have shown similar accuracy for these modalities [33].

This chapter focuses on MRI of osteochondral lesions and will present MRI techniques required to demonstrate these lesions. It will describe MR imaging findings of osteochondral lesions and gradings, focus on the differential diagnosis of osteochondral lesions, and present findings associated with the repair of osteochondral abnormalities.

3.2 MR Imaging Technique of the Ankle

As previously mentioned, MRI of the ankle is challenging and imaging techniques need to be optimized to directly visualize osteochondral

T.M. Link, MD, PhD (✉)
Department of Radiology and Biomedical Imaging,
University of California, San Francisco, CA, USA
e-mail: thomas.link@ucsf.edu

P. Vavken, MD • V. Valderrabano, MD, PhD
Orthopaedic Department, University Hospital
of Basel, Basel, Switzerland
e-mail: patrick.vavken@usb.ch;
victor.valderrabano@usb.ch

C.N. van Dijk, J.G. Kennedy (eds.), *Talar Osteochondral Defects*,
DOI 10.1007/978-3-642-45097-6_3, © ESSKA 2014

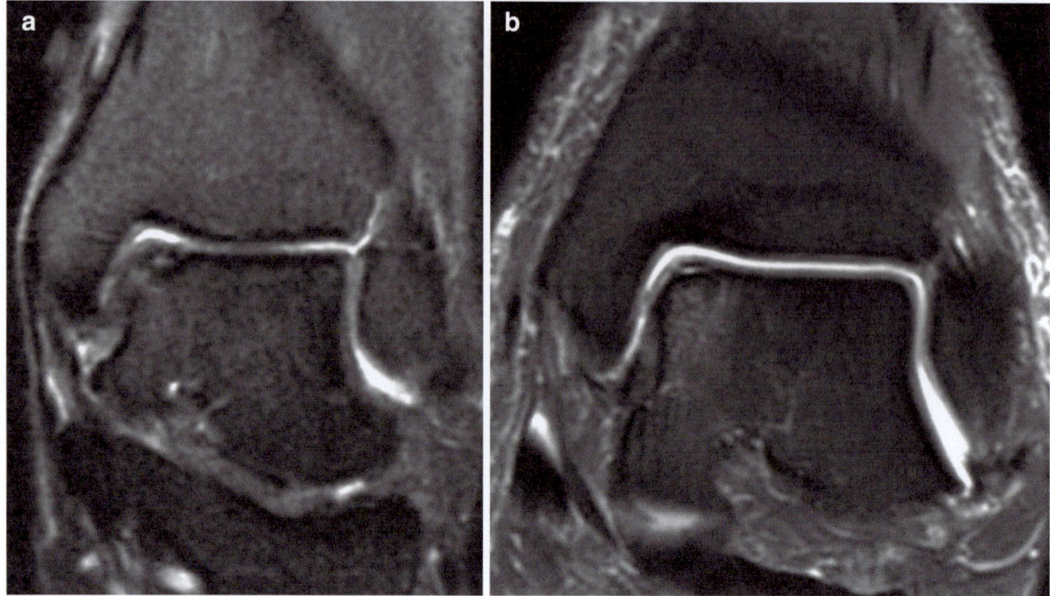

Fig. 3.1 Comparison of image quality using 1.5 and 3 T MRI. Osteochondral lesion at the talar dome in both images (fat saturated intermediate-weighted fast spin echo sequence). The 3T image (**b**) shows better delineation of the cartilage, more detail and is less blurry than the 1.5T image (**a**). Differences are due to the higher signal-to-noise ratio at 3T

lesions. Imaging should be performed at high field systems operating at 1.5 or 3 T field strength; previous studies have shown that 3 T systems provide superior image contrast and cartilage visualization [1, 2] (Fig. 3.1). In addition, adequate surface coils need to be used, ideally multichannel coils that provide parallel imaging capabilities. So-called chimney coils are available that were specifically tailored for the ankle and provide reproducible positioning of the ankle joint; alternatively knee surface coils can be used which provide high SNR. However, they require that the ankle joint is positioned in an extended position, which may not be well reproducible.

In addition to the hardware, the choice of adequate imaging sequences is critical. Usually spin-echo sequences are used; these include fluid-sensitive intermediate-weighted fast spin-echo sequences as well as non-fat-saturated T1-weighted and proton-density-weighted sequences. Fat-saturated intermediate-weighted fast spin-echo sequences provide information on the cartilage layer, the bone marrow, the tendons, and the ligaments at the same time. The advantage of fat saturation includes better visualization of the bone marrow edema pattern and less chemical shift artifacts at the interface between the cartilage and bone marrow. The workhorse sequences are 2D fast spin-echo sequences and they are usually the main part of a standard routine imaging protocol [19, 21]. Table 3.1 shows representative sequences used for clinical imaging of the ankle at 1.5 and 3.0 T.

In addition, thin section 3D sequences have been introduced to allow for better visualization of the cartilage layer. Among these, 3D fast spin-echo sequences have been found to be particularly useful [12, 28, 29] (Fig. 3.2). Using 3D fast spin-echo sequences provides isotropic datasets of the ankle, which can be reconstructed in any imaging plane, e.g., from a sagittal source image dataset, coronal and axial sequences can be generated. The advantage over standard 2D fast spin-echo sequences is the decrease of partial volume effects, allowing better depiction of subtle cartilage defects. A number of other 3D

Table 3.1 Standard clinical sequences and sequence parameters for ankle imaging

Sequence	Field strength	TR (ms)	TE (ms)	Flip angle	NEX	ETL	Matrix (pixels)	FOV (cm)	BW (kHz)	ST (mm)
axT1	3.0 T	675	15.7	90	2	5	384×256	12	31.25	3
	1.5 T	600	10	90	2	3	256×192	12	31.25	3
axT2	3.0 T	4,500	42	90	2	16	512×256	12	31.25	3
	1.5 T	4,000	40	90	2	12	320×224	12	16.67	3
sagT1	3.0 T	675	15.4	90	2	4	384×256	12	31.25	3
	1.5 T	625	23.5	90	2	4	384×224	12	16.67	3
sagIR	3.0 T	3,700	68	90	2	15	320×160	12	31.25	3
	1.5 T	3,400	68	90	2	8	256×192	12	16.67	3
corIM	3.0 T	4,000	16.7	90	4	9	384×256	10×8	31.25	2
	1.5 T	4,000	15.5	90	3	12	384×224	10×8	16.67	2

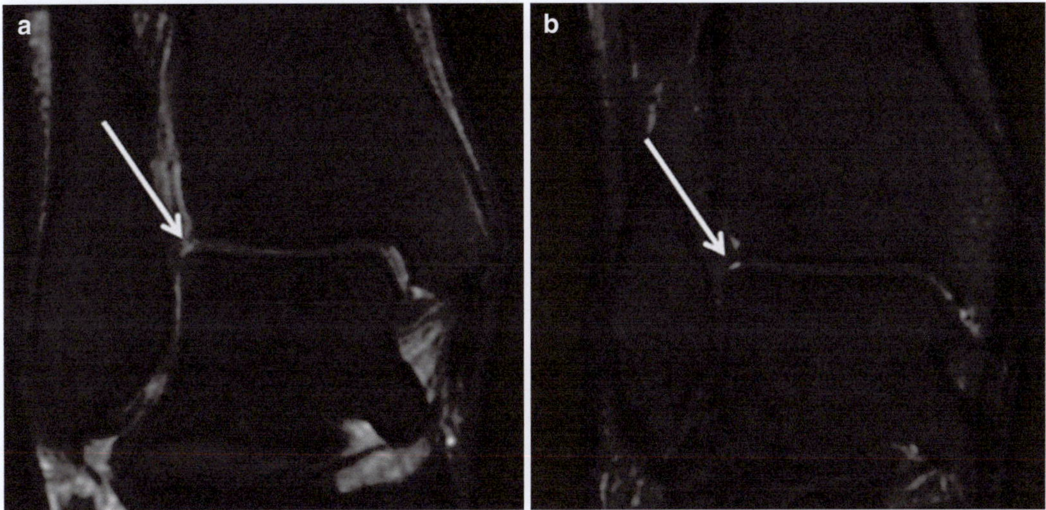

Fig. 3.2 Standard fat saturated intermediate-weighted fast spin echo sequence (**a**) and thin Section 3 D fast spin echo CUBE sequence (**b**). Note higher detail in the CUBE sequence, which better depicts full thickness cartilage defect at the medial talar dome (*arrows*)

sequences based on gradient echoes have also been developed, such as balanced steady-state free precession (bSSFP), iterative decomposition of water and fat with echo asymmetry, and least-squares estimation combined with spoiled gradient echo (IDEAL-SPGR) and multiecho in steady-state acquisition (MENSA) sequences. A recent study, however, found that 3D fast spin-echo sequences may be superior to those in visualizing cartilage and associated bone marrow changes [7].

Short-tau inversion recovery (STIR) sequences have also been used at the ankle as they are very fluid sensitive and provide excellent depiction of bone marrow abnormalities. In addition, they reduce magic angle effects, thus optimizing evaluation of the ankle tendons [31]. Contrast media are usually not required for imaging of the ankle but have been suggested previously to improve evaluation of the viability of osteochondral lesions and osteochondral autograft transfer systems [18].

3.3 MR Imaging Findings in Osteochondral Lesions

Common etiologies for osteochondral lesions of the talus are acute or chronic intra-articular injuries, and most frequently they are related to sports injuries. MRI is usually performed after an ankle sprain, which does not improve over time or if locking or catching occurs. Standard radiographs not infrequently are normal at the time of the injury, and they may also be negative on subsequent studies. Radiographic findings, which are suspicious for osteochondral injury, may be subchondral lucency or a small fracture fragment. CT and MRI are second-line imaging techniques. While CT has a high spatial resolution and is excellent for identifying small bony lesions, MRI has the advantage of directly visualizing cartilage and of identifying bone bruises and microfractures, which may not be visualized with CT. MRI provides information on cartilage defects and bone marrow abnormalities, but because of the limited cartilage thickness, MRI is challenging and the MRI technique needs to be adequately chosen as outlined above.

The initial classification of osteochondral lesions was based on radiographs and developed by Berndt and Harty in 1959 [3]. This is still widely used, and additional MRI-based classifications have been developed [9, 22, 32]. The original Berndt and Harty Stage I represents an area of osteochondral compression, Stage II a partially loose fragment, Stage III a completely detached fragment without displacement, and Stage IV a completely detached and displaced fragment. A grade 0 has been added, which is an x-ray-negative but MRI-positive lesion [4]. Scranton and others have added a Stage V to describe lesions with deep cystic changes [30].

In 2003, Mintz et al. proposed an MRI grading system of osteochondral lesions [22], which represents a modification of the arthroscopic grading system of the ankle proposed by Cheng et al. [8]. This system differentiates 6 grades: grade 0 is normal; grade 1 represents a hyperintense but morphologically

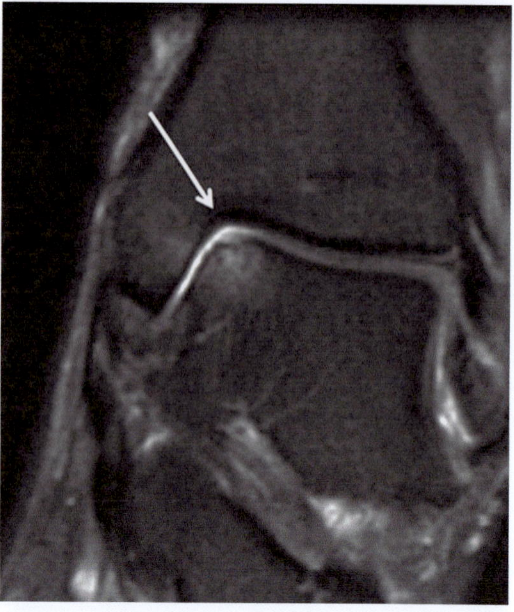

Fig. 3.3 Coronal fat-saturated intermediate weighted fast spin echo sequence demonstrating an osteochondral lesion at the medial talar dome (*arrow*). There is increase in signal of the cartilage and irregularity of the underlying bone, but the cartilage surface appears intact and there are no defects

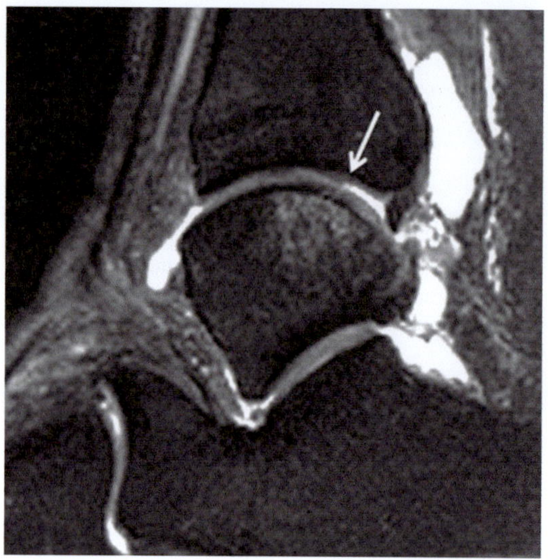

Fig. 3.4 Sagittal fat-saturated dual echo steady state (DESS) sequence demonstrating an osteochondral injury at the talus. There is cartilage fissuring (*arrow*) with underlying bone marrow edema pattern (bone bruise)

intact cartilage surface (Fig. 3.3); grade 2, a fibrillation or fissures not extending to bone (Fig. 3.4); grade 3, a flap or exposed bone (Fig. 3.5); grade 4, a loose undisplaced fragment (Fig. 3.6), and grade 5, a displaced fragment (Fig. 3.7).

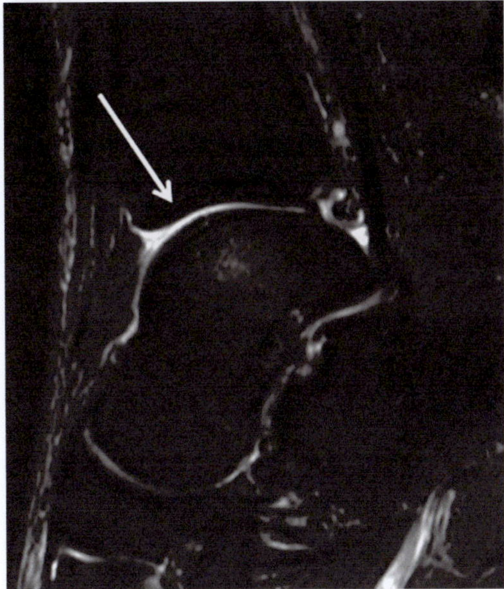

Fig. 3.5 Sagittal fat-saturated intermediate weighted fast spin echo sequence showing an osteochondral lesion with a cartilage flap, a partially separated layer of cartilage with delamination (*arrow*) and underlying mild bone marrow edema pattern

Other MRI-based classification systems include these by Taranow et al. [32] and Hepple et al. [9]. Taranow et al. [32] differentiated a grade 1 with subchondral compression/bone bruise appearing as high signal on T2-weighted images (Fig. 3.4), a grade 2 with subchondral cysts that are not seen acutely (arise from grade 1), a grade 3 with a partially separated or detached fragments in situ (Fig. 3.6), and a grade 4 with displaced fragments (Fig. 3.7). Hepple et al. [9] developed a six-grade classification, where grade 1 consists of articular cartilage damage only, grade 2a of a cartilage injury with underlying fracture and surrounding bony edema, grade 2b of a cartilage lesion without surrounding bony edema, grade 3 of a detached but undisplaced fragment (Fig. 3.6), grade 4 of a detached and displaced fragment (Fig. 3.7), and grade 5 of subchondral cyst formation (Fig. 3.8).

Modified Outerbridge and Noyes classifications have been used to classify focal cartilage lesions in MR images [11, 24–27]. These classifications differentiate cartilage with abnormal signal and/or swelling, focal cartilage lesions less and more than 50 % of the cartilage thickness, as well as full thickness cartilage lesions. Differentiating cartilage lesions less and more than 50 %, however,

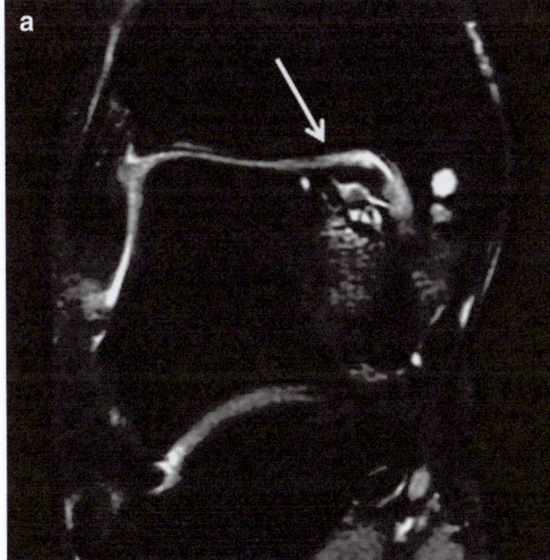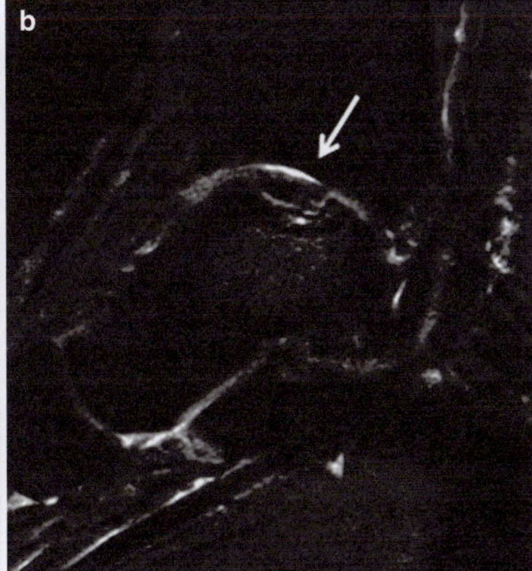
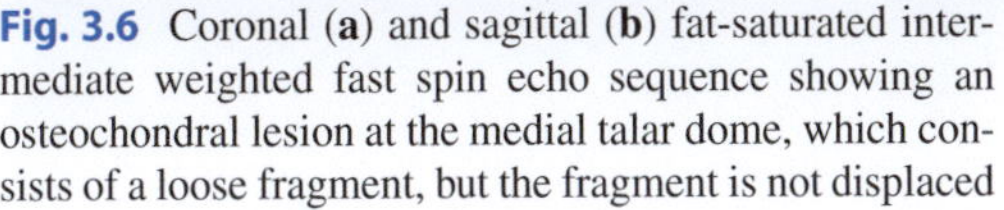

Fig. 3.6 Coronal (**a**) and sagittal (**b**) fat-saturated intermediate weighted fast spin echo sequence showing an osteochondral lesion at the medial talar dome, which consists of a loose fragment, but the fragment is not displaced (*arrows*). Fluid between the bony fragment and the adjacent bone and adjacent bone marrow edema pattern is also depicted

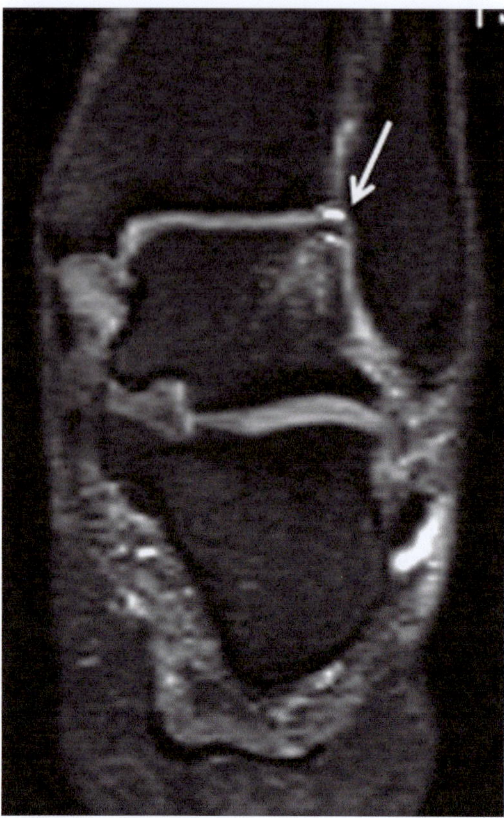

Fig. 3.7 Coronal fat-saturated dual echo steady state (DESS) sequence demonstrates an osteochondral injury at the lateral aspect of the talar dome with a mildly displaced osteochondral fragment (*arrow*)

may be challenging at the ankle because the cartilage is very thin and additional chemical shift artifacts at the interface between cartilage and bone may obscure the deeper layers of the cartilage. The International Cartilage Repair Society (ICRS) classification is also used; it is based on the Outerbridge classification and differentiates 4 grades as above with additional subgrades [13].

Previous studies have analyzed the accuracy of MRI for osteochondral lesions and found high specificities and good sensitivities [10, 22]. Joshy et al. [10] showed 100 % specificity for the diagnosis of osteochondral lesions; however, the sensitivity was lower at 83.3 %. Mintz et al. [22] analyzed 54 individuals who underwent ankle arthroscopy and found that MRI correctly identified all 40 osteochondral lesions and all 14 normal ankles. MRI correctly graded 33 of 40 (83 %) of the osteochondral lesions using the previously described 5-point scale. Of the remaining seven lesions, all were identified within one grade. Collapsing all grades into disease-negative status (grades 0 and 1) and disease-positive status (grades 2, 3, 4, and 5) yielded sensitivity of 95 %, specificity of 100 %, negative predictive value of 88 %, and positive predictive value of 100 %. It should be noted, however, that Verhagen and coworkers found, contrary to their hypothesis,

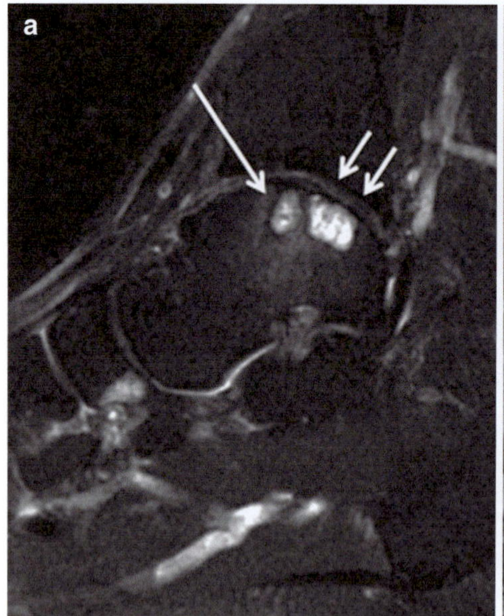
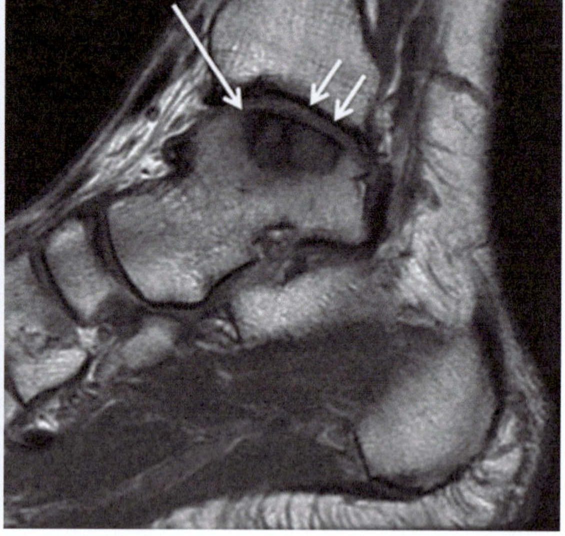

Fig. 3.8 Sagittal fat-saturated intermediate weighted (**a**) and T1-weighted (**b**) fast spin echo sequences of the ankle showing large cystic, subchondral changes underlying the cartilage (*large arrows*) with irregularity and thinning of the overlying cartilage (*small arrows*)

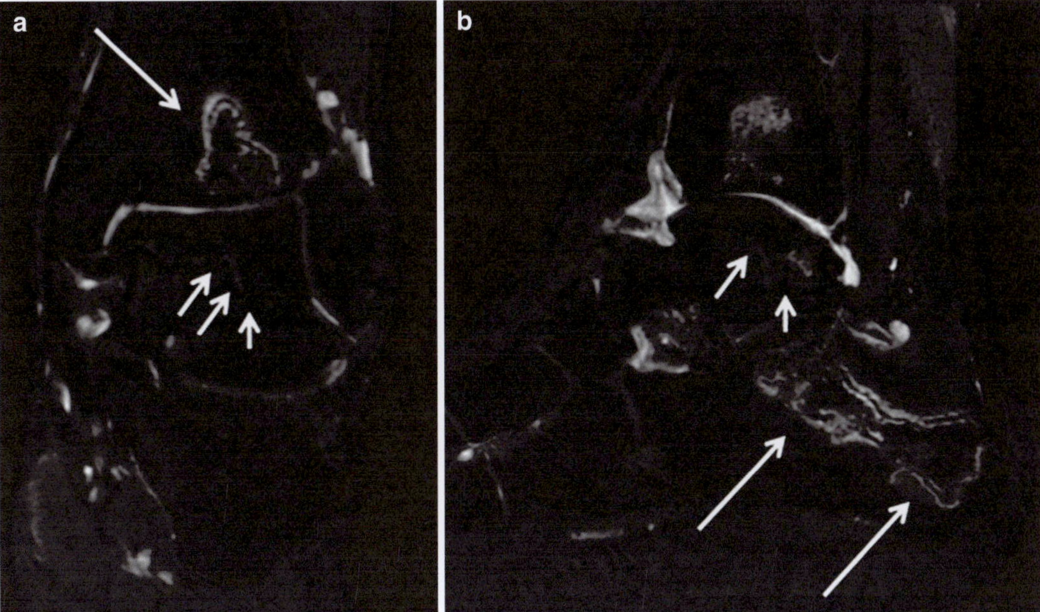

Fig. 3.9 Coronal (**a**) and sagittal (**b**) fat-saturated intermediate weighted fast spin echo sequences demonstrating multiple bone infarcts in the distal tibia, ankle and calcaneus (*large arrows*). The large subchondral bone marrow infarct/avascular necrosis in the talus mimics an osteochondral lesion (*small arrows*)

that conventional MRI did not prove to be better than high-resolution multidetector helical CT for the detection or exclusion of osteochondral lesions [33].

It should be noted that osteochondral lesions are also found in the setting of osteoarthritis, inflammatory and septic arthritis, as well as bone infarcts (Fig. 3.9) and arthropathies such as hemophilic osteoarthropathy. These disease entities have characteristic MRI patterns that include more generalized abnormalities involving the cartilage, bone marrow, and synovium. Changes are usually more severe than those found in focal osteochondral lesions and usually are accompanied by secondary degenerative changes. Also the management of these lesions will be different and affected by the underlying disease process.

Stress-related changes of the bone marrow can be observed in athletes and dancers. These T2 bright bone marrow signal abnormalities are usually subtle and not well circumscribed as shown in Fig. 3.10. There are no deformities and cartilage abnormalities associated with these lesions, and they are usually reversible with reduced

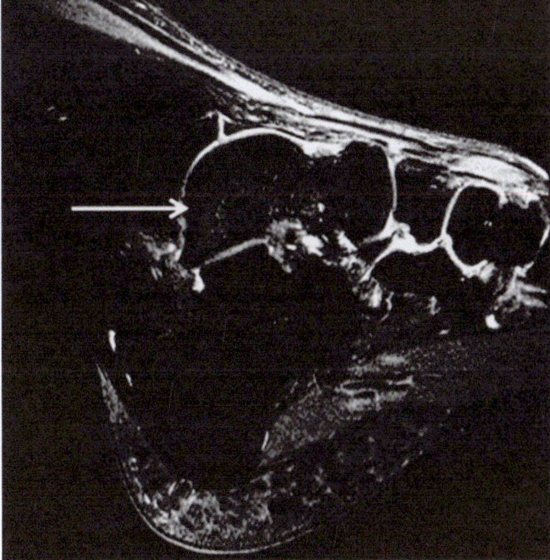

Fig. 3.10 Sagittal fat-saturated intermediate weighted fast spin echo sequence shows bone marrow edema pattern in the talus (*arrow*) consistent with a stress reaction in a professional dancer. No associated cartilage abnormalities or bone deformity

weight-bearing activities but may progress to stress fractures and eventually also to osteochondral lesions.

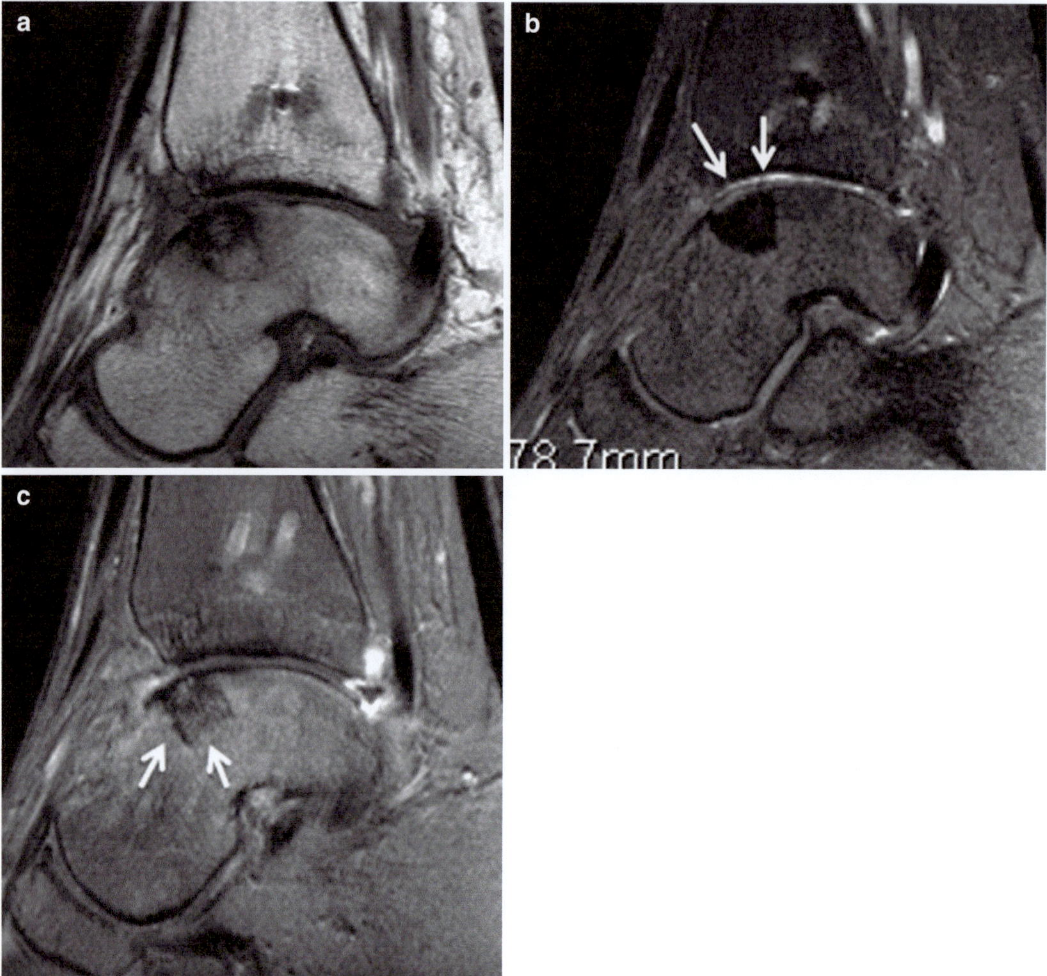

Fig. 3.11 Sagittal T1-weighted (**a**), fat-saturated fluid sensitive (**b**) and fat-saturated T1-weighted (**c**) gadolinium-enhanced spin echo sequences demonstrate an osteochondral autograft transfer system (OATS) or mosaicplasty. The cartilage covering the bone plug is intact and well integrated (*arrows* in (**b**)). However, the bone plug is low in signal and shows only limited contrast enhancement (*arrows* in (**c**)) consistent with limited viability of the bone plug

3.4 MR Imaging Findings in Cartilage Repair

Multiple management options are available for osteochondral lesions including nonsurgical treatment, debridement, drilling, surgical excision, and curettage. Cartilage repair procedures include osteochondral autograft, microfracture, and autologous chondrocyte implantation; MRI has been used to assess the morphological outcome of these procedures at the ankle noninvasively [14, 15]. Also an MRI-based classification system has been developed to evaluate and grade these procedures semiquantitatively; this system was named Magnetic Resonance Observation of Cartilage Repair Tissue (MOCART) scoring system [34]. While this grading system has been mostly used for the knee, it has also been adapted for evaluating cartilage repair procedures at the ankle [15]. It differentiates and grades different aspects including (1) the degree of defect repair and defect filling, (2) integration with the border zone, (3) quality of repaired tissue surface, (4) adhesions, and (5) synovitis. Figure 3.11 shows sagittal images of the ankle joint after an osteochondral autograft transfer procedure, with good defect repair and filing, integration of the border zone, intact cartilage surface, and mild synovitis. The low signal intensity of the bone and decreased contrast enhancement is consistent with limited viability of the implanted bone cores.

A previous study correlating 1.5 T MRI-based MOCART scores with second-look arthroscopic findings found that the degree of defect repair and filling showed congruent results in 59 % of the cases [15]. For the surface of the repaired tissue, the results were in agreement in 89 % cases. The results, however, were limited for the assessment of the integration of the border zone, with substantial disagreement in the abnormal cases. The authors acknowledge this limitation and suggest that imaging at 3 T may have improved these results. Kuni et al. [14] correlated 1.0 T MR imaging findings in 22 patients undergoing microfracture at the ankle joint with clinical findings. Similar to previous studies, they found limited correlation between MR and clinical findings [18, 20], and in particular in patients with the worst clinical outcome and persisting severe pain, they were not able to identify any common MR imaging characteristics. However, they did find significant differences in the clinical scores between patients with a persisting or new bone marrow edema pattern compared to those without a bone marrow edema pattern at the follow-up, suggesting that a persistent or new bone marrow edema pattern may be associated with worse clinical outcome.

3.5 Conclusion and Future Developments

MRI is the best available imaging modality to visualize cartilage directly, and advances in imaging over the last 10 years have greatly improved imaging of challenging anatomic structures such as the ankle cartilage. In addition, MRI provides sensitive information on bone marrow and synovial abnormalities. Compared to arthroscopy as a standard of reference, MRI performs well in diagnosing and grading osteochondral lesions.

However, it should be noted that MRI does not perform as well in assessing the success of cartilage repair procedures, and in particular, the correlation between clinical findings and MRI findings is limited. MRI and CT have demonstrated similar accuracy for detecting symptomatic talar OCD. For preoperative planning, multidetector helical CT may provide better information.

With improvement in morphological MR imaging including higher spatial resolution sequences and 3 T MRI, better diagnosis and monitoring of osteochondral lesions and associated repair will be achieved. Also new sequences for quantitative assessment of the cartilage matrix, such as T1rho, T2, and dGEMRIC, may provide additional insights in the collagen structure and proteoglycan content of the cartilage [5, 6, 16, 17, 19, 23]. These may in the future provide a better marker to determine the prognosis of osteochondral lesions and associated repair but also to more sensitively monitor changes in cartilage degeneration.

Conflict of Interests The author has no current conflict of interests with the products presented.

References

1. Barr C, Bauer JS, Malfair D, Ma B, Henning TD, Steinbach L, Link TM. MR imaging of the ankle at 3 Tesla and 1.5 Tesla: protocol optimization and application to cartilage, ligament and tendon pathology in cadaver specimens. Eur Radiol. 2007;17:1518–28.
2. Bauer J, Barr C, Steinbach L, Malfair D, Krug R, Ma C, Link T. Imaging of the articular cartilage of the ankle at 3.0 and 1.5 Tesla. Eur Radiol Suppl. 2006;16(S1):238.
3. Berndt AL, Harty M. Transchondral fractures (osteochondritis dissecans) of the talus. J Bone Joint Surg Am. 1959;41–A:988–1020.
4. Bowman M. Osteochondral Lesions of the talus and occult fractures of the foot and ankle. In: Schon LC, Porter DA, editors. Baxter's the foot and ankle in sport. Philadelphia: Elsevier; 2007. p. 293–338.
5. Burstein D, Velyvis J, Scott KT, Stock KW, Kim YJ, Jaramillo D, Boutin RD, Gray ML. Protocol issues for delayed Gd(DTPA)(2-)-enhanced MRI (dGEMRIC) for clinical evaluation of articular cartilage. Magn Reson Med. 2001;45:36–41.
6. Burstein D, Gray M. New MRI techniques for imaging cartilage. J Bone Joint Surg Am. 2003;85–A Suppl 2:70–7.

7. Chen CA, Kijowski R, Shapiro LM, Tuite MJ, Davis KW, Klaers JL, Block WF, Reeder SB, Gold GE. Cartilage morphology at 3.0T: assessment of three-dimensional magnetic resonance imaging techniques. J Magn Reson Imaging. 2010;32:173–83.

8. Cheng MS, Ferkel RD, Applegate GR, editors. Osteochondral lesions of the talus: a radiologic and surgical comparison. Annual Meeting of the Academy of Orthopaedic Surgeons, New Orleans, 16–21 Feb 1995.

9. Hepple S, Winson IG, Glew D. Osteochondral lesions of the talus: a revised classification. Foot Ankle Int. 1999;20:789–93.

10. Joshy S, Abdulkadir U, Chaganti S, Sullivan B, Hariharan K. Accuracy of MRI scan in the diagnosis of ligamentous and chondral pathology in the ankle. Foot Ankle Surg. 2010;16:78–80.

11. Kijowski R, Blankenbaker DG, Davis KW, Shinki K, Kaplan LD, De Smet AA. Comparison of 1.5- and 3.0-T MR imaging for evaluating the articular cartilage of the knee joint. Radiology. 2009;250:839–48.

12. Kijowski R, Davis KW, Woods MA, Lindstrom MJ, De Smet AA, Gold GE, Busse RF. Knee joint: comprehensive assessment with 3D isotropic resolution fast spin-echo MR imaging–diagnostic performance compared with that of conventional MR imaging at 3.0 T. Radiology. 2009;252:486–95.

13. Kleemann RU, Krocker D, Cedraro A, Tuischer J, Duda GN. Altered cartilage mechanics and histology in knee osteoarthritis: relation to clinical assessment (ICRS Grade). Osteoarthritis Cartilage. 2005;13:958–63.

14. Kuni B, Schmitt H, Chloridis D, Ludwig K. Clinical and MRI results after microfracture of osteochondral lesions of the talus. Arch Orthop Trauma Surg. 2012;132:1765–71.

15. Lee KT, Choi YS, Lee YK, Cha SD, Koo HM. Comparison of MRI and arthroscopy in modified MOCART scoring system after autologous chondrocyte implantation for osteochondral lesion of the talus. Orthopedics. 2011;34:e356–62.

16. Li X, Han ET, Busse RF, Majumdar S. In vivo T(1rho) mapping in cartilage using 3D magnetization-prepared angle-modulated partitioned k-space spoiled gradient echo snapshots (3D MAPSS). Magn Reson Med. 2008;59:298–307.

17. Li X, Cheng J, Lin K, Saadat E, Bolbos RI, Jokbe B, Ries MD, Horvai A, Link TM, Majumdar S. Quantitative MRI using T(1rho) and T(2) in human osteoarthritic cartilage specimens: correlation with biochemical measurements and histology. Magn Reson Imaging. 2011;29:324–34.

18. Link TM, Mischung J, Wortler K, Burkart A, Rummeny EJ, Imhoff AB. Normal and pathological MR findings in osteochondral autografts with longitudinal follow-up. Eur Radiol. 2006;16:88–96.

19. Link TM, Stahl R, Woertler K. Cartilage imaging: motivation, techniques, current and future significance. Eur Radiol. 2007;17:1135–46.

20. Link TM. Correlations between joint morphology and pain and between magnetic resonance imaging, histology, and micro-computed tomography. J Bone Joint Surg Am. 2009;91 Suppl 1:30–2.

21. Link TM. MR imaging in osteoarthritis: hardware, coils, and sequences. Magn Reson Imaging Clin N Am. 2010;18:95–110.

22. Mintz DN, Tashjian GS, Connell DA, Deland JT, O'Malley M, Potter HG. Osteochondral lesions of the talus: a new magnetic resonance grading system with arthroscopic correlation. Arthroscopy. 2003;19:353–9.

23. Mosher TJ, Dardzinski BJ. Cartilage MRI T2 relaxation time mapping: overview and applications. Semin Musculoskelet Radiol. 2004;8:355–68.

24. Noyes FR, Stabler CL. A system for grading articular cartilage lesions at arthroscopy. Am J Sports Med. 1989;17:505–13.

25. Potter HG, Linklater JM, Allen AA, Hannafin JA, Haas SB. Magnetic resonance imaging of articular cartilage in the knee. An evaluation with use of fast-spin-echo imaging. J Bone Joint Surg Am. 1998;80:1276–84.

26. Recht MP, Resnick D. Magnetic resonance imaging of articular cartilage: an overview. Top Magn Reson Imaging. 1998;9:328–36.

27. Recht MP, Goodwin DW, Winalski CS, White LM. MRI of articular cartilage: revisiting current status and future directions. AJR Am J Roentgenol. 2005;185:899–914.

28. Ristow O, Steinbach L, Sabo G, Krug R, Huber M, Rauscher I, Ma B, Link TM. Isotropic 3D fast spin-echo imaging versus standard 2D imaging at 3.0 T of the knee-image quality and diagnostic performance. Eur Radiol. 2009;19:1263–72.

29. Ristow O, Stehling C, Krug R, Steinbach L, Sabo G, Ambekar A, Huber M, Link TM. Isotropic 3-dimensional fast spin echo imaging versus standard 2-dimensional imaging at 3.0 T of the knee: artificial cartilage and meniscal lesions in a porcine model. J Comput Assist Tomogr. 2010;34:260–9.

30. Scranton Jr PE, McDermott JE. Treatment of type V osteochondral lesions of the talus with ipsilateral knee osteochondral autografts. Foot Ankle Int. 2001;22:380–4.

31. Srikhum W, Nardo L, Karampinos DC, Melkus G, Poulos T, Steinbach LS, Link TM. Magnetic resonance imaging of ankle tendon pathology: benefits of additional axial short-tau inversion recovery imaging to reduce magic angle effects. Skeletal Radiol. 2013;42:499–510.

32. Taranow WS, Bisignani GA, Towers JD, Conti SF. Retrograde drilling of osteochondral lesions of the medial talar dome. Foot Ankle Int. 1999;20:474–80.

33. Verhagen RA, Maas M, Dijkgraaf MG, Tol JL, Krips R, van Dijk CN. Prospective study on diagnostic strategies in osteochondral lesions of the talus. Is MRI superior to helical CT? J Bone Joint Surg Br. 2005;87:41–6.

34. Welsch GH, Mamisch TC, Quirbach S, Zak L, Marlovits S, Trattnig S. Evaluation and comparison of cartilage repair tissue of the patella and medial femoral condyle by using morphological MRI and biochemical zonal T2 mapping. Eur Radiol. 2009;19:1253–62.

Diagnosis of Osteochondral Defects of the Talus by Computerized Tomography (CT) and Single-Photon Emission Computed Tomography (SPECT-CT)

4

Mies A. Korteweg, Martin Wiewiorski,
Geert J. Streekstra, Klaus Strobel,
Victor Valderrabano, and Mario Maas

Take-Home Points

- *In diagnosing osteochondral defects, MRI and CT have similar diagnostic accuracies. CT is faster, better for preoperative planning, cheaper and allows the ankle to be depicted in various anatomical positions in a 3D manner.*
- *CT enables clear delineation of the true osteochondral defect, will not overcall the size due to bone marrow edema (as seen on MRI), and helps assessing the extent of the osseous defect in the presence of cystic defects.*
- *CT in plantar flexion facilitates the surgical choice of an anterior or posterior approach for arthroscopy.*
- *CT arthrography detects cartilaginous defects and can therefore aid in detection of early-stage osteochondral defects.*
- *SPECT-CT discriminates active from nonactive osteochondral defects, which can aid the clinician in treatment planning.*

M.A. Korteweg, MD, PhD • M. Maas, MD, PhD (✉)
Department of Radiology, Academic Medical Center,
University of Amsterdam, Amsterdam,
The Netherlands
e-mail: m.a.korteweg@amc.uva.nl;
m.maas@amc.uva.nl

M. Wiewiorski, MD • V. Valderrabano, MD, PhD
Orthopaedic Department, University Hospital
of Basel, Basel, Switzerland
e-mail: martin.wiewiorski@usb.ch;
victor.valderrabano@usb.ch

G.J. Streekstra, PhD
Department of Radiology, Academic Medical Center,
University of Amsterdam, Amsterdam,
The Netherlands
e-mail: g.j.streekstra@amc.uva.nl

K. Strobel, MD, PhD
LA Nuklearmedizin/Radiologie, Luzerner
Kantonsspital, Luzern, Switzerland
e-mail: klaus.strobel@luks.ch

4.1 Imaging with Radiation

4.1.1 Plain Radiography

When a patient with deep ankle pain is suspected to have an osteochondral defect (OCD) of the talus, it is common to first perform conventional diagnostic tests before proceeding to the computerized tomography (CT) or magnetic resonance imaging (MRI). Even though conventional radiographs are often negative when performed directly following initial injury, other important pathology such as a fracture can be ruled out. Standard conventional radiographic imaging of the ankle consists of two views: the so-called mortise and lateral views. A mortise is a rectangular cavity prepared to receive a tenon

C.N. van Dijk, J.G. Kennedy (eds.), *Talar Osteochondral Defects*,
DOI 10.1007/978-3-642-45097-6_4, © ESSKA 2014

which together form a mortise-and-tenon joint. The weight-bearing mortise view (the fibula and distal tibia form a mortise) is made with the ankle in 10–20° internal rotation, enabling clear visualization of the lateral and medial clear space of the upper ankle joint as well as the talar dome. On the mortise view, the lateral malleolus is in the same coronal plane as the medial malleolus.

The weight-bearing lateral view is useful for delineation of the posterior aspect of the tibia, potential loose bodies, or other causes of ankle pain caused by osseous structures such as anterior tibiotalar spurs and/or an os trigonum.

Apart from these commonly performed views, other additional radiographic images can be performed. For better visualization of the talar dome, a mortise view in plantar flexion can be performed. This weight-bearing plantar flexion view is made by providing a 4 cm heel rise, which facilitates an improved delineation of the posterior aspect of the talus.

However, even with additional plain radiographs, conventional radiographic imaging can miss up to 50 % of the OCDs [8]. Therefore, the main purpose of performing conventional radiographs is for excluding other causes of acute and chronic ankle pain such as fractures and impingement. Additionally, even if an OCD is detected on plain radiographs, further imaging is often needed, as the extent and location of the OCD are of primary importance for the prognosis and choice of treatment. Both MRI and CT can visualize the defect in three dimensions. Each imaging modality has advantages and disadvantages. Therefore, either one of these modalities is the preferred next diagnostic step. Currently it is up to the experience and preference of the orthopedic surgeon to decide which technique to use for diagnosing OCDs [6].

4.2 CT Imaging

4.2.1 CT Technique

Modern day CT scanners are multi-slice helical systems. The patient moves continuously through the scanner (gantry) in which one or several beams are positioned that spin around and produce X-ray photons to make standard transversal views. The photons are attenuated by the patient, yet when they pass through the patient, they retain a certain level of energy (frequency) which is detected by the detectors inside the scanner. The difference in attenuation is tissue specific. By means of computer analysis, these raw data are mathematically analyzed before being back-projected onto a matrix using a reconstruction algorithm. In this computer-process reconstruction, "kernels" tailored to specific tissues are added. Kernels are also referred to as "filters" or "algorithms" with bone or soft tissue being often-used examples of kernels. A bone kernel is more sensitive to high frequencies, and therefore bone filter images are ideal for diagnosing bone pathologies but contain more noise. Soft tissue kernels "roll off" more high frequencies and therefore have less noise, lower resolution, and more soft tissue contrast. It is preferred to use images that are reconstructed using both kernels.

Afterward, using a fixed data set, the window and level values (the gray scale) of an image can be adjusted at any time, as with many forms of digital data. One should be aware of the fact that this is a post-processing action, and in this way different from using different kernels. Reformatting of the existing transversal data into other imaging planes, for example, coronal and sagittal slices, can also be performed after the data set has been acquired. The reformatted data however has lower spatial resolution, if scanned at a less than 16-slice CT scanner. Actual 3D images can be reconstructed from the data using volume and surface rendering.

The quality of an image depends on the signal and contrast to noise ratios. Several factors influence the amount of signal or contrast in an image. For example, more signal can be achieved by increasing the milliamperes (mAs) (the number of photons), but this also increases the radiation dose. Secondly, a larger pixel size also leads to more signal in that pixel. This is similar to increasing the slice thickness, as more photons will be present in each slice. However, increasing both pixel size and slice width lowers the spatial resolution. Bone kernels (filters) are only sensitive to high frequencies and therefore have lower contrast to noise ratios than images made with soft tissue kernels. Larger patients attenuate more X-rays, resulting in the detection of fewer photons by the detector, which also reduces the signal and contrast to noise ratio.

The quality of an image can be reduced by artifacts. CT artifacts can be caused by movement, by bone itself, or can result from metal implants. In the case of bone, which has a similar effect as hardware, this artifact is called beam hardening. Beam hardening is caused by the fact that the attenuation of bone is greater than that of soft tissue. Having passed through bone, the average energy of an X-ray beam becomes greater (more hard). The beam is hardened to different extents which influences the reconstruction algorithm and results in artifacts. This effect can be diminished by increasing the slice thickness.

Partial volume averaging occurs when a voxel (3D pixel) contains several different tissues. The contents of the voxel are averaged by the computer analysis, which as a result can lead to misinterpretations of an image. To reduce partial volume averaging, thinner slices can be used. To avoid misinterpretations, the scan should be viewed in different reconstructed positions.

4.2.2 CT Imaging of an OCD

To visualize an OCD, an adequate scan protocol should be available. Common X-ray beam settings for an ankle CT are 130 kV with 75 mA with an exposure time of approximately 1 s. The field of view (FOV) should contain the entire ankle. Thin section images with a maximum 1 mm slice thickness should be derived; ideally 0.3 mm slice thickness is used. The ankle should be scanned with a bone kernel to achieve the desired high, submillimeter, resolution. Additionally a soft tissue kernel reconstruction should be performed.

This provides lower resolution, but the contrast between tissues is increased, thereby providing a better image of the soft tissues.

An OCD can have various dimensions. The size of the smallest OCD which can be visualized measures 0.3–1.0 mm; this is constrained by the scan resolution applied. An OCD can consist of cortex irregularities and/or cystic changes of the subchondral bone. The cortex irregularities are depicted by a non-smooth border of the talus or tibia. The white cortical line can be interrupted or have a dented appearance. The cortical irregularities are indicative of overlying cartilaginous defects. The cystic appearances in the subchondral bone consist of lucent areas depicted as dark gray directly underneath the irregular cortex. In larger OCDs, the overlying cortex and cartilage have disappeared, and a cortical defect is seen. In these cases, it is important to have a close look at the joint to possibly identify the missing bony structure from the defect which might have become a loose body. Fragmentation and detachment of small bony structures can be better visualized with CT than with MRI.

In case of a CT arthrography, the cartilaginous defect will be filled with the intra-articular-injected contrast material. *The excellent image contrast between intra-articular-injected iodinated contrast, cartilage, and cortex on CT arthrography facilitates an easy detection of even small, only cartilaginous, OCDs* (see Sect. 4.2.4). Surrounding bone marrow edema, which is often a key finding on MRI, is not easily depicted on CT scan. This does not hamper visibility of the OCD [3] but is a merit of CT since true delineation of the OCD is guaranteed. Sometimes edema is visible on CT; the bone can appear more dense, corresponding to an increase of fluid at that site.

By acquiring high spatial resolution 3D CT data sets, which frequently consist of 0.3 mm thick slices, small osseous details can be detected (Fig. 4.1). To avoid partial volume effects, every image should always be looked at in two views. Because of the nearly isotropic resolution of the CT, multi-planar reformatting (MPR) quality can

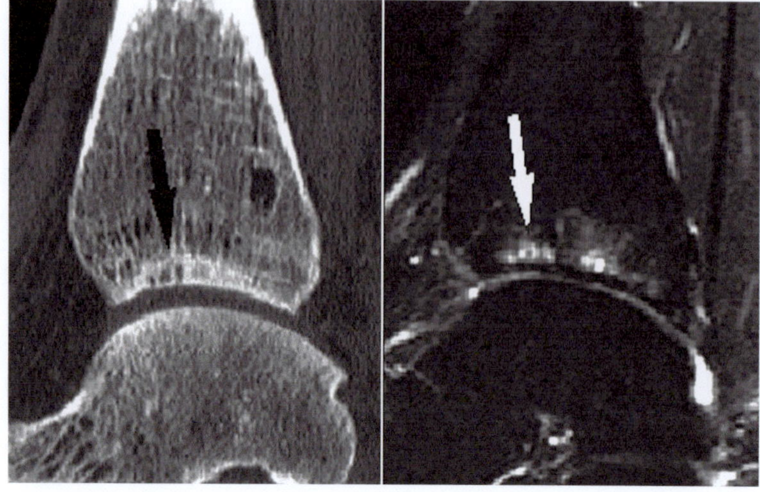

Fig. 4.1 Sagittal CT image (*right*) depicting small cystic changes in the tibial plafond (*arrows*). The defect is more clearly seen but overestimated on the fat-suppressed T2-weighted sagittal MR image (*left*)

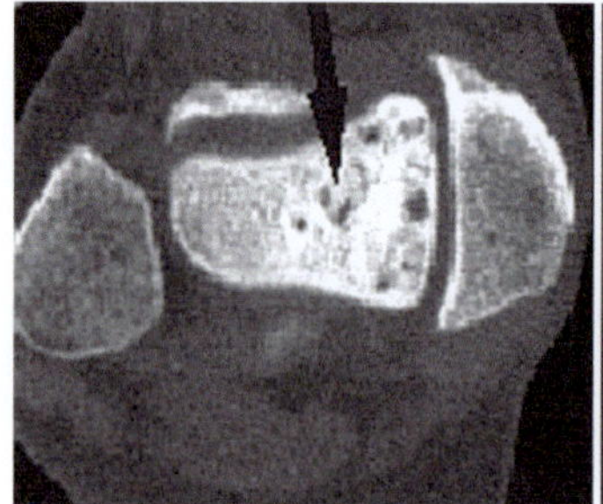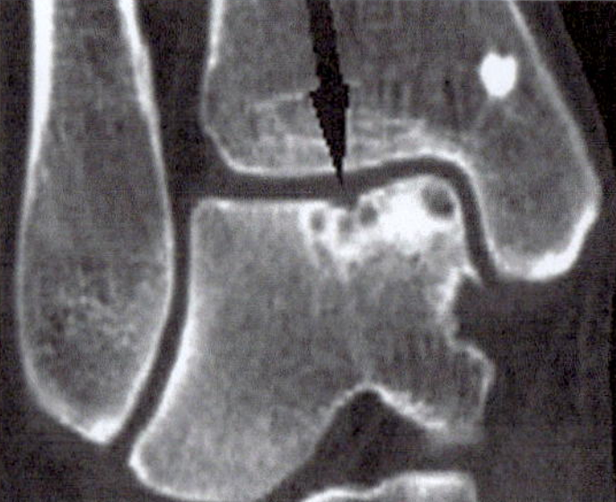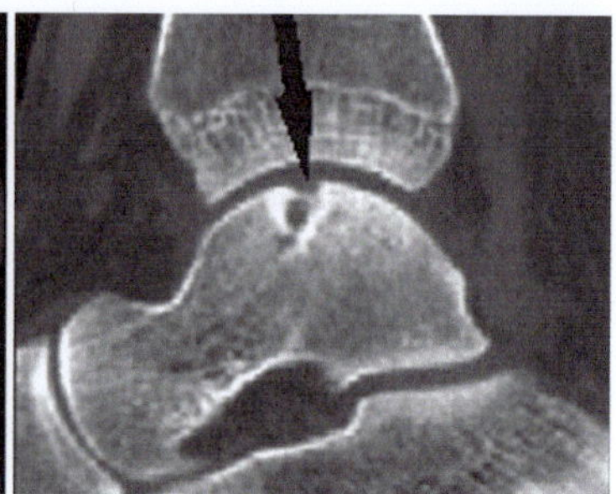

Fig. 4.2 CT image of a multicystic osteochondral defect (*arrow*) located medial in the talar dome. The CT image is reformatted in three planes; from *right* to *left*, the original axial plane and the coronal and sagittal reformatted plane, respectively. The cortex is disrupted, indicating instability

be performed in any desired plane without loss of image quality. To obtain a clear view of the extent and location of the defect, three orthogonal imaging planes are recommended. The anatomical position of the defects can often be most clearly visualized on a coronal or sagittal MPR image (Fig. 4.2). Not only can the extent of the defect be determined, but additional defects, such as kissing lesions in the tibia plafond, can also be visualized clearly.

Even though CT is not ideal for depicting soft tissues, these tissues are also in the field of view. A data set made with a soft tissue kernel should be part of the standard imaging protocol. Especially with optimal adjustment of the window and level, these tissues can be visualized and screened for pathology. Therefore, soft tissue swelling, such as focal synovitis, areas of ligamentous disruption like deep parts of the deltoid ligament, and supernumerary muscles and soft tissue masses (lipomas, cysts) can be seen on CT.

A frequently asked question is as follows: MRI is often considered the imaging modality of choice for imaging OCDs; as MRI can visualize cartilage and CT cannot, why should in fact CT scans be used? Verhagen et al. answered this question by performing a prospective study on diagnostic strategies in OCDs of the talus. In this study they found that 41 % of OCDs of the ankle were missed on radiography, with arthroscopy as gold standard. Furthermore, both CT (non-contrast, multi-detector with multi-planar reformatted images) and routine MRI performed similar to arthroscopy. It was shown that MRI had the highest sensitivity (96 %), but CT was more specific (99 %) [3]. Clinical implementation of this research might be to perform a CT if radiography is positive for an OCD and to perform an MRI, followed by CT to plan surgery, in case of negative radiography.

4.2.3 Advantages of CT

The use of CT is superior in the detection of OCDs as compared to conventional radiography [12, 13, 16]. Imaging of OCDs in the ankle by multi-detector computed tomography (CT) has several other benefits.

An advantage of CT is that additional bony pathologies which could influence treatment, such as (undercalled) fractures, osteophytes, loose bodies, ossicles, osteoarthritis, bony coalitions, transient osteoporosis, or osteonecrosis, can be detected, especially when two sides are compared. Verhagen also showed that a CT scan provides better visibility of cortical outlines and lower risk for overestimation of the OCD in comparison with MRI which often overcalls the extent of the defect due to the clearly visible bone marrow edema [13] on MRI.

As compared to MRI in particular, CT scans have the advantage that the ankle can be placed in various positions. As no coil is needed to image the ankle, a CT scan of the ankle can also be performed in plantar flexion. This is beneficial as this can aid the surgeon in deciding which operative approach should be chosen. This position is comparable to the X-ray of the ankle in plantar flexion, but with more detail and in three dimensions. With the aid of a preoperative CT scan in plantar flexion, the surgeon can make a reliable and accurate assessment preoperatively of the arthroscopic location of the defects. Bergen et al. concluded in a prospective blinded study that there is an excellent correlation between the CT and arthroscopic location of the OCDs [1]. This can be used to determine the method of surgery, whether an anterior approach is feasible.

Next, compared to MRI, CT scans are performed very fast and at submillimeter resolution. A standard MRI scan of the ankle lasts approximately 30 min with at most 2 mm resolution, whereas a CT scan of the ankle is performed within 1 min while providing very detailed, often submillimeter, images. Fast imaging reduces motion artifacts. Mainly due to the shorter scan time, less manpower is needed per patient. Consequently a CT scan is cheaper than an MRI scan of the ankle. Furthermore CT scans can be used for the imaging of OCDs of patients with contraindications for MRI, i.e., claustrophobia and metal implants (e.g., ICDs and neurostimulators). CT can easily be used for follow-up of OCDs treated both conservatively as well as surgically. After surgery the boney healing response can be monitored well by CT. The formations of callus, the progressive sclerosis of a defect, and periosteal reaction are depicted well by CT.

Another advantage of CT above MRI is that if desired both ankles can be imaged at once. Scanning both ankles at the same time is beneficial. It does not hamper image quality or significantly increase radiation burden yet provides the opportunity to compare both bony and soft tissues of both ankles. Imaging the other ankle provides an anatomical comparison in the same scan time as one ankle.

A new technique that is explored is a weight-bearing cone beam CT of the ankle. This new device allows the assessment of a small FOV, of only one ankle, yet adds weight bearing as a potential important tool in analysis of chronic ankle pain. Its use in patients with an OCD needs to be studied.

4.2.4 CT Arthrography

CT scans can only depict cartilage indirectly, as it mainly visualizes bone. However, cartilage can be depicted more accurately with CT arthrography. For CT arthrography, negative or positive contrast could be applied with, respectively, water or iodinated contrast material in a single or double method, with or without additional air. Iodinated contrast material provides better contrast than water in respect to cartilage, thereby achieving more reliable delineation of the cartilage pathology. Therefore, preferably positive contrast material is used for CT arthrography. A single contrast method, without the additional injection of air, is most often used.

For this procedure, iodinated contrast is injected intra-articularly in the tibiotalar joint, with fluoroscopic guidance (Fig. 4.3a). The preferred approach of the joint is anterior, placing the needle between the extensor hallucis longus tendon and the extensor digitorum tendon while avoiding the dorsalis pedis artery. Contrast injected intra-articularly will quickly spread throughout the joint. More contrast can be added if there is communication with the posterior subtalar joint or the flexor hallucis tendon. If the patient reports a sensation of tension in the joint, the injection is terminated. For the ankle this most often occurs after approximately 5 ml.

CT arthrography has been reported to be just as good or even better than MR arthrography for the detection of cartilage pathology [4, 10]. The intrinsic combination of high-resolution CT imaging and indirect cartilage mapping with detailed imaging of the cartilaginous defects makes CT arthrography powerful (Fig. 4.3b, c). The disadvantage of CT arthrography is that it is an invasive procedure, which as any invasive procedure can cause complications and side effects such as hemorrhage and infection.

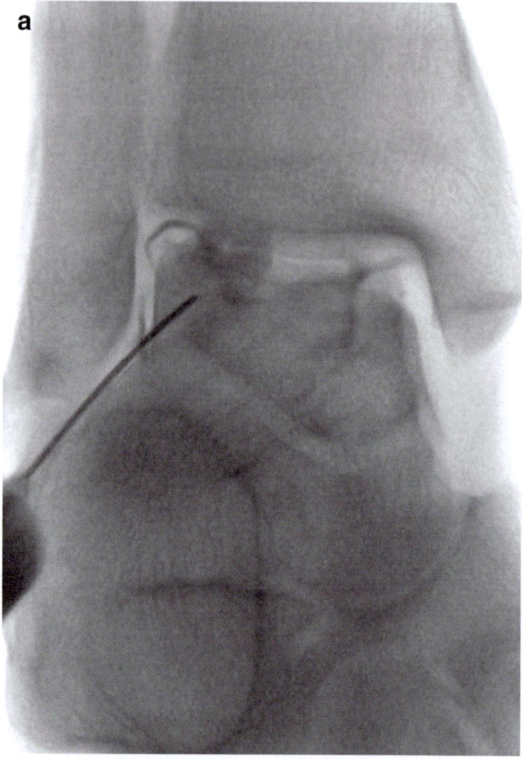

Fig. 4.3 Images of a 34-year-old male patient with pain in the right upper ankle joint. The upper ankle joint space was filled with contrast media under fluoroscopic guidance (**a**). Late-phase SPECT-CT arthrography coronal (**b**) and sagittal images (**c**) show an osteochondral defect with multiple small bony fragments in the medial part of the talus and increased perifocal activity. The cartilage layer is well preserved without larger cartilage defects. No loose bodies were observed. Patient was treated with Pridie drilling

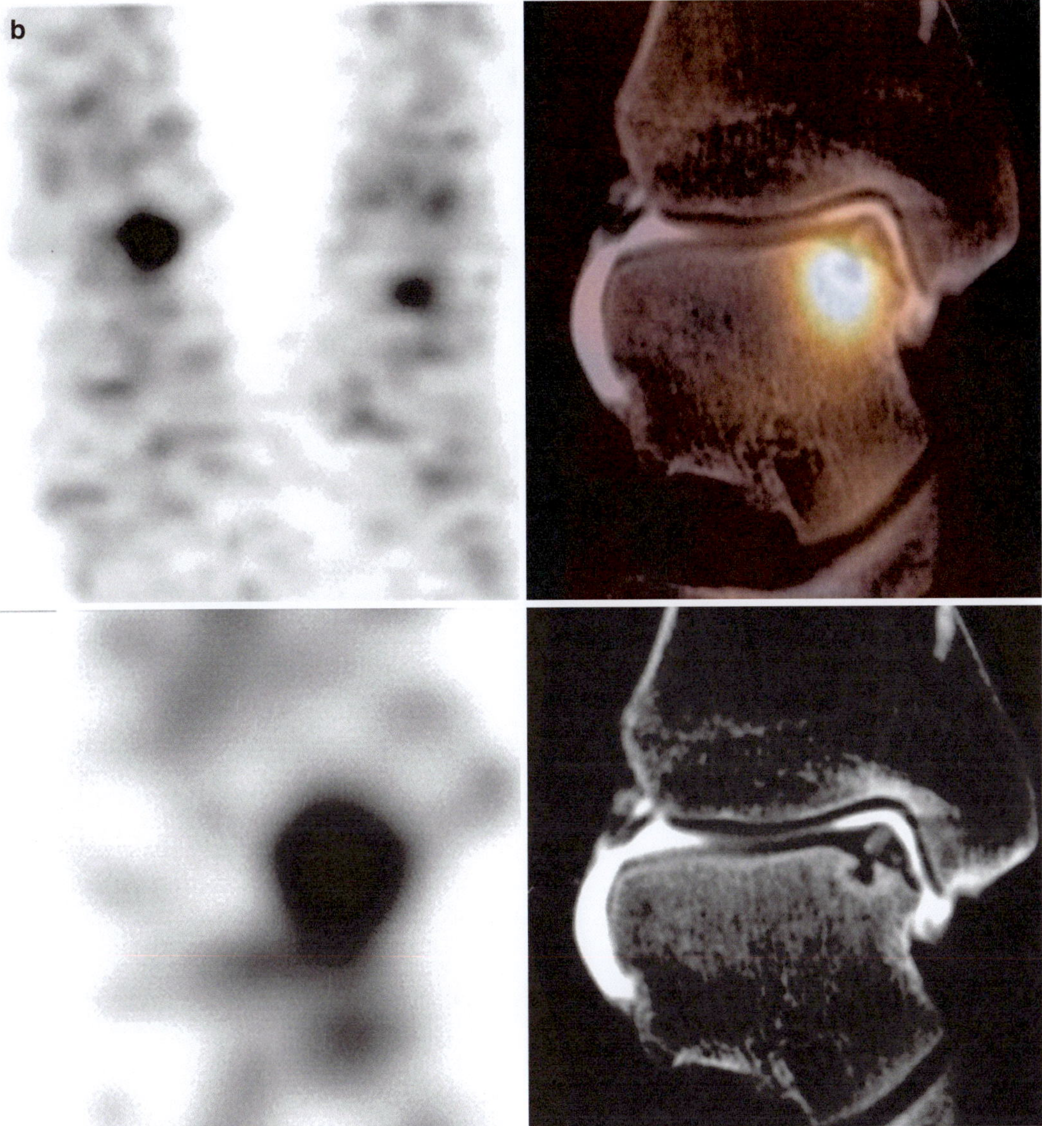

Fig. 4.3 (continued)

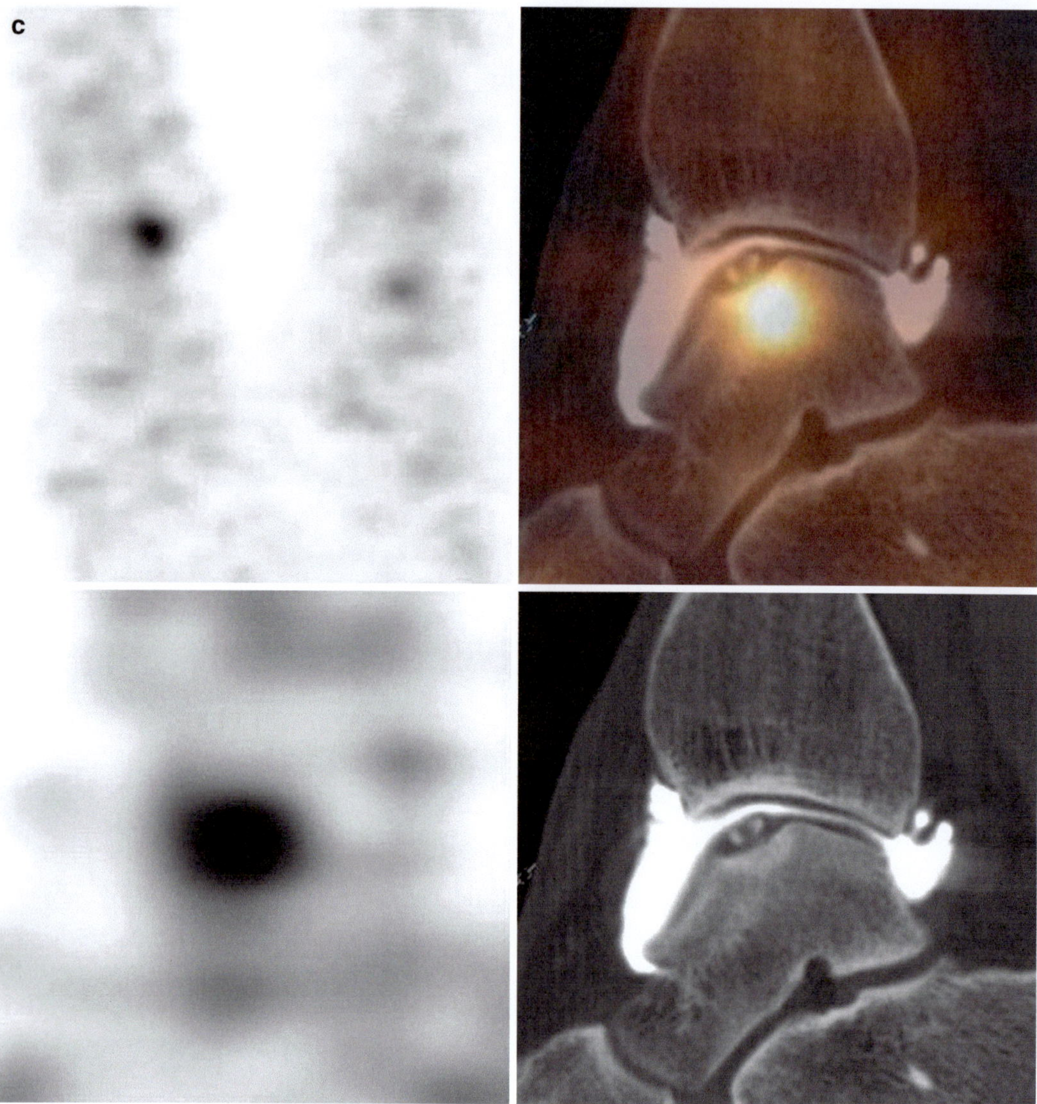

Fig. 4.3 (continued)

4.2.5 Staging Systems

In recent years several OCD classification systems have been designed in an attempt to aid in prognosis and therapeutic planning of the defects. Two of these often-used radiologic staging systems are mentioned below. As various clinicians may use different classification systems, it is advised for the radiologist to describe the appearance of the OCD as well, to prevent possible misunderstandings. In general, it is important for radiologists, surgeons, and other clinicians to use the same terminology so that each person knows what is meant by a certain description or stage of a disease. The sole use of a classification system in radiology reports should be discouraged as this leads to loss of information which could be important to the surgeon.

More than 50 years ago, in 1959, Berndt and Harty designed a classification system for transchondral fractures (OCDs) in the talus based on

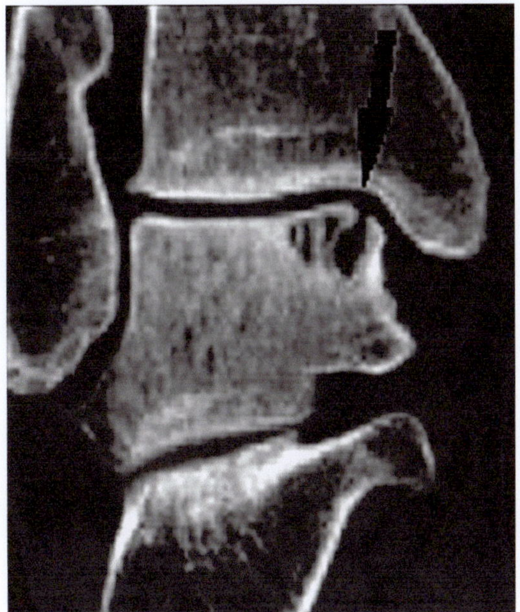

Fig. 4.4 Coronal CT image of a multicystic osteochondral defect (*arrow*), located medial in the talar dome. Stage 2 lesion, according to Ferkel classification system, with a large subchondral cystic component with a small defect in the cortical bone. The cortex is disrupted, indicating instability

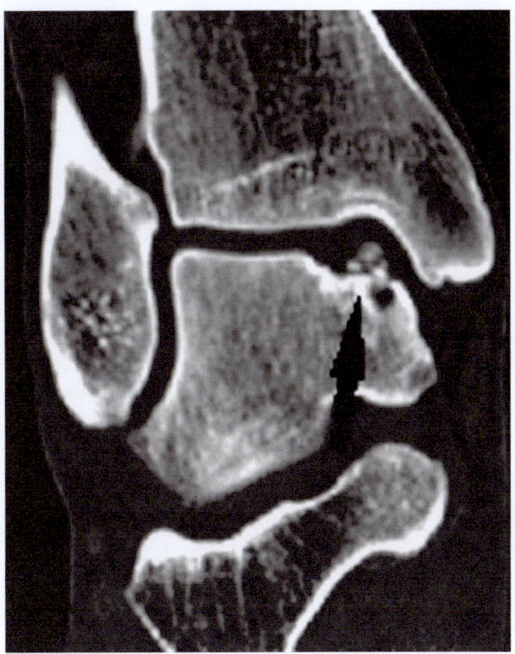

Fig. 4.5 Coronal CT image of a stage 3, according to Ferkel classification system, osteochondral defect in the medial talar dome consisting of a completely detached but non-displaced loose fragment (*arrow*)

conventional radiographs [2]. For this classification, refer to Chap. 1. In stages 1 and 2, a cystic defect with an intact roof or a minor disruption of the talar roof or tibial plafond can be noted (Fig. 4.4). These stages are difficult to detect by conventional radiographic imaging. However, these stages can also be overlooked on CT imaging, as the bony changes can be very subtle. CT imaging has the highest sensitivity and specificity for stage 3 and 4 defects. CT imaging plays an important role in the delineation of defects that may present with loose fragments (Fig. 4.5).

Ferkel et al. developed an OCD classification system for CT-based staging on the Berndt and Harty system [5]. For this classification also, see Chap. 1.

There are several arthroscopic-based staging systems which often lack a correlation with diagnostic imaging methods and are therefore primarily used by surgeons. These systems should not be extrapolated to stage OCDs on imaging modalities. Since arthroscopic classification systems are based on arthroscopy, only the superficial defects are described as the surgeon cannot visualize deeper lying pathology.

4.2.6 Pitfalls of Imaging

An additional OCD in the directly opposing tibia plafond is called a kissing defect (Fig. 4.6) [11]. These lesions are quite rare and can be overlooked by any diagnostic modality or arthroscopy, due to the satisfaction of search principle [13]. These defects should not be mistaken for osteoarthritis, in which case there also should be joint space narrowing, increased sclerosis, and bone formation. It is important to mention these kissing defects, as the treatment plan needs to be adapted to these findings.

Postoperative analysis of an OCD can be difficult due to the various operative treatment procedures as well as the disruption of the normal anatomical architectures of the tibiotalar joint. This can lead to misinterpretation of the

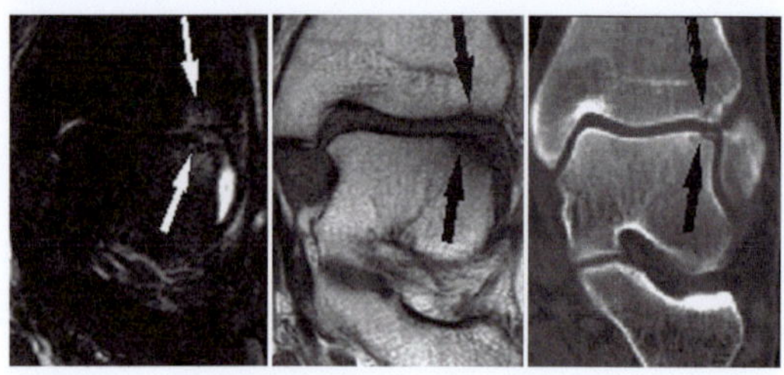

Fig. 4.6 A kissing osteochondral defect, stage 2 according to Ferkel, medially in the talar dome and the tibial plafond (*arrow*) on (from *right* to *left*) coronal fat-suppressed T2-weighted MR image, T1-weighted MR image, and CT. Due to the high spatial resolution of CT (0.3 mm slice thickness), the small cystic defects are depicted

images. Providing detailed information, concerning the used operative techniques and treatment, will aid the radiologist in accurate image interpretation.

4.2.7 Disadvantages of CT Imaging

Disadvantages of CT imaging are the radiation dose patients acquire, the fact that cartilage cannot be visualized directly, less clear visualization of soft tissues, and non-weight-bearing conditions.

Concerning the first disadvantage mentioned, the average effective radiation dose acquired of a CT scan of the ankle is 0.07 millisievert (mSv). This radiation dose is very low compared to the annual effective background dose for the Netherlands, which is 2.5 mSv, and for a citizen of Denver, Colorado, USA, which is 6 mSv. Also compared to a hip or shoulder CT scan, which amounts to an effective radiation dose of 3.09 and 2.06 mSv, respectively [3], the radiation dose of an ankle CT scan is low.

Regarding the second disadvantage mentioned, CT cannot visualize cartilage directly, but CT arthrography is capable of discerning cartilage defects by injection of a contrast medium in the joint. Various studies have shown that by using CT arthrography, cartilage thickness can be measured indirectly just as well or even better than by using MR arthrography [4, 10]. See Sect. 4.2.4.

Thirdly, as mentioned previously soft tissues can be visualized by CT. However, MRI is superior for the visualization of bone marrow edema and has higher contrast for the depiction of soft tissue imaging. Nevertheless, CT has been proven to be just as effective in the detection of OCDs [13].

Contrary to conventional imaging, for CT examination and for the majority of the MRI examinations, patients are required to lie in a supine or prone position; thereby, no pressure is applied on the ankle joint. Therefore, CT images are currently all non-weight-bearing views.

4.3 SPECT-CT

4.3.1 SPECT-CT, Rationale and Basic Science

One of the potential disadvantages of the previously described static CT technology might be that it does not necessarily reveal biological activity directly. Even the indirect signs of increased or decreased metabolic activity such as hyper- or hypointensity on MRI or changes in density on planar radiographs are only indicative of underlying processes and typically occur with some delay after the onset of a problem. Planar technetium-labeled skeletal scintigraphy has been the preferred method to monitor biological, metabolic osseous activity, yet at the expense of spatial resolution. While the latter might not be a concern in screening for pathology or stress fractures, it poses a severe problem in areas of complex anatomy with numerous potential sources of pain, such as the foot and ankle. Combining single-photon emission computed tomography (SPECT) and CT merges the high sensitivity of scintigraphy for increased bone turnover with the high spatial resolution of CT (Fig. 4.3b) and allows reliable evaluation of osseous defects and the metabolic activity of the adjacent tissues at the same time.

While this is all true in theory, these assumptions have to be tested and confirmed scientifically. The first and most pressing issue in imaging is reliability, i.e., if the findings and interpretation of an imaging study are consistent and reproducible. Pagenstert et al. assessed the inter- and intra-observer correlation of SPECT-CT and compared them to SPECT alone, CT alone, non-fused SPECT, and CT studies in 20 patients with refractory postoperative foot pain [9]. The average age was 47 years (range 27–59), consisting of 11 women and 9 men. Interobserver correlation was, ranked highest to lowest, 0.92 for SPECT-CT, 0.83 for SPECT and CT, 0.8 for CT, and 0.69 for bone scans alone. The intra-observer correlation for independent assessors was, again ranked highest to lowest, 0.87 for SPECT-CT, 0.71 for CT, 0.66 for bone scans, and 0.64 for SPECT and CT.

The next important question is validity, i.e., if SPECT-CT really shows what we want it to show. In most cases that is simply pain. Wiewiorski et al. showed that in patients with chronic ankle pain, a CT-guided injection of bupivacaine (1.5 %, 5 cc) to the point of highest SPECT-CT intensity enabled an immediate drop on the visual analog pain scale of more than 50 %. These findings are in strong support of the ability of SPECT-CT to accurately locate a pain source [14].

In comparing impact of imaging on therapeutic planning, Leumann et al. compared effectiveness of SPECT-CT and MRI in patients with a known talar OCD. They found that offering both imaging studies to treating orthopedists changed treatment recommendations in 52 % of cases, mostly toward regenerative treatment options such as cartilage repair [7].

4.3.2 Advantages of SPECT-CT

One clear advantage of SPECT-CT is the fusion of structural information with data on metabolic activity. As the studies described above have shown, these data are valid and reliable, and there is strong evidence that SPECT-CT is indeed able to accurately identify the location that generates the pain, even in the complex anatomy of the foot and ankle.

Another advantage is that the addition of SPECT-CT to conventional images has shown substantial impact on clinical decision-making. Thus, while SPECT-CT is by no means a first-line technique, patients with complicated injuries and long-standing foot and ankle problems without a clear treatment regimen will benefit from SPECT-CT.

A further technical advantage is that SPECT-CT can be used for patients with implanted hardware. Especially in postoperative situations, such as nonunion, malunion, or adjacent joint degeneration after open reposition and internal fixation, SPECT-CT is a valuable tool for patients that cannot undergo an MRI.

Last but not least, current SPECT-CT uses osteoblast-specific tracers, but in the future other tracers, such as for tenocytes, might be available and help in the diagnosis of tendon/ligament to bone healing in such situations as ankle sprains, but also in anterior cruciate ligament reconstruction or rotator cuff repair.

4.3.3 Disadvantages of SPECT-CT

The important drawback of SPECT-CT is the radiation burden. Following guidelines from the American College of Radiology (ACR) [15], it is stated that technetium-99m bone scan of the ankle on itself provides an adult effective dose estimate range of 1–10 mSv, to which the CT scan dose needs addition. Special concern for this radiation is the pediatric population for which the pediatric effective dose estimate range is 0.3–3 mSv [15].

A second disadvantage of SPECT-CT is the potential for false-positive findings. It is crucial to first study the whole body scan to see if the area of interest actually stands out from the remainder of the skeleton in terms of uptake before studying fused, focused images. Also, in postoperative situations bone scans might show increased uptake as part of the physiological remodeling processes. An experienced assessor will be able to differentiate these, but it requires all clinical information while interpreting a study.

Another disadvantage is the cost and required level of infrastructure. SPECT-CT is, today, certainly a tool for larger hospitals or academic centers with both radiologist and nuclear medicine experts. Costs are high, both in terms of equipment and per study. Tracers have to be administered hours before the actual imaging session, which translates into an increased period of in-hospital stay compared to MRI or CT. Last but not least, current tracer uptake is not as specific as the CT in terms of spatial resolution and not 100 % selective for osteoblast activity. This potentially complicates SPECT-CT interpretation in situations of closely adjacent defects.

Conclusion

So where does this leave the team of clinicians in charge of the patient with chronic ankle pain suspected for an OCD of the tibiotalar joint? Which imaging steps are most beneficial, with the least radiation burden, and are most cost-effective? In order to evaluate suggested imaging modalities, it can be supportive to check the advice given by the radiologic community of expert musculoskeletal radiologists in the USA. On the website of the ACR (www.acr.org), the appropriateness criteria are listed concerning various clinical conditions among which is chronic ankle pain [16]. Conventional radiography is suggested as a first step. If the radiograph is negative, plain MRI is suggested as the next most appropriate step. The other imaging options; MR arthrography, CT arthrography or plain CT are considered possibly appropriate next steps if the radiograph is negative. For evaluation of an OCD, we prefer CT scan over MRI as CT is superior for preoperative planning. The use of SPECT-CT is not yet advised, also because of costs and radiation-related aspects.

Conflict of Interests The author has no current conflict of interests with the products presented.

References

1. van Bergen CJA, Tuijthof GJM, Blankevoort L, Maas M, Kerkhoffs GM, van Dijk CN. Computed tomography of the ankle in full plantar flexion: a reliable method for preoperative planning of arthroscopic access to osteochondral defects of the talus. Arthroscopy. 2012;288:985–92.
2. Berndt AL, Harty M. Transchondral fractures (osteochondritis dissecans) of the talus. J Bone Joint Surg Am. 1959;41–A:988–1020.
3. Biswas D, Bible JE, Bohan M, Simpson AK, Whang PG, Grauer JN. Radiation exposure from musculoskeletal computerized tomographic scans. J Bone Joint Surg Am. 2009;91:1882–9.
4. El-Khoury GY, Alliman KJ, Lundberg HJ, Rudert MJ, Brown TD, Saltzman CL. Cartilage thickness in cadaveric ankles: measurement with double contrast multi-detector row CT arthrography versus MR imaging. Radiology. 2004;233:768–73.
5. Ferkel RD, Sgaglione NA, Del Pixxo W. Arthroscopic treatment of osteochondral lesions of the talus: technique and results. Orthop Trans. 1990;14:172.
6. Ferkel RD, Van Dijk CN, Younger A. Osteochondral lesions of the talus: current treatment dilemmas. Instructional course lectures. 2013; Unpublished paper presented at the American Association of Orthopaedic Surgeons annual meeting 2013, Chicago, Illinois, USA.
7. Leumann A, Valderrabano V, PLaass C, Rasch H, Studler U, Hintermann B, Pagenstert GI. A novel imaging method for osteochondral lesions of the talus- comparison of SPECT-CT with MRI. Am J Sports Med. 2011;39:1095–101.
8. Loomer R, Fisher C, Lloyd-Smith R, Sisler J, Cooner T. Osteochondral lesions of the talus. Am J Sports Med. 1993;21:13–9.
9. Pagenstert GI, Barg A, Leumann AG, Rasch H, Müller-Brand J, Hintermann B, Valderrabano V. SPECT-CT imaging in degenerative joint disease of the foot and ankle. J Bone Joint Surg Br. 2009;91:1191–6.
10. Schmid MR, Pfirrmann CWA, Hodler J, Vienne P, Zanetti M. Cartilage lesions in the ankle joint: comparison of MR arthrography and CT arthrography. Skeletal Radiol. 2003;32:259–65.
11. Sijbrandij ES, van Gils APG, Louwerens JW, de Lange EE. Posttraumatic subchondral bone contusions and fractures of the talotibial joint: occurrence of "kissing" lesions. AJR Am J Roentgenol. 2000;175:1007–10.
12. Stone JW. Osteochondral lesions of the talar dome. J Am Ac Orthop Surg. 1996;4:63–73.
13. Verhagen RAW, Maas M, Dijkgraaf MGW, Tol JL, Krips R, van Dijk CN. Prospective study on diagnostic strategies in osteochondral lesions of the talus: is MRI superior to helical CT? J Bone Joint Surg Br. 2005;87-B:41–6.
14. Wiewiorski M, Pagenstert G, Rasch H, Jacob AL, Valderrabano V. Pain in osteochondral lesions. Foot Ankle Int. 2011;4:92–9.
15. www.acr.org/media/ACR/Documents/AppCriteria/Diagnostic/ChronicAnklePain.pdf.16.
16. Zinman C, Wolfson N, Reis ND. Osteochondritis of the dome of the talus. J Bone Joint Surg Am. 1988;70:1017–9.

Diagnosis of Osteochondral Defects by Arthroscopy

5

David E. Oji, David A. McCall, Lew C. Schon,
and Richard D. Ferkel

> **Take-Home Points**
> - *Arthroscopic classification of chondral defect can be done by the Ferkel or the International Cartilage Repair Society (ICRS) classification.*
> - *CT, MRI, and arthroscopy all have high sensitivity and specificity in diagnosing an osteochondral defect.*
> - *Arthroscopy has the advantage of directly visualizing and identifying the chondral defect.*
> - *Negative radiographs, CT, and MRI do not necessarily rule out an osteochondral defect.*
> - *Osteochondral defects can be characterized by location, size, depth, stability, displacement, containment, and type of lesion.*

D.E. Oji, MD (✉)
Division of Foot and Ankle, Department
of Orthopaedics, Medstar Union Memorial Hospital,
Johnston Professional Building, Baltimore, MD, USA
e-mail: david.oji@jhmi.edu

D.A. McCall, MD
Department of Orthopaedic Surgery,
Southern California Orthopedic Institute,
University of California,
Los Angeles/Van Nuys, CA, USA
e-mail: dmccall@scoi.com

L.C. Schon, MD
Department of Orthopaedics,
Medstar Union Memorial Hospital,
Baltimore/Washington, DC, USA

Division of Foot and Ankle, Johns Hopkins School
of Medicine & Georgetown School of Medicine, Johns
Hopkins University, Baltimore/Washington, DC, USA
e-mail: lewschon@comcast.net

R.D. Ferkel, MD
Department of Orthopaedic Surgery,
University of California Los Angeles,
Los Angeles, CA, USA

Southern California Orthopedic Institute,
Van Nuys, CA, USA
e-mail: rferkel@scoi.com

5.1 Introduction

Chondral lesions of the talus can be a potential cause of long-term debilitation. Although advanced studies such as magnetic resonance imaging (MRI) and computed tomography (CT) have been shown to be very sensitive and specific in identifying these defects, a negative study cannot definitively rule out osteochondral defects (OCDs) [13, 25]. In a patient who continues to be symptomatic in the setting of negative imaging studies, a diagnostic ankle arthroscopy may be needed for the most accurate diagnosis. With the development of improved instrumentation and technology, ankle arthroscopy has evolved to become a useful tool for both diagnosis and treatment of osteochondral defects. More importantly, arthroscopic management of osteochondral defects can reduce the morbidity associated with surgical approaches such as an ankle arthrotomy and malleolar osteotomy.

C.N. van Dijk, J.G. Kennedy (eds.), *Talar Osteochondral Defects*,
DOI 10.1007/978-3-642-45097-6_5, © ESSKA 2014

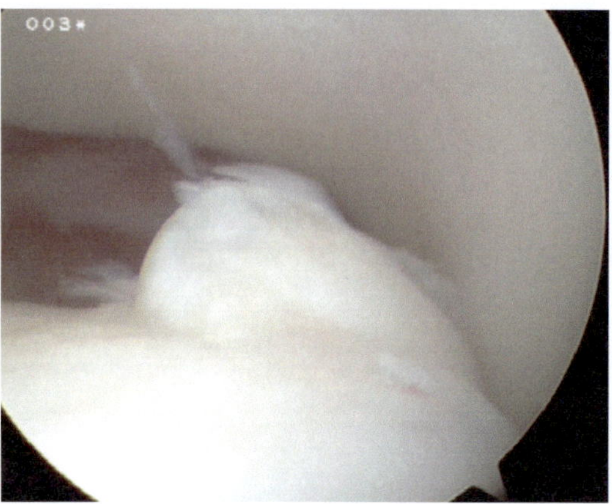

Fig. 5.1 Arthroscopic stage D medial talar dome lesion in a right ankle

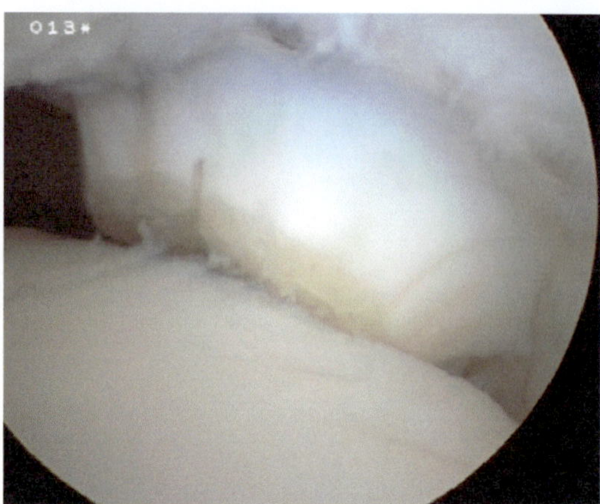

Fig. 5.2 Arthroscopic stage F medial talar dome lesion in a right ankle

5.2 Classification

There are many classification systems to describe OCDs based on imaging studies such as the Berndt and Harty based on radiographs [2], Hepple [11] and Anderson [1] classification based on MRI findings, and the CT-based Ferkel and Sgaglione classification [7]. Pritsch and co-workers were the first to develop an arthroscopic classification based on the overlying cartilage [20]. The classification is as follows:

- Grade I: Intact, firm, shiny cartilage
- Grade II: Intact but soft cartilage
- Grade III: Frayed cartilage

Ferkel and Cheng expanded this system in 1995 to include chondromalacia and displaced osteochondral lesions [8] (Figs. 5.1 and 5.2):

- Grade A: Smooth, intact cartilage, but soft or ballottable
- Grade B: Rough surface
- Grade C: Fibrillations/fissures
- Grade D: Flap present or bone exposed
- Grade E: Loose, undisplaced fragment
- Grade F: Displaced fragment

Taranow and co-workers in 1999 used a dual approach using MRI for preoperative evaluation and then arthroscopy for final staging to classify OCDs [26].

In addition to classification systems based on talar lesions, the International Cartilage Repair Society (ICRS) developed a standardized classification system for evaluating cartilage injuries based on the depth and area of damage [3] (Fig. 5.3):

- Grade 0: Normal cartilage
- Grade 1: Superficial lesions with soft indentation and/or superficial fissures
- Grade 2: Abnormal cartilage with lesions extending down to <50 % of cartilage depth
- Grade 3: Severely abnormal with cartilage defects extending down >50 % of cartilage with four subgroups:
  - 3a: Defects that do not extend to the calcified layer
  - 3b: Defects that extend to the calcified layer
  - 3c: Defects down to but not through the subchondral bone plate
  - 3d: Blistering of the cartilage
- Grade 4: Severely abnormal full thickness defects:
  - 4a: Penetrating subchondral bone but not the full diameter of defect
  - 4b: Penetrating subchondral bone the full diameter of defect

5.3 Comparison of Imaging Versus Arthroscopic Diagnostic Techniques

The clinical decision to obtain an MRI or CT to evaluate for possible OCD after a thorough physical examination and baseline radiographs is determined by a number of factors. However, there is debate regarding the optimal imaging modality to evaluate an OCD. Verhagen and co-workers

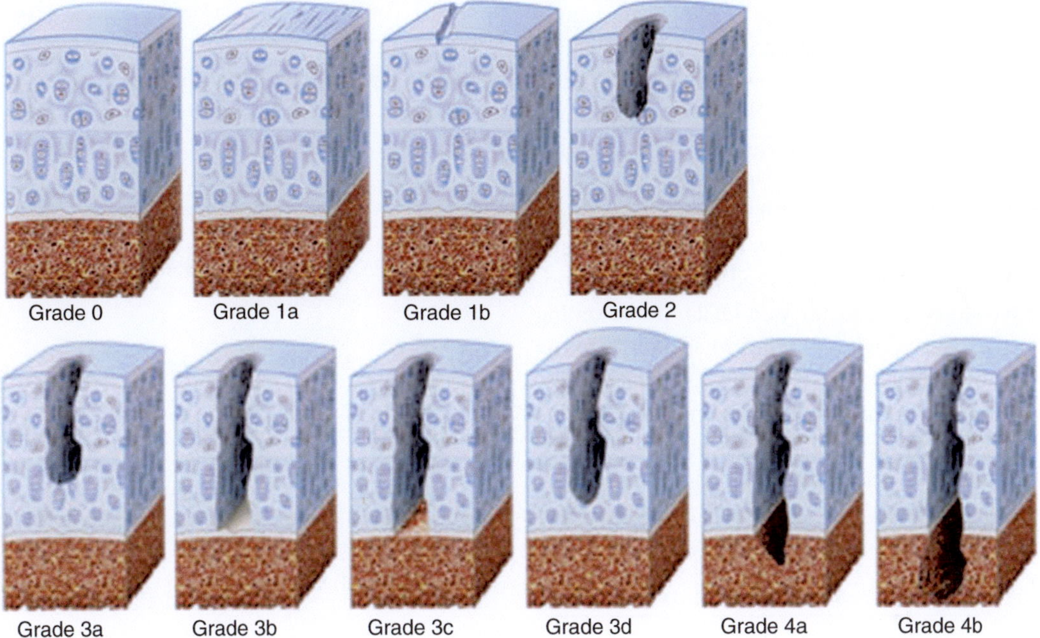

Fig. 5.3 ICRS classification

investigated the utility of MRI, CT, and arthroscopy in the diagnosis of OCDs [29]. Although all three modalities were found to be superior to physical examination and radiographs alone, there was no statistical significance between MRI, CT, and diagnostic arthroscopy in detecting or excluding an OCD. Sensitivity and specificity for detecting an OCD with arthroscopy in this study were 100 and 97 %, respectively. The sensitivity and specificity values for MRI were 96 and 96 % and 81 and 99 % for CT.

The capability of MRI and arthroscopy to identify and exclude chondral defects of the talus has been compared previously [13]. However, when MRI findings did not correlate with arthroscopic findings, it was found that MRI tended to overgrade the lesion severity, especially with subchondral edema [13, 16]. Moreover, MRI's predilection to detect subchondral changes as opposed to superficial lesions might result in missing surface defects [24].

As opposed to MRI, arthroscopy has the advantage of being able to directly visualize and identify a surface OCD. However, one drawback to arthroscopy is its inability to potentially identify a subchondral lesion with intact surface cartilage [15].

O'Neill and co-workers assessed the accuracy of the radiologist and orthopedic surgeon readings of MRI in patients with ankle instability [18]. The physician's preoperative readings were compared to intraoperative findings. Interestingly, the radiologist and orthopedic surgeon only identified 39 and 45 % of chondral lesions, respectively. In a separate study, 38 % of chondral lesions were missed by MRI [24].

These articles question the accuracy of preoperative MRI for evaluating for chondral defects. O'Neill and co-workers indicated that almost all of the unidentified chondral defects were full thickness that warranted microfracture and were not necessarily large or deep lesions. This again indicates the difficulty of identifying superficial lesions in a region known for a thin layer of cartilage compared to other joints such as the knee [23]. The difficulties in detecting these defects were attributed to studies with low-powered magnets [12, 17, 25], differences in patient positioning [22], variability in the radiologist skills [18], and differences in imaging sequences [9, 19, 21]. These problems can be commonly encountered in the general orthopedic community who may not have access to a musculoskeletal radiologist or 1.5 or 3.0 T MRI. As a result, many OCDs can be missed.

In the past, the value of diagnostic ankle arthroscopy in the setting of a patient with no definitive diagnosis has been questioned [27, 28]. However, the study by O'Neill, Van Aman, and Guyton suggests the difficulty in identifying OCDs with MRI alone. Their study suggests a more common scenario for community orthopedic surgeons without access to a musculoskeletal radiologist or a high-powered magnet with various sequences to identify an OCD. In the setting of a patient with a high clinical suspicion for an OCD, especially if considering a separate procedure such as a modified Brostrom to treat ankle instability, a diagnostic ankle arthroscopy may be warranted to accurately diagnose and treat patients.

5.4 Indications and Contraindications for Arthroscopic Diagnosis of Osteochondral Defect

As written by Drs. Ferkel and Hommen, "arthroscopic examination of the ankle and foot provides the opportunity to directly visualize and evaluate articular cartilage and soft tissue pathology [6]." If the index of suspicion for an OCD is high in the setting of negative imaging studies, and surgery is already planned to treat a separate pathology, a diagnostic ankle arthroscopy may be warranted to evaluate and treat a possible OCD. There are several possible etiologies for OCDs to include macrotrauma, repetitive microtrauma, ankle instability, and idiopathic avascular necrosis of the talus. As indicated above by O'Neill and co-workers, only 39 % of chondral lesions were identified by MRI in the setting of ankle instability [18].

Contraindications for a diagnostic ankle arthroscopy include localized soft tissue infection which could potentially cause intra-articular dissemination and severe degenerative joint disease where adequate range of motion and joint distraction cannot be achieved for joint visualization [6].

Table 5.1 Twenty-one-point ankle arthroscopic examination [5]

Location	Point of examination
Anterior ankle	1. Deltoid ligament
	2. Medial gutter
	3. Medial talus
	4. Central talus
	5. Lateral talus
	6. Talofibular articulation trifurcation
	7. Lateral gutter
	8. Anterior gutter
Central ankle	9. Mediocentral tibiotalus
	10. Middle tibiotalus
	11. Lateral tibiotalus
	12. Capsular reflection of FHL
	13. Transverse tibiofibular ligament
	14. Posterior inferior tibiofibular ligament
Posterior ankle	15. Medial gutter
	16. Medial talus
	17. Central talus
	18. Lateral talus
	19. Talofibular articulation
	20. Lateral gutter
	21. Posterior gutter, FHL, flexor hallucis longus

5.5 Arthroscopic Evaluation of an Osteochondral Defect

Arthroscopic evaluation of the articular surface should be done in a systematic manner to carefully evaluate the cartilage defect. This allows one to document the arthroscopic findings in a reproducible fashion, to accurately diagnose any potential intra-articular pathology, and to improve the quality of future clinical studies of the ankle arthroscopy patient population. A systematic 21-point ankle arthroscopic examination is used to ensure no pathology is missed [5]. The 21-point examination consists of three phases: the eight-point anterior examination, the six-point central examination, and the seven-point posterior examination (Table 5.1). The eight-point anterior examination includes the deltoid ligament, medial gutter, medial talus, central talus, lateral talus, talofibular articulation (trifurcation of the talus, tibia, and fibula), lateral gutter, and anterior gutter. The six-

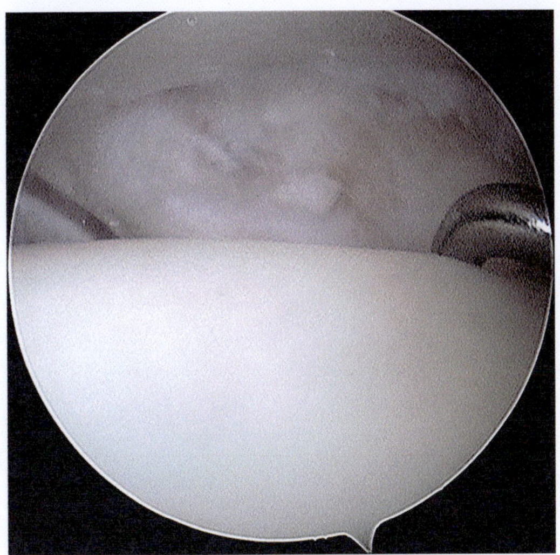

Fig. 5.4 Talar dome with no chondral defect

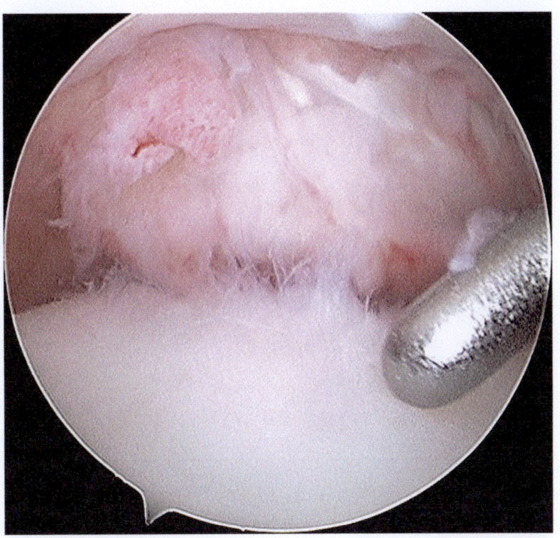

Fig. 5.5 OCD demonstrating a roughened surface and ICRS grade 2 changes

point central examination is performed by maneuvering the arthroscope through the notch of Harty. The notch of Harty is an anatomic elevation of the anteromedial distal tibia. The central examination includes the medial central tibiotalus, middle tibiotalus, lateral tibiotalus, capsular reflection of the FHL tendon, transverse tibiofibular ligament, and posterior inferior tibiofibular ligament. The seven-point posterior examination includes the medial gutter, medial talus, central talus, lateral talus, talofibular articulation, lateral gutter, and posterior gutter. Generally, the combination of the anteromedial, anterolateral, and posterolateral portals allows excellent visualization of the entire joint.

An arthroscopic probe can be used through the working portal to manipulate the OCD and document the characteristics. The most basic of these are the location, size, and depth of the defect. Location of the OCD should be described in both the sagittal (anterior, central, or posterior) and coronal plane (lateral, central, or medial). The size of the defect is similarly important to document considering lesions greater than or equal to 1.5 cm^2 have a higher failure rate with reparative techniques [4, 10, 14, 15]. Depth of the defect is defined by whether the OCD is a superficial lesion affecting only the cartilage; is it affecting both the cartilage and underlying subchondral bone; is there a subchondral defect with

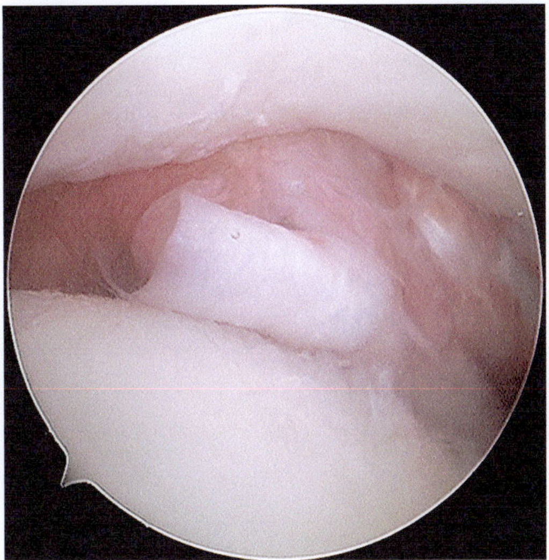

Fig. 5.6 Chondral defect with a large superficial flap and fissures present at the base

intact overlying cartilage; or is there a cystic defect greater than 7 mm [5]. Superficial lesions can be further characterized by whether its surface is soft versus rough, are fibrillations or fissures present, and whether a flap is present or is bone exposed as described in the Ferkel Arthroscopic Classification [7]. The depth of the defect can also be evaluated by using the ICRS grading system [3] (Figs. 5.4, 5.5, 5.6, 5.7, 5.8, and 5.9).

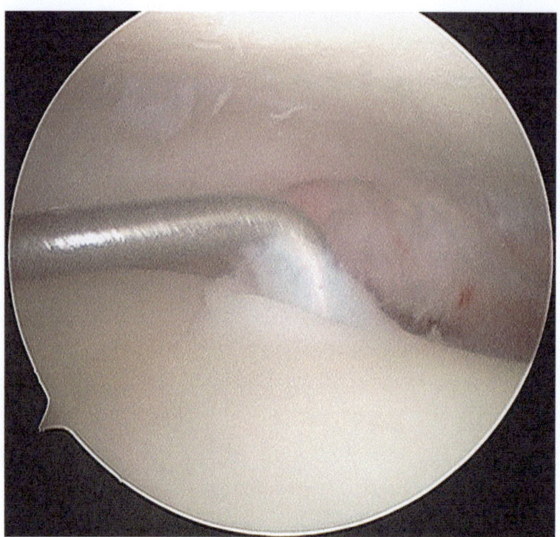

Fig. 5.7 Chondral defect with a small superficial flap and fissure

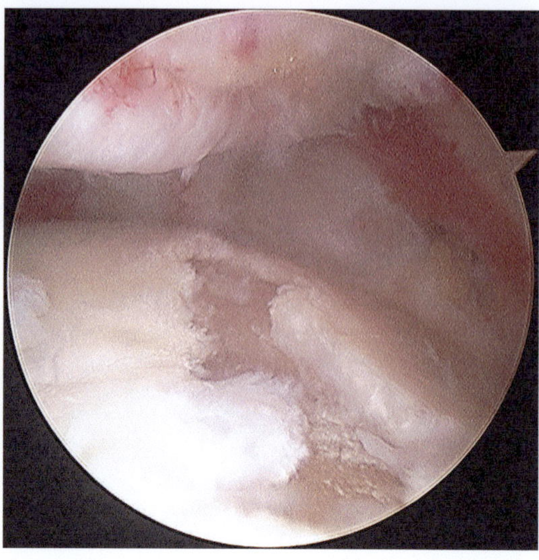

Fig. 5.9 A transverse anterior full thickness grade 4 OCD extending from the medial to lateral aspect of the talar dome

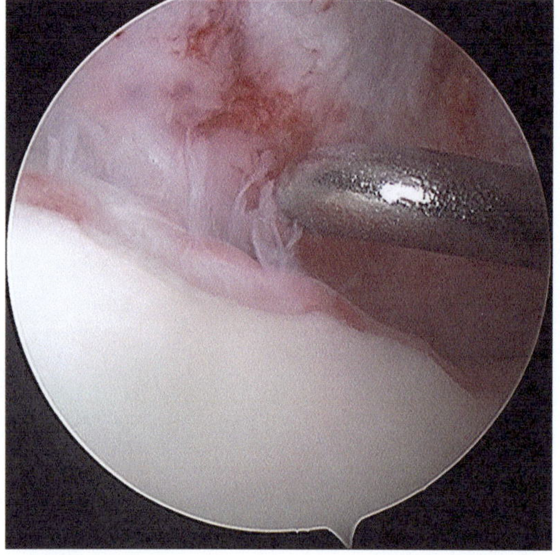

Fig. 5.8 A full thickness ICRS grade 4 unconstrained shoulder defect

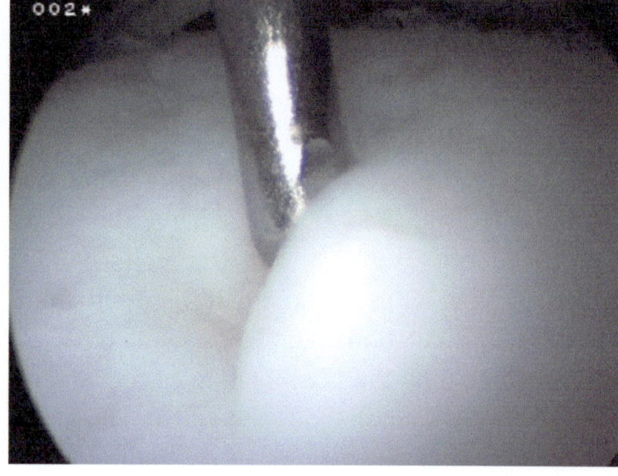

Fig. 5.10 Surrounding zone classification I: blistering with thickening of cartilage layer

In addition, OCDs can be characterized by whether it is a stable versus unstable defect, if the fragment is displaced, and whether the OCD is a contained or uncontained shoulder lesion [15].

Finally, a mention of the zone around the OCD should be included. Although the ICRS has a stage 3d which includes blistering of the surface cartilage, we have seen varying degrees of adjacent cartilage changes that warrant description and that may be present with ICRS stages other than 3. In this regard, we use a surrounding zone classification using roman numerals: I bulging and thickening of cartilage but no delamination; II bulging with fragile, friable connection with subchondral bone; and III complete delamination (Figs. 5.10, 5.11, and 5.12). All of these characteristics can help determine what intervention is best suited for the type of OCD (Table 5.2).

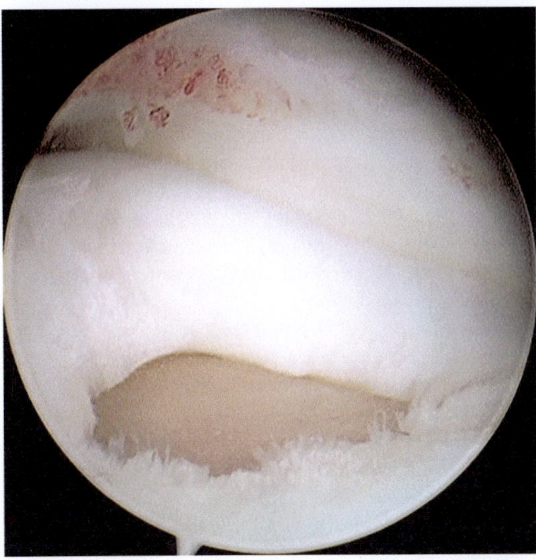

Fig. 5.11 Surrounding zone classification II: bulging with fragile, friable connection with subchondral bone

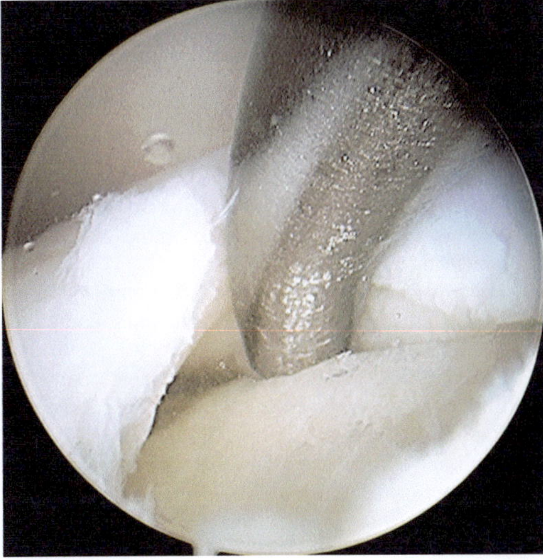

Fig. 5.12 Surrounding zone classification III: complete delamination

Table 5.2 Characteristics to describe an osteochondral defect arthroscopically

1. Location of defect:
   (a) Sagittal plane
       (i) Lateral
       (ii) Central
       (iii) Medial
   (b) Coronal plane
       (i) Anterior
       (ii) Central
       (iii) Posterior
2. Size of defect:
   (a) <1.5 cm^2 or <15 mm in greatest diameter
   (b) ≥1.5 cm^2 or ≥15 mm in greatest diameter
3. Depth of lesion:
   (a) Superficial defect involving only the cartilage
       (i) Is the surface soft or ballottable?
       (ii) Is the surface rough?
       (iii) Are fibrillations or fissures present?
   (b) Does the lesion involve the chondral and subchondral bone?
   (c) Subchondral lesion with intact overlying cartilage
   (d) Cystic defect >7 mm
   (e) ICRS grade
4. Stability of the defect:
   (a) Stable
   (b) Unstable
5. Fragment displacement:
   (a) Non-displaced
   (b) Displaced
6. Containment of lesion:
   (a) Contained
   (b) Unconstrained shoulder lesion
7. Surrounding zone classification:
   (a) I: Blistering with thickening of cartilage layer
   (b) II: Bulging with fragile, friable connection with subchondral bone
   (c) III: Complete delamination

Conclusion

Clinical suspicion of an osteochondral defect should be worked up with radiographs, MRI, and/or a CT scan. However, not all studies, especially MRIs, are of the same quality. In a patient with high clinical suspicion for a defect but with negative advanced imaging, a diagnostic arthroscopy may be warranted. In evaluating an osteochondral defect with arthroscopy, it is important to characterize the osteochondral defect by type, location, size, depth, displacement, stability, and containment. All of these characteristics can affect what type of surgical management may be needed and help determine prognosis after treatment.

Conflict of Interests The author has no current conflict of interests with the products presented.

References

1. Anderson IF, Crichton KJ, Grattan-Smith T, Cooper RA, Brazier D. Osteochondral fractures of the dome of the talus. J Bone Joint Surg Am. 1989;71: 1143–52.
2. Berndt AL, Harty M. Transchondral fractures (osteochondritis dissecans) of the talus. J Bone Joint Surg Am. 1959;41-A:988–1020.
3. Brittberg M, Winalski CS. Evaluation of cartilage injuries and repair. J Bone Joint Surg Am. 2003;85-A Suppl 2:58–69.
4. Choi WJ, Park KK. Osteochondral lesions of the talus: is there a critical defect size for poor outcome. Am J Sports Med. 2009;37(10):1974–80.
5. Ferkel RD. Arthroscopic surgery: foot and ankle. Philadelphia: JB Lippincott; 1996.
6. Ferkel RD, Hommen J. editors. Arthroscopy of the foot and ankle. In: Coughlin MJ, Mann RA, Saltzman CL editors. Surgery of the foot and ankle. 8th ed. Mosby: Philadelphia; 2007. p. 1641–726.
7. Ferkel RD, Sgaglione N, DelPizzo W. Arthroscopic treatment of osteochondral lesions of the talus: long-term results. Orthop Trans. 1990;14:172–3.
8. Ferkel RD, Zanotti RM, Komenda GA. Arthroscopic treatment of chronic osteochondral lesions of the talus: long term results. Am J Sports Med. 2008;36(9): 1750–2.
9. Friemert B. Diagnosis of chondral lesions of the knee joint: can MRI replace arthroscopy? A prospective study. Knee Surg Sports Traumatol Arthrosc. 2004;12(1):58–64.
10. Giannini S, Vannini F. Operative treatment of osteochondral lesions of the talar dome: current concepts review. Foot Ankle Int. 2004;25(3):168–75.
11. Hepple S, Winson IG, Glew D. Osteochondral lesions of the talus: a revised classification. Foot Ankle Int. 1999;20(12):789–93.
12. Kuikka PI. Sensitivity of routine 1.0-Tesla magnetic resonance imaging versus arthroscopy as gold standard in fresh traumatic chondral lesions of the knee in young adults. Arthroscopy. 2006;22(10):1033–9.
13. Lee KB. A comparison of arthroscopic and MRI findings in staging of osteochondral lesions of the talus. Knee Surg Sports Traumatol Arthrosc. 2008;16(11):1047–51.
14. Lee KB, Bai LB. Second-look arthroscopic findings and clinical outcomes after microfracture for osteochondral lesions of the talus. Am J Sports Med. 2009;37(10):63–70.
15. McGahan PJ, Pinney SJ. Current concept review: osteochondral lesions of the talus. Foot Ankle Int. 2010;31(1):90–101.
16. Mintz DN. Osteochondral lesions of the talus: a new magnetic resonance grading system with arthroscopic correlation. Arthroscopy. 2003;19(4):353–9.
17. Mori R. Clinical significance of magnetic resonance imaging (MRI) for focal chondral lesions. Magn Reson Imaging. 1999;17(8):1135–40.
18. O'Neill PJ, Van Aman SE, Guyton GP. Is MRI adequate to detect lesions in patients with ankle instability? Clin Orthop Relat Res. 2010;468(4):1115–9.
19. Potter HG. Magnetic resonance imaging of articular cartilage in the knee. An evaluation with use of fast-spin-echo imaging. J Bone Joint Surg Am. 1998;80(9):1276–84.
20. Pritsch M, Horoshovski H, Farine I. Arthroscopic treatment of osteochondral lesions of the talus. J Bone Joint Surg Am. 1986;68(6):862–5.
21. Recht MP. Abnormalities of articular cartilage in the knee: analysis of available MR techniques. Radiology. 1993;187(2):473–8.
22. Schneck CD. MR imaging of the most commonly injured ankle ligaments. Part I. Normal anatomy. Radiology. 1992;184(2):499–506.
23. Sugimoto K. Cartilage thickness of the talar dome. Arthroscopy. 2005;21(4):401–4.
24. Takao M. Arthroscopic assessment for intra-articular disorders in residual ankle disability after sprain. Am J Sports Med. 2005;33(5):686–92.
25. Tan TC. MR imaging of articular cartilage in the ankle: comparison of available imaging sequences and methods of measurement in cadavers. Skeletal Radiol. 1996;25(8):749–55.
26. Taranow WS, Bisignani GA, Towers JD, et al. Retrograde drilling of osteochondral fragments of the talar dome. Foot Ankle Int. 1999;20:474–80.
27. van Dijk CN, Scholte D. Arthroscopy of the ankle joint. Arthroscopy. 1997;13(1):90–6.
28. van Dijk CN, Verhagen RA, Tol JL. Arthroscopy for problems after ankle fracture. J Bone Joint Surg Br. 1997;79(2):280–4.
29. Verhagen RA. Prospective study on diagnostic strategies in osteochondral lesions of the talus. Is MRI superior to helical CT? J Bone Joint Surg Br. 2005;87(1):41–6.

Preoperative Planning for Osteochondral Defects

6

Inge C.M. van Eekeren, Arthur J. Kievit, and C. Niek van Dijk

Take-Home Points
- *The preoperative planning depends on the type of surgery, while the type of surgery also depends on the preoperative planning.*
- *Preoperative planning consists of physical examination, standard radiographs, CT scan, MRI scan, plantarflexed CT scans, and in some cases a 3D CT reconstruction.*

6.1 Introduction

For operative treatment of talar osteochondral defects (OCD), several surgical treatment options are available [14]. Each surgical technique has its specific indication [11]. Debridement and bone marrow stimulation is the first treatment of choice in primary defects <15 mm in diameter. Large cystic lesions can be treated by retrograde drilling. Fixation is for large lesions, most often posttraumatic. Secondary treatment options are osteochondral autograft transfer (OATS), HemiCAP, and autologous chondrocyte implantation (ACI). In case of malalignment, a sliding calcaneal osteotomy can be indicated. For each treatment, a careful preoperative planning is needed.

6.2 Type of Treatment

The type of treatment is predominantly determined by the size and location of the lesion, age of the patient, and alignment as well as dealing with a primary or secondary lesion.

- Size of lesion: if the lesion is smaller than 15 mm in diameter, the primary choice of surgical treatment is bone marrow stimulation. This treatment option can also be considered for secondary lesions. In case of primary larger lesions, fixation or retrograde drilling should be considered. For secondary lesions, OATS, HemiCAP, allograft, or ACI can be indicated depending on the location of the lesion, preference, and experience of the surgeon. Each of these procedures has their specific pearls and pitfalls.
- Age of the patient: for bone marrow stimulation, older age is correlated with a slightly less successful outcome. For adolescent patients, a more conservative approach is usually recommended. In case of surgery, consider fixation as a first step.

I.C.M. van Eekeren, MD, PhD (✉)
A.J. Kievit, MD, PhD
Department of Orthopaedic Surgery,
Orthopaedic Research Centre Amsterdam,
Academic Medical Center, University of Amsterdam,
Amsterdam, The Netherlands
e-mail: i.c.vaneekeren@amc.uva.nl;
a.j.kievit@amc.uva.nl

C.N. van Dijk, MD, PhD
Department of Orthopaedic Surgery and Traumatology,
Academic Medical Center, University of Amsterdam,
Amsterdam, The Netherlands
e-mail: c.n.vandijk@amc.uva.nl

C.N. van Dijk, J.G. Kennedy (eds.), *Talar Osteochondral Defects*,
DOI 10.1007/978-3-642-45097-6_6, © ESSKA 2014

- Alignment: in case of malalignment, one should consider realignment surgery by means of a sliding calcaneal osteotomy. Usually this is a secondary treatment option.
- Primary/secondary lesion: primary lesions are mostly treated by bone marrow stimulation or in case of a large fragment and younger age by fixation. For a large cystic lesion, one must consider retrograde drilling. As secondary treatment options, bone marrow stimulation can be performed in defects <15 mm in diameter. OATS, HemiCAP, allograft, or ACI are also options for secondary lesions.

6.3 Preoperative Planning

When the diagnosis of an osteochondral defect has been made, nonoperative treatment has failed, and the type of treatment has been decided upon, preoperative planning starts. The preoperative planning starts with the history of the patient and physical examination [7]. Concerning physical examination, the range of motion of the ankle joint is important. In maximal plantar flexion, the lesion moves anterior. In case of normal plantar flexion, 90–95 % of talar OCD can be treated by means of anterior arthroscopy. By forced plantar flexion, these lesions can be brought into the anterior or central third of the talar dome. Soft tissue distraction is an alternative to forced plantar flexion. Some surgeons prefer a combination of plantar flexion and distraction. Joint stability is important. In case of slight to mild anterior drawer, the anterior approach to these lesions gets easier. Alignment of the ankle and hindfoot must be checked by measuring the calcaneocrural angle [9]. Standard radiographs are usually insufficient for preoperative planning. Multislice helical computed tomography (CT) and magnetic resonance imaging (MRI) have demonstrated similar accuracy for detection of an osteochondral talar defect [13]. For preoperative planning, however, a CT scan is preferred, because it visualizes the exact location and size of the lesion [2]. An additional CT scan in full plantar flexion (only sagittal reconstruction is needed) can be made to determine if the lesion is accessible by anterior arthroscopy with the foot in plantar flexion [12]. In Fig. 6.1, a flowchart is displayed of factors of importance for the preoperative planning.

6.3.1 Bone Marrow Stimulation (BMS)

In the physical examination, special attention is given to the range of motion (regarding dorso- and in particular plantar flexion) and laxity of the ankle joint in order to determine the accessibility of the defect. In case of a normal plantar flexion, 90–95 % of the lesions can be treated by means of anterior arthroscopy. An additional CT scan in full plantar flexion can be made to determine if the lesion is accessible by means of anterior arthroscopy without fixed distraction or if a posterior approach is indicated.

6.3.2 Fixation

In adolescents in (sub)acute situations, or other primary cases, in which the fragment is 15 mm or larger, fixation of the fragment should be considered [10]. Preoperative planning consists of localization of the defect on CT. It is important to plan the approach and to fine-tune it to the choice of fixation technique, i.e., screw, absorbable fixation, or fibrin glue [3, 4, 8]. Most medial lesions can be approached by anterior arthrotomy. In case of doubt we advice to make a preoperative CT scan in forced plantar flexion with sagittal reconstruction. If the anterior 50 % of the lesion comes in front of the anterior distal tibia, an anterior arthrotomy can be performed. In more posterior lesions, a medial malleolar osteotomy is needed. For lateral lesions, an oblique fibular osteotomy can be necessary when the defect is located posterior. In other cases standard anterolateral incision is sufficient [5, 6]. In most patients detachment of the anterior talofibular ligament (ATFL) (and calcaneofibular ligament (CFL)) is needed in order to dislocate the talus anterior. After fixation of the fragment, the ligaments are reconstructed.

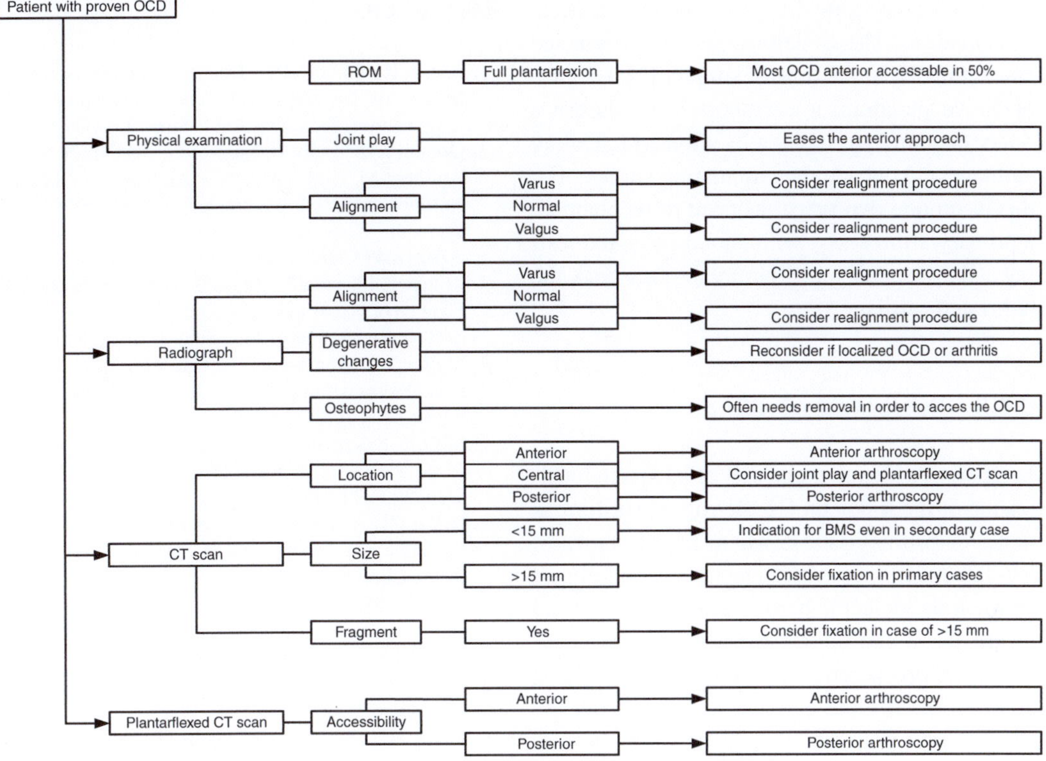

Fig. 6.1 Factors of importance for preoperative planning of operative talar OCD treatment

6.3.3 Sliding Calcaneal Osteotomy

Most important in the preoperative planning is the detection of the amount of malalignment of the ankle by means of physical examination, standard weight-bearing X-rays, and alignment views. Correction of the deformity is usually between 5 and 10 mm displacement.

6.3.4 Implant: HemiCAP, Osteochondral Autograft Transfer (OATS), and Allograft

For preoperative planning, however, a CT scan is preferred, because it visualizes the exact location and size of the lesion [2]. A CT is required for size and location, and curvation of the talus can be checked by a 3D reconstruction. Specific for the OATS procedure, it is important to check the ipsilateral knee for any pathology. An allograft has to be matched before operation, while the exact fit of a metal implant and OATS are determined intraoperatively.

6.3.5 Autologous Chondrocyte Implantation (ACI)

Preoperatively a CT scan is made to evaluate the size and location of the defect. The defect should be focal, contained, and preferably more than 1.5 cm in diameter or 1 cm^2 [7]. Preoperatively contraindications to ACI (bipolar lesions ("kissing lesions") and diffuse degenerative joint changes) need to be diagnosed on preoperative X-ray as well as on CT scan. Skeletal malalignment and ligamentous instability should be diagnosed preoperatively with adequate physical examination. These deformities are corrected concomitantly at the time of surgery [1]. For preoperative planning, it is important to choose a donor chondrocyte site at a location with healthy cartilage and outside the articulating surface. For this technique two surgeries need to be planned: a primary arthroscopy with chondrocyte harvesting and a secondary arthrotomy to place back the cultivated cartilage.

6.3.6 Retrograde Drilling

Preoperative planning consists of adequate localization of the lesion on CT. Retrograde drilling is done for primary OCDs when there is more or less intact cartilage with a large subchondral cyst or when the defect is hard to reach via the usual anterolateral and anteromedial portals as diagnosed on preoperative CT. For medial lesions, arthroscopic drilling can take place through the sinus tarsi. For lateral lesions, the cyst is approached from anteromedial.

Conclusion

After diagnosis of an osteochondral defect, a decision has to be made on how to treat the patient. When nonoperative treatment is unsuccessful, there are several surgical treatment options. The preoperative planning depends on the type of surgery, while the type of surgery depends also on the preoperative planning. Preoperative planning can consist of physical examination, standard radiographs, CT scan, MRI scan, a plantarflexed CT scan, and in some cases a 3D CT reconstruction.

Conflict of Interest The author has no current conflict of interests with the products presented

References

1. Bazaz R, Ferkel RD. Treatment of osteochondral lesions of the talus with autologous chondrocyte implantation. Tech Foot Ankle Surg. 2004;3:45–52.
2. Gomoll AH, Madry H, Knutsen G, van Dijk N, Seil R, Brittberg M, et al. The subchondral bone in articular cartilage repair: current problems in the surgical management. Knee Surg Sports Traumatol Arthrosc. 2010;18:434–47.
3. Kumai T, Takakura Y, Kitada C, Tanaka Y, Hayashi K. Fixation of osteochondral lesions of the talus using cortical bone pegs. J Bone Joint Surg Br. 2002;84:369–74.
4. Mallon WJ, Wombwell JH, Nunley JA. Intra-articular talar fractures: repair using the Herbert bone screw. Foot Ankle. 1989;10:88–92.
5. Muir D, Saltzman CL, Tochigi Y, Amendola N. Talar dome access for osteochondral lesions. Am J Sports Med. 2006;34:1457–63.
6. Navid DO, Myerson MS. Approach alternatives for treatment of osteochondral lesions of the talus. Foot Ankle Clin. 2002;7:635–49.
7. Reilingh ML, van Bergen CJ, van Dijk CN. Diagnosis and treatment of osteochondral defects of the ankle. South Afr Orthop J. 2009;8:44–50.
8. Shea MP, Manoli A. Osteochondral lesions of the talar dome. Foot Ankle. 1993;14:48–55.
9. Stiehl JB, Inman V. In: Stiehl JB, editor. Inman's joints of the ankle. 2 ed. Baltimore: Williams & Wilkins; 1999.
10. Stone JW. Osteochondral lesions of the talar dome. J Am Acad Orthop Surg. 1996;4:63–73.
11. van Bergen CJ, de Leeuw PA, van Dijk CN. Treatment of osteochondral defects of the talus. Rev Chir Orthop Reparatrice Appar Mot. 2008;94:398–408.
12. van Bergen CJ, Tuijthof GJ, Blankevoort L, Maas M, Kerkhoffs GM, van Dijk CN. Computed tomography of the ankle in full plantar flexion: a reliable method for preoperative planning of arthroscopic access to osteochondral defects of the talus. Arthroscopy. 2012;28:985–92.
13. Verhagen RA, Maas M, Dijkgraaf MG, Tol JL, Krips R, van Dijk CN. Prospective study on diagnostic strategies in osteochondral lesions of the talus. Is MRI superior to helical CT? J Bone Joint Surg Br. 2005;87:41–6.
14. Zengerink M, Struijs PA, Tol JL, van Dijk CN. Treatment of osteochondral lesions of the talus: a systematic review. Knee Surg Sports Traumatol Arthrosc. 2010;18:238–46.

Mark E. Easley and Samuel B. Adams Jr.

Take-Home Points

- *Posterolateral osteochondral lesions of the talus (OLTs) represent approximately 5 % of all OLTs.*
- *With current arthroscopic techniques, most posterolateral OLTs may be readily managed arthroscopically.*
- *Should the posterolateral OLT fail to respond to or not be amenable to arthroscopic management, secondary reconstructive procedures including osteochondral transfer, ACI, juvenile allograft cartilage implantation, or structural allograft reconstruction may be considered.*
- *While some advanced autologous chondrocyte or juvenile allograft cartilage implantations may be performed arthroscopically, most secondary reconstructive procedures warrant exposure via one of the following surgical approaches: (1) posterolateral arthrotomy, (2) Achilles tendon-splitting approach, (3) anterior or anterolateral arthrotomy with or without ligament release, (4) anterior or antero-lateral arthrotomy with anterolateral distal tibial osteotomy, or (5) anterolateral arthrotomy with distal fibular osteotomy.*

7.1 Introduction

Whereas lateral osteochondral lesions of the talus (OLT) were reported to commonly occur at the anterolateral aspect of the talar dome [11, 12, 14, 23, 24, 72], more recent reports suggest that lateral OLTs occur most commonly at the central portion of the lateral talar dome [19, 43]. Elias and coworkers demonstrated that while centrolateral OLTs were far more common than anterolateral or posterolateral OLTs, the frequency of posterolateral OLTs was 5 % compared to other OLTs, twice that of anterolateral OLTs [19]. Posterolateral OLTs tend to involve smaller surface area than anterolateral OLTs but greater surface area than centrolateral OLTs. The depth for posterolateral OLTs is relatively shallow compared to OLTs in other zones of the talar dome but involves a considerable amount of the talus when considering the relative height of the talar body compared to the height in the central or anterior portion of the talar dome.

Surgical management of OLTs is relatively well defined. Current surgical options include:

Options That Do Not Resurface, Only Promote Fibrocartilage Formation:

M.E. Easley, MD (✉) • S.B. Adams Jr. MD
Department of Orthopaedic Surgery,
Duke University Medical Center, Durham, NC, USA
e-mail: mark.e.easley@duke.edu;
samuel.adams@dm.duke.edu

C.N. van Dijk, J.G. Kennedy (eds.), *Talar Osteochondral Defects*,
DOI 10.1007/978-3-642-45097-6_7, © ESSKA 2014

1. Debridement (open versus arthroscopic)
2. Abrasion arthroplasty/chondroplasty (open versus arthroscopic)
3. Arthroscopic drilling
4. Microfracture
5. Retrograde drilling

Options Intended to Resurface with Hyaline Cartilage:

1. Osteochondral transfer
2. (Matrix-induced) autologous chondrocyte implantation
3. Particulated juvenile cartilage implantation
4. Synthetic/recombinant resurfacing techniques
5. Structural allograft

Traditionally, options that do not resurface but simply promote fibrocartilage formation are initially considered for OLTs. However, some authors suggest that certain types of OLTs respond less favorably to these non-resurfacing options; these types of OLTs include:

1. Large OLTs
2. OLTs that disrupt the subchondral architecture of the talar shoulder
3. OLTs associated with subchondral cysts
4. OLTs that have failed prior treatment with non-resurfacing options

In these situations, resurfacing procedures may be favored.

7.2 Arthroscopic Access to the Posterolateral Talar Dome

7.2.1 Patient in the Supine Position

Traditional methods of distraction allow sufficient access to most areas of the talar dome via anteromedial and anterolateral portals so that OLT debridement and microfracture techniques are possible. Becher and Thermann reported successful arthroscopic microfracture of lateral OLTs but did not provide detail of the sagittal position for the lateral OLTs [10]. Ferkel and coworkers reported on long-term results of arthroscopic treatment of OLTs in 50 patients, but their comprehensive series did not include any posterolateral lesions [23]. However, these authors commented that the posterolateral portal

allows for access to posterolateral OLTs [22, 23]. Chuckpaiwong and coworkers suggested that microfracture of lateral OLTs trended toward successful outcome, but the authors did not distinguish lateral lesions based on the lateral OLT's sagittal plane position [15].

Arthroscopy typically affords access to any OLT, including posterolateral OLTs. Feiwell and Frey demonstrated in a cadaveric model, with a simulated supine patient position and using joint distraction, that using various combinations of the anteromedial, anterolateral, and posterolateral portals the entire talar dome could be visualized and accessed with arthroscopic curettes, including the posterolateral talar dome [20, 21]. These investigators noted that the lateral talar articular surface could not be accessed by any combination of these standard arthroscopic portals. Although joint distraction improves ankle joint visualization and access [20, 21, 23, 44], it may potentially lead to traction neuralgia, also when trying to access posterolateral OLTs [16, 17].

With the patient in the supine position, arthroscopic visualization and access of OLTs via traditional anteromedial and anterolateral portals without joint distraction are limited to the anterior 48 % of the lateral talar dome, even with the ankle in maximum plantar flexion [75, 76]. Van Bergen and coworkers confirmed this with CT scan analysis of fully plantar flexed ankles and noted that this access depended on the patient's ankle plantar flexion and was independent of joint laxity [75]. Several authors have recommended arthroscopy for OLTs in the anterior half of the talar dome but open approaches for the posterior half of the talar dome [34, 40, 50, 64].

Voto and coworkers suggested that the addition of a trans-Achilles posterior portal could be safely used to enhance posterior talar dome visualization and access [78]. Since Voto and coworkers' description of a dedicated posterior portal, several other investigators have studied optimal arthroscopic access to the posterior ankle. Maffulli and coworkers describe double posteromedial portals that may be added to routine anterior ankle arthroscopy with the patient in the supine position [5]. The authors note that the procedure is safe, allows satisfactory access to the posterior talar dome to manage OLTs, and is readily learned. Two different investigations tout the advantages of coaxial portals, immediately posterior to the medial malleolus (anterior to the posterior tibial tendon) and fibula (anterior or posterior to the peroneal tendons), utilized with the patient in the supine position [1, 79]. Coaxial portals are removed from neurovascular structures at risk, allow for large working space since the instrument and arthroscope are opposite one another, and do not require extensive debridement of the posterior ankle ligaments for visualization. The posterolateral talar dome may be readily visualized and accessed via coaxial portals.

7.2.2 Patient in the Prone Position

Even though the authors touting coaxial portals cite the risks of dedicated posteromedial and posterolateral portals such as (1) close proximity to the neurovascular structures, (2) interference between arthroscope and instruments, and (3) need to remove many of the posterior ankle ligaments to allow adequate ankle access, several authors have reported that dedicated posterior ankle portals used with the patient in the prone position are safe [49, 54, 71, 80]. Since Van Dijk and coworkers' original description [77], dedicated posterior ankle arthroscopy with the patient in the prone position has gained traction as a safe method to visualize and access the posterior ankle, including the posterolateral talar dome [9, 49, 54, 66, 80]. In fact, some authors suggest that the advantages to dedicated posterior ankle arthroscopy warrant addressing combined anterior and posterior ankle pathology by repositioning the patient intraoperatively; Scholten and van Dijk suggest that posterior ankle pathology may be addressed with the patient prone and two dedicated posterior ankle portals after which the patient is turned supine to address anterior ankle pathology with traditional anterior portals [67]. Hampton and coworkers recently provided a technique tip in which combined anterior, lateral, and posterior ankle procedures, including anterior and posterior ankle arthroscopy, may be performed with the patient in a lateral decubitus position and without the need

for repositioning during surgery [39]. To improve arthroscopic access to the posterior ankle and posterolateral OLTs, Beals and coworkers report a minimally invasive distraction technique that was safely employed for 14 patients undergoing prone posterior ankle arthroscopy [9] (Beals).

7.3 Retrograde Drilling

When arthroscopy reveals that the cartilage cap is intact over the defect noted on preoperative imaging studies, then retrograde drilling with or without bone grafting may be considered [73]. The access to the posterolateral talar dome for retrograde drilling may be more challenging than lesions in other areas of the talar dome, but it should be possible in most cases, particularly when a microvector guide is used to target the defect. Computer navigation techniques have been described for retrograde drilling of OLTs; while only case reports for medial talar dome lesions have been reported, advances in this technology may eventually be applied to the posterolateral talar dome [36, 55].

7.4 Open (Non-arthroscopic) Access to the Posterolateral Talar Dome

7.4.1 Overview

Arthroscopy may safely reach all areas of the talar dome, including the posterolateral surface; however, not all recommended procedures for OLTs may be possible arthroscopically. Schuman and coworkers suggested that posterior OLTs may be drilled via standard anterior arthroscopy portals when the ankle is in maximum plantar flexion [68]. While this may be possible using a relatively small diameter drill bit, perpendicular access with larger diameter chisels used for osteochondral transfer may not be feasible. Currently described procedures for resurfacing including osteochondral transfer, ACI, and structural allograft reconstruction are simply not possible via arthroscopy and require open procedures.

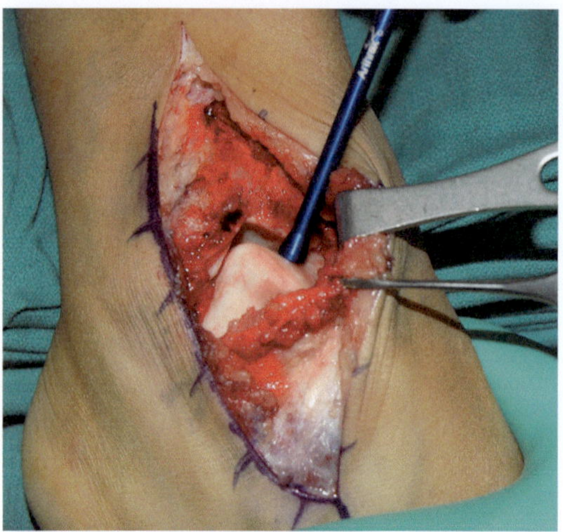

Fig. 7.1 Posterolateral OLT exposure with ATFL release, talar plantar flexion, and inversion to allow perpendicular access for osteochondral transfer

7.4.2 Arthrotomy

Osteochondral transfer, structural allograft reconstruction, and ACI typically require extensile exposure, and osteochondral transfer also necessitates perpendicular access to the OLT. Scranton and coworkers observed that perpendicular access to lateral OLTs was possible in all cases in their series without lateral malleolar osteotomy, suggesting that all lateral OLTs could be accessed via ATFL release, anterior talar subluxation, and plantar flexion, irrespective of sagittal plane position of the OLT [69] (Fig. 7.1). These authors did not make specific reference to posterolateral OLTs. Flick and Gould proposed carefully gouging the anteromedial tibial plafond to improve access to the medial talar dome [24]. Assenmacher and coworkers described similar access but added a limited plafondplasty in which the anterior margin of the tibia corresponding to the OLT in the coronal plane is removed without damaging the native tibial cartilage [7]. In a recent cadaveric study, Peters and coworkers demonstrated that via an anterolateral arthrotomy and plantar flexion perpendicular access was possible to 53 % of the lateral talar dome [59]. When these same investigators performed a $10 \times 10 \times 8$ mm plafondplasty in the anterior distal tibia, perpendicular access increased to 81 % in the sagittal plane.

While limited (non-perpendicular) posterior access was possible beyond 81 %, these authors noted that the posterior 11 % of the lateral talar dome was completely inaccessible.

The posterolateral approach has been described between the peroneal and Achilles tendon or through the peroneal tendon sheath, with the latter approach necessitating anterior subluxation of the peroneal tendons [47, 50, 56, 70]. The sural nerve must be protected and carefully retracted laterally during this approach, to limit the risk of sural nerve injury. The flexor hallucis longus tendon should be identified and retracted medially to fully expose the posterolateral talar dome. Ankle dorsiflexion greatly enhances talar dome exposure [56]. Kreuz and coworkers utilized the posterolateral approach through the peroneal tendon sheath for osteochondral transfer; with the ankle dorsiflexed, these surgeons were able to access a posterolateral OLT without the need for osteotomy [47].

Patzkowski and coworkers, using a cadaveric model, confirmed that an Achilles tendon-splitting approach affords greater exposure to the posterior talar dome than a posterolateral approach, particularly with the ankle in dorsiflexion [58]. The authors suggested that the Achilles tendon-splitting approach offers similar access to the posterolateral talar dome as the posterolateral approach. While these authors' investigation does not directly study access for treatment of OLTs, their conclusions imply that greater dissection into the gastrocnemius and/or soleus musculature may be required for perpendicular access to the posterolateral talar dome when using the tendon-splitting approach.

7.4.3 Extensile Exposures to the Posterolateral Talar Dome

Several authors describe more extensive tibial osteotomies to access the posterior ankle, including the posterolateral talar dome [45, 46, 63, 74]. Sammarco and coworkers describe an anterior tibial wedge osteotomy that corresponds to the coronal plane position of the OLT, allowing perpendicular access to the posterior talar dome, including the posterolateral aspect of the talus [63]. Kreuz and coworkers modified this technique to take less bone but afford the same access to the posterior talus; however, these authors only described their technique for the posteromedial talar dome [45, 46]. Tochigi and coworkers, in a technique tip article, suggested that access to the centrolateral talar dome may be improved with an anterolateral tibial plafond osteotomy, where an osteochondral block resembling that of a juvenile Tillaux fragment is reflected via an anterolateral ankle arthrotomy [74]. Through an anterior or anterolateral approach, a 1×1.5 cm anterolateral fragment of the distal tibial plafond (at Chaput's tubercle) is mobilized using a combination of reciprocating saw and osteotome and reflected on the anterior inferior syndesmotic ligament. After the posterolateral OLT has been managed, the anterolateral bone block is reduced and secured with screw fixation. Al-Shaikh and coworkers described using an anterolateral arthrotomy in 5 of 6 patients with lateral OLTs to gain satisfactory perpendicular access for osteochondral transfer; in the sixth patient, the authors report using a lateral malleolar osteotomy to gain perpendicular access [4]. Little detail was provided with respect to how the lateral malleolar osteotomy was performed.

Perpendicular access has been the focus of several recent investigations, including ones dedicated to the lateral talar dome [25, 53, 62]. Muir and coworkers suggested that an average of 80 % of lateral OLTs may have perpendicular access without osteotomy [53]. Via a 6 mm anterolateral arthrotomy lateral to the peroneus tertius, 36 % of the lateral talar dome in the sagittal plane, 54 % of the talar dome in the coronal plane, and 28 % of the entire talar dome are exposed for perpendicular access, respectively. These authors observed that an anterolateral osteotomy [74] adds a mean 22 % to sagittal plane exposure via an anterolateral arthrotomy, with 62 % of the talar dome in the sagittal plane, 36 % in the coronal plane, and 35 % of the entire talar dome accessible for perpendicular access. A posterolateral arthrotomy affords 37 % of the talar dome in the sagittal plane, 37 % in the coronal plane, and 12 % of the entire talar dome,

respectively. A fibular osteotomy, performed after repair of the anterolateral tibial osteotomy in the cadaveric model, afforded 100 % access to the talar dome in the sagittal plane, 52 % in the coronal plane, and 43 % of the entire talar dome, respectively.

Whereas Muir and coworkers' study comprehensively analyzed access to the entire talar dome, Garras and coworkers' investigation focused on the perpendicular access to the posterolateral talar dome [25]. These authors observed in their cadaver model that sagittal plane exposure to the lateral talar dome averaged: 43 % with anterolateral arthrotomy and ATFL release, 68.5 % with anterolateral tibial osteotomy, 88 % with fibular osteotomy, 91 % with fibular osteotomy and ATFL release, and 95 % with fibular osteotomy and combined ATFL and CFL release [25]. Rush and coworkers, also using a cadaveric model, observed that temporary invasive distraction with an external fixator afforded greater sagittal plane/posterior access to the lateral talar dome than anterolateral arthrotomy or anterolateral tibial osteotomy alone and afforded greatest posterolateral talar dome perpendicular access when combined with the anterolateral tibial osteotomy [62]. In an attempt to limit vascular compromise to the lateral ankle, Ove and coworkers demonstrated that the posterolateral talar dome may be fully accessed via a medial malleolar osteotomy; however, this was without consideration for perpendicular access [57].

Ray and Coughlin [61] reported using Gatellier's description of a distal fibular osteotomy [26] to access a posterolateral OLT. Ly and Fallat [51] and Draper and Fallat [18] also described this technique for improving access for surgical treatment of posterolateral talar OLTs. These authors describe an oblique fibular osteotomy that resembles the fracture pattern of a Weber B ankle fracture (Fig. 7.2a, b). With the osteotomy originating from the joint line and directed laterally and superiorly to exit in the lateral fibular cortex approximately 2–3 cm proximal to the joint line, the syndesmotic ligaments are preserved. The osteotomy is secured with lag screw(s) if possible and stabilized with a lateral neutralization plate; the

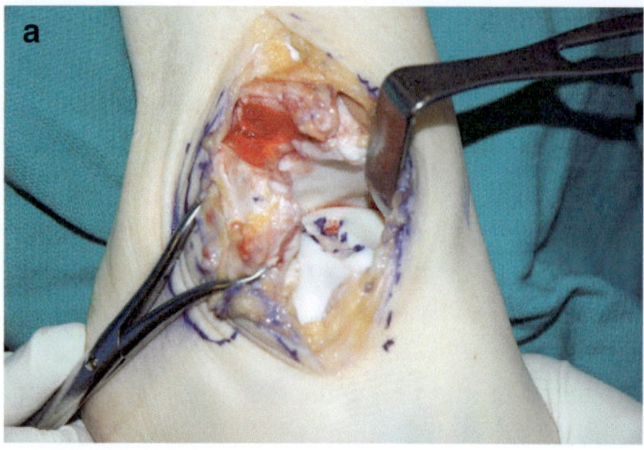 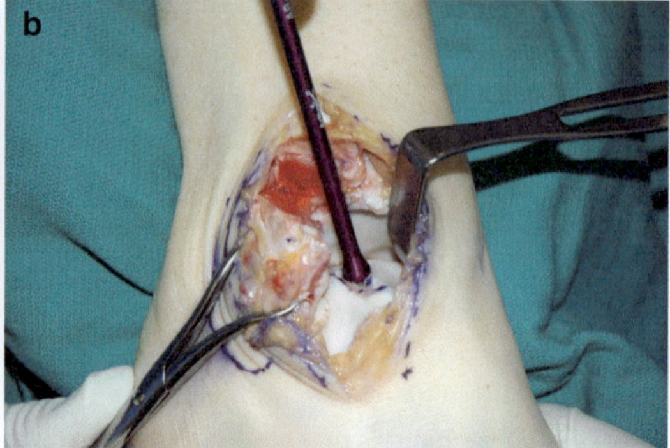

Fig. 7.2 Posterolateral OLT exposure with ATFL release and fibular osteotomy to gain perpendicular access for osteochondral transfer. (**a**) Exposure after ATFL release and oblique fibular osteotomy. (**b**) Sizing guide for perpendicular access

screw holes may be predrilled prior to the osteotomy to facilitate anatomic reduction. Hansen [41] and Allen and DiGiovanni [6] described a fibular window to access the lateral talar dome. With this technique a 3 cm intercalated segment of fibula is osteotomized and reflected posteriorly on a soft tissue pedicle, thereby creating perpendicular access to the lateral talar dome, including the posterolateral articular surface. The anterior aspect of the interosseous membrane and anterior inferior tibiofibular ligaments need to be released to reflect the intercalated fibular segment. Upon completion of the cartilage procedure, the ligaments are repaired, and the osteotomy is stabilized with lateral plate fixation; the fibula may be predrilled prior to osteotomy to facilitate anatomic reduction, and a syndesmotic screw fixation may be considered to optimize stabilization.

Autologous chondrocyte implantation (ACI) traditionally requires an extensile exposure, occasionally necessitating lateral distal tibial or distal fibular osteotomy [27, 29, 32, 65]. Giannini and coworkers reported favorable outcomes using ACI for OLTs with long-term follow-up [27, 29]. The authors reported performing ACI for lateral OLTs through a lateral arthrotomy with fibular osteotomy but offer no detail of where on the talar dome the lateral lesion was located in the sagittal plane and provide little detail of the surgical exposure. Likewise, Schneider and coworkers accessed five lateral OLTs with fibular osteotomy to perform MACI but provided no specifics regarding exact location of the OLT in the sagittal plane or how the osteotomy was performed [65].

Structural allograft reconstruction generally requires extensile exposure. Several authors have published results of talar allograft reconstructions for voluminous OLTs [2, 35, 37, 38, 60]. Gross and coworkers' series of nine patients only included medial talar allograft reconstructions [37]. Hahn and coworkers' series included three lateral talar structural allograft reconstructions, including one posterolateral OLT reconstruction [38]. These authors reported using the fibular window technique described by Hansen and Allen and DiGiovanni [6, 41]. Raikin described three cases of lateral talar dome structural allograft reconstruction, exposing the lateral talar dome via an extensile anterior approach in two cases and a lateralized ankle arthrotomy with distal fibular osteotomy in the third case [60]. He used the anterior extensile approach to perform a hemi-talus reconstruction (entire replacement of talar dome in the sagittal plane) and the fibular osteotomy for a location-specific OLT to preserve uninvolved cartilage. Raikin did not provide detail of the specific technique for fibular osteotomy and did not define if the location-specific lateral OLT was posterolateral on the talar dome. Adams and coworkers reported using a distal fibular osteotomy for structural allograft reconstruction of a lateral OLT and also did not provide detail of the sagittal plane position of the lateral OLT or the specific technique used for fibular osteotomy [2]. Gortz and coworkers reported 6 of 11 structural

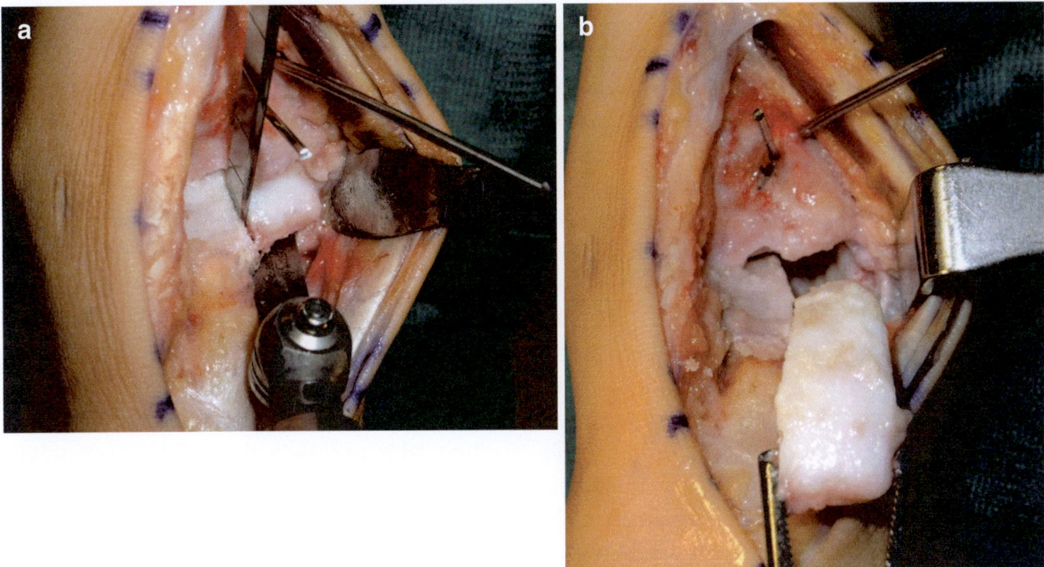

Fig. 7.3 Extensile anterior ankle arthrotomy for large lateral OLT. (**a**) Microsagittal saw excision of the lateral aspect of the talus, including the massive OLT. (**b**) Extraction of the lateral aspect of the talus, including the OLT

allograft reconstructions being for lateral OLTs [35]. These authors performed all shell allograft reconstructions through an extensile anterior ankle approach, with joint distraction but without malleolar osteotomy (Fig. 7.3a, b). No specific detail was provided with respect to sagittal plane position of the lateral OLTs.

7.5 Modern Resurfacing Techniques Not Requiring Extensile Exposures

Giza and coworkers described performing matrix-induced ACI (MACI) for OLTs [33]. The investigators harvested cartilage from the margin of the OLT at the time of initial arthroscopic inspection/debridement, culturing the chondrocytes, imbedding the cells in a collagen membrane, and then implanting this graft into the prepared OLT via an arthrotomy at a second surgery. The authors enhanced exposure with ankle plantar flexion and a limited plafondplasty originally described by Assenmacher and coworkers [7] in which the anterior margin of the tibia is removed without damaging the native tibial cartilage. While the authors described treating lateral OLTs with this technique via an anterolateral

arthrotomy without malleolar osteotomy, they did not include detail about the sagittal plane location of the lateral OLT and if posterolateral OLT could be accessed via this technique.

Recent reports suggest that juvenile allograft cartilage implantation may be an attractive alternative to osteochondral transfer and ACI [3, 13, 42, 48]. Juvenile allograft cartilage implantation does not require perpendicular access and may be implanted via relatively limited open approaches to treat OLTs failing to respond to primary arthroscopic management.

Giannini and coworkers reported that results for ACI or MACI performed arthroscopically may match those reported via the open technique [8, 28, 31]. The technique involves harvesting cartilage from the ankle during a first-stage arthroscopic inspection/debridement of the OLT, culturing these chondrocytes, embedding the chondrocytes in a scaffold, and then implanting the chondrocyte-seeded scaffold in the OLT during a second arthroscopy. The authors offer no detail regarding posterolateral OLTs being treated with this technique.

More recently, Giannini and coworkers presented a 4-year follow-up on patients treated with a one-step bone marrow-derived cell transplantation for OLTs [30]. The authors describe positioning the patient prone for bone marrow, aspirating bone marrow from the iliac crest, mixing the bone marrow concentrate with hyaluronic acid or collagen powder, and implanting the bone marrow "paste" in the prepared OLT arthroscopically. The authors note that nine lateral OLTs were treated by this method but do not offer detail about the location of the lateral OLTs in the sagittal plane.

Giannini and coworkers suggest that the arthroscopic ACI and MACI procedures carry less morbidity than their open technique [30, 31]. Magnan and coworkers also describe favorable outcome with a two-stage arthroscopic MACI technique for OLTs, using traditional arthroscopic techniques with the patient in the supine position [52]. These investigators treated seven centrolateral OLTs; their series did not include posterolateral OLTs. Early experience suggests that the juvenile allograft cartilage implantation may be performed arthroscopically [48]. Scholten and coworkers suggest that dedicated posterior ankle arthroscopy may allow better access to the posterior ankle than open techniques and affords a more rapid recovery [66]. Given that experience that has been gained in dedicated posterior arthroscopy, it seems that arthroscopic ACI, MACI, bone marrow-derived cell transplantation, and juvenile allograft cartilage implantation would lend themselves well to addressing posterolateral OLTs via posterior portals. This may be particularly applicable to the bone marrow-derived cell transplantation where Giannini and coworkers describe turning the patient supine to perform arthroscopic cell transplantation through traditional anterior portals after the patient is initially positioned prone for bone marrow aspiration [31].

Conclusion

Posterolateral OLTs represent approximately 5 % of all OLTs and with current arthroscopic techniques are readily managed arthroscopically. Should the posterolateral OLT fail to respond to or not be amenable to arthroscopic management, secondary reconstructive procedures including osteochondral transfer, ACI, juvenile allograft cartilage implantation, or structural allograft reconstruction may be considered. While some advanced autologous chondrocyte or juvenile allograft cartilage implantations may be performed arthroscopically, most secondary reconstructive procedures warrant exposure via one of the following surgical approaches: (1) posterolateral arthrotomy, (2) Achilles tendon-splitting approach, (3) anterior or anterolateral arthrotomy with or without ligament release, (4) anterior or anterolateral arthrotomy with anterolateral distal tibial osteotomy, or (5) anterolateral arthrotomy with distal fibular osteotomy.

Conflict of Interests The author has no current conflict of interests with the products presented.

References

1. Acevedo JI, Busch MT, Ganey TM, Hutton WC, Ogden JA. Coaxial portals for posterior ankle arthroscopy: an anatomic study with clinical correlation on 29 patients. Arthroscopy. 2000;16(8):836–42.
2. Adams Jr SB, Viens NA, Easley ME, Stinnett SS, Nunley 2nd JA. Midterm results of osteochondral lesions of the talar shoulder treated with fresh osteochondral allograft transplantation. J Bone Joint Surg Am. 2011;93(7):648–54.
3. Adams Jr SB, Yao J, Schon LC. Particulated juvenile cartilage allograft transplantation for the treatment of osteochondral lesions of the talus. Tech Foot Ankle Surg. 2011;10(2):92–8.
4. Al-Shaikh RA, Chou LB, Mann JA, Dreeben SM, Prieskorn D. Autologous osteochondral grafting for talar cartilage defects. Foot Ankle Int. 2002;23(5):381–9.
5. Allegra F, Maffulli N. Double posteromedial portals for posterior ankle arthroscopy in supine position. Clin Orthop Relat Res. 2010;468(4):996–1001.
6. Allen SD, DiGiovanni CW. Distal fibular window osteotomy for exposure of lateral talar osteochondral lesions. Tech Foot Ankle Surg. 2003;2(2):129–34.
7. Assenmacher JA, Kelikian AS, Gottlob C, Kodros S. Arthroscopically assisted autologous osteochondral transplantation for osteochondral lesions of the talar dome: an MRI and clinical follow-up study. Foot Ankle Int. 2001;22(7):544–51.
8. Battaglia M, Vannini F, Buda R, Cavallo M, Ruffilli A, Monti C, et al. Arthroscopic autologous chondrocyte

implantation in osteochondral lesions of the talus: mid-term T2-mapping MRI evaluation. Knee Surg Sports Traumatol Arthrosc. 2011;19(8):1376–84.

9. Beals TC, Junko JT, Amendola A, Nickisch F, Saltzman CL. Minimally invasive distraction technique for prone posterior ankle and subtalar arthroscopy. Foot Ankle Int. 2010;31(4):316–9.

10. Becher C, Thermann H. Results of microfracture in the treatment of articular cartilage defects of the talus. Foot Ankle Int. 2005;26(8):583–9.

11. Berndt AL, Harty M. Transchondral fractures (osteochondritis dissecans) of the talus. J Bone Joint Surg Am. 1959;41–A:988–1020.

12. Berndt AL, Harty M. Transchondral fractures (osteochondritis dissecans) of the talus. J Bone Joint Surg Am. 2004;86–A(6):1336.

13. Bleazey S, Brigido SA. Reconstruction of complex osteochondral lesions of the talus with cylindrical sponge allograft and particulate juvenile cartilage graft: provisional results with a short-term follow-up. Foot Ankle Spec. 2012;5(5):300–5.

14. Canale ST, Belding RH. Osteochondral lesions of the talus. J Bone Joint Surg Am. 1980;62(1):97–102.

15. Chuckpaiwong B, Berkson EM, Theodore GH. Microfracture for osteochondral lesions of the ankle: outcome analysis and outcome predictors of 105 cases. Arthroscopy. 2008;24(1):106–12.

16. de Leeuw PA, Golano P, Clavero JA, van Dijk CN. Anterior ankle arthroscopy, distraction or dorsiflexion? Knee Surg Sports Traumatol Arthrosc. 2010;18(5):594–600.

17. Dowdy PA, Watson BV, Amendola A, Brown JD. Noninvasive ankle distraction: relationship between force, magnitude of distraction, and nerve conduction abnormalities. Arthroscopy. 1996;12(1):64–9.

18. Draper SD, Fallat LM. Autogenous bone grafting for the treatment of talar dome lesions. J Foot Ankle Surg. 2000;39(1):15–23.

19. Elias I, Zoga AC, Morrison WB, Besser MP, Schweitzer ME, Raikin SM. Osteochondral lesions of the talus: localization and morphologic data from 424 patients using a novel anatomical grid scheme. Foot Ankle Int. 2007;28(2):154–61.

20. Feiwell LA, Frey C. Anatomic study of arthroscopic portal sites of the ankle. Foot Ankle. 1993;14(3):142–7.

21. Feiwell LA, Frey C. Anatomic study of arthroscopic debridement of the ankle. Foot Ankle Int. 1994;15(11): 614–21.

22. Ferkel RD. Arthroscopic surgery: the foot and ankle. In: Ferkel RD, editor. Arthroscopic surgery: the foot and ankle. Philadelphia: JB Lippincott; 1999. p. 145–69.

23. Ferkel RD, Zanotti RM, Komenda GA, Sgaglione NA, Cheng MS, Applegate GR, et al. Arthroscopic treatment of chronic osteochondral lesions of the talus: long-term results. Am J Sports Med. 2008;36(9): 1750–62.

24. Flick AB, Gould N. Osteochondritis dissecans of the talus (transchondral fractures of the talus): review of

the literature and new surgical approach for medial dome lesions. Foot Ankle. 1985;5(4):165–85.

25. Garras DN, Santangelo JA, Wang DW, Easley ME. A quantitative comparison of surgical approaches for posterolateral osteochondral lesions of the talus. Foot Ankle Int. 2008;29(4):415–20.

26. Gatellier J. The juxtoretroperoneal route in the operative treatment of fracture of the malleolus with posterior margin fragment. Gynecol Obstret. 1931;52:67–70.

27. Giannini S, Battaglia M, Buda R, Cavallo M, Ruffilli A, Vannini F. Surgical treatment of osteochondral lesions of the talus by open-field autologous chondrocyte implantation: a 10-year follow-up clinical and magnetic resonance imaging T2-mapping evaluation. Am J Sports Med. 2009;37 Suppl 1:112S–8.

28. Giannini S, Buda R, Cavallo M, Ruffilli A, Cenacchi A, Cavallo C, et al. Cartilage repair evolution in post-traumatic osteochondral lesions of the talus: from open field autologous chondrocyte to bone-marrow-derived cells transplantation. Injury. 2010; 41(11):1196–203.

29. Giannini S, Buda R, Grigolo B, Vannini F. Autologous chondrocyte transplantation in osteochondral lesions of the ankle joint. Foot Ankle Int. 2001;22(6):513–7.

30. Giannini S, Buda R, Vannini F, Cavallo M, Grigolo B. One-step bone marrow-derived cell transplantation in talar osteochondral lesions. Clin Orthop Relat Res. 2009;467(12):3307–20.

31. Giannini S, Buda R, Vannini F, Di Caprio F, Grigolo B. Arthroscopic autologous chondrocyte implantation in osteochondral lesions of the talus: surgical technique and results. Am J Sports Med. 2008;36(5):873–80.

32. Giannini S, Vannini F. Operative treatment of osteochondral lesions of the talar dome: current concepts review. Foot Ankle Int. 2004;25(3):168–75.

33. Giza E, Sullivan M, Ocel D, Lundeen G, Mitchell ME, Veris L, et al. Matrix-induced autologous chondrocyte implantation of talus articular defects. Foot Ankle Int. 2010;31(9):747–53.

34. Gobbi A, Francisco RA, Lubowitz JH, Allegra F, Canata G. Osteochondral lesions of the talus: randomized controlled trial comparing chondroplasty, microfracture, and osteochondral autograft transplantation. Arthroscopy. 2006;22(10):1085–92.

35. Gortz S, De Young AJ, Bugbee WD. Fresh osteochondral allografting for osteochondral lesions of the talus. Foot Ankle Int. 2010;31(4):283–90.

36. Gras F, Marintschev I, Muller M, Klos K, Lindner R, Muckley T, et al. Arthroscopic-controlled navigation for retrograde drilling of osteochondral lesions of the talus. Foot Ankle Int. 2010;31(10):897–904.

37. Gross AE, Agnidis Z, Hutchison CR. Osteochondral defects of the talus treated with fresh osteochondral allograft transplantation. Foot Ankle Int. 2001;22(5): 385–91.

38. Hahn DB, Aanstoos ME, Wilkins RM. Osteochondral lesions of the talus treated with fresh talar allografts. Foot Ankle Int. 2010;31(4):277–82.

39. Hampton CB, Shawen SB, Keeling JJ. Positioning technique for combined anterior, lateral, and posterior ankle and hindfoot procedures: technique tip. Foot Ankle Int. 2010;31(4):348–50.

40. Hankemeier S, Muller EJ, Kaminski A, Muhr G. 10-year results of bone marrow stimulating therapy in the treatment of osteochondritis dissecans of the talus. Unfallchirurg. 2003;106(6):461–6.

41. Hansen Jr ST. The fibular window. Functional reconstruction of the foot and ankle. Philadelphia: Lippincott Williams & Wilkins; 2000. p. 496–7.

42. Hatic 2nd SO, Berlet GC. Particulated juvenile articular cartilage graft (DeNovo NT Graft) for treatment of osteochondral lesions of the talus. Foot Ankle Spec. 2010;3(6):361–4.

43. Hembree WC, Wittstein JR, Vinson EN, Queen RM, Larose CR, Singh K, et al. Magnetic resonance imaging features of osteochondral lesions of the talus. Foot Ankle Int. 2012;33(7):591–7.

44. Kelberine F, Frank A. Arthroscopic treatment of osteochondral lesions of the talar dome: a retrospective study of 48 cases. Arthroscopy. 1999;15(1):77–84.

45. Kreuz PC, Lahm A, Haag M, Kostler W, Konrad G, Zwingmann J, et al. Tibial wedge osteotomy for osteochondral transplantation in talar lesions. Int J Sports Med. 2008;29(7):584–9.

46. Kreuz PC, Steinwachs M, Edlich M, Kaiser T, Mika J, Lahm A, et al. The anterior approach for the treatment of posterior osteochondral lesions of the talus: comparison of different surgical techniques. Arch Orthop Trauma Surg. 2006;126(4):241–6.

47. Kreuz PC, Steinwachs M, Erggelet C, Lahm A, Henle P, Niemeyer P. Mosaicplasty with autogenous talar autograft for osteochondral lesions of the talus after failed primary arthroscopic management: a prospective study with a 4-year follow-up. Am J Sports Med. 2006;34(1):55–63.

48. Kruse DL, Ng A, Paden M, Stone PA. Arthroscopic De Novo NT((R)) juvenile allograft cartilage implantation in the talus: a case presentation. J Foot Ankle Surg. 2012;51(2):218–21.

49. Lijoi F, Lughi M, Baccarani G. Posterior arthroscopic approach to the ankle: an anatomic study. Arthroscopy. 2003;19(1):62–7.

50. Loomer R, Fisher C, Lloyd-Smith R, Sisler J, Cooney T. Osteochondral lesions of the talus. Am J Sports Med. 1993;21(1):13–9.

51. Ly PN, Fallat LM. Trans-chondral fractures of the talus: a review of 64 surgical cases. J Foot Ankle Surg. 1993;32(4):352–74.

52. Magnan B, Samaila E, Bondi M, Vecchini E, Micheloni GM, Bartolozzi P. Three-dimensional matrix-induced autologous chondrocytes implantation for osteochondral lesions of the talus: midterm results. Adv Orthop. 2012;2012:942174.

53. Muir D, Saltzman CL, Tochigi Y, Amendola N. Talar dome access for osteochondral lesions. Am J Sports Med. 2006;34(9):1457–63.

54. Nickisch F, Barg A, Saltzman CL, Beals TC, Bonasia DE, Phisitkul P, et al. Postoperative complications of posterior ankle and hindfoot arthroscopy. J Bone Joint Surg Am. 2012;94(5):439–46.

55. O'Loughlin PF, Kendoff D, Pearle AD, Kennedy JG. Arthroscopic-assisted fluoroscopic navigation for retrograde drilling of a talar osteochondral lesion. Foot Ankle Int. 2009;30(1):70–3.

56. Orr JD, Dutton JR, Fowler JT. Anatomic location and morphology of symptomatic, operatively treated osteochondral lesions of the talus. Foot Ankle Int. 2012;33(12):1051–7.

57. Ove PN, Bosse MJ, Reinert CM. Excision of posterolateral talar dome lesions through a medial transmalleolar approach. Foot Ankle. 1989;9(4):171–5.

58. Patzkowski JC, Kirk KL, Orr JD, Waterman BR, Kirby JM, Hsu JR. Quantification of posterior ankle exposure through an achilles tendon-splitting versus posterolateral approach. Foot Ankle Int. 2012;33(10):900–4.

59. Peters PG, Parks BG, Schon LC. Anterior distal tibia plafondplasty for exposure of the talar dome. Foot Ankle Int. 2012;33(3):231–5.

60. Raikin SM. Fresh osteochondral allografts for large-volume cystic osteochondral defects of the talus. J Bone Joint Surg Am. 2009;91(12):2818–26.

61. Ray RB, Coughlin EJ. Osteochondritis dissecans of the talus. J Bone Joint Surg. 1947;29:697–706.

62. Rush JK, Kirk K, Kirby J, Hsu J. Lateral talar dome access utilizing temporary invasive distraction. Foot Ankle Int. 2010;31(3):236–41.

63. Sammarco GJ, Makwana NK. Treatment of talar osteochondral lesions using local osteochondral graft. Foot Ankle Int. 2002;23(8):693–8.

64. Saxena A, Eakin C. Articular talar injuries in athletes: results of microfracture and autogenous bone graft. Am J Sports Med. 2007;35(10):1680–7.

65. Schneider TE, Karaikudi S. Matrix-Induced Autologous Chondrocyte Implantation (MACI) grafting for osteochondral lesions of the talus. Foot Ankle Int. 2009;30(9):810–4.

66. Scholten PE, Sierevelt IN, van Dijk CN. Hindfoot endoscopy for posterior ankle impingement. J Bone Joint Surg Am. 2008;90(12):2665–72.

67. Scholten PE, van Dijk CN. Combined posterior and anterior ankle arthroscopy. Case Rep Orthop. 2012;2012:693124.

68. Schuman L, Struijs PA, van Dijk CN. Arthroscopic treatment for osteochondral defects of the talus. Results at follow-up at 2 to 11 years. J Bone Joint Surg Br. 2002;84(3):364–8.

69. Scranton Jr PE, Frey CC, Feder KS. Outcome of osteochondral autograft transplantation for type-V cystic osteochondral lesions of the talus. J Bone Joint Surg Br. 2006;88(5):614–9.

70. Seil R, Rupp S, Pape D, Dienst M, Kohn D. Approach to open treatment of osteochondral lesions of the talus. Orthopade. 2001;30(1):47–52.

71. Sitler DF, Amendola A, Bailey CS, Thain LM, Spouge A. Posterior ankle arthroscopy: an anatomic study. J Bone Joint Surg Am. 2002;84–A(5):763–9.

72. Stone JW. Osteochondral lesions of the talar dome. J Am Acad Orthop Surg. 1996;4(2):63–73.

73. Taranow WS, Bisignani GA, Towers JD, Conti SF. Retrograde drilling of osteochondral lesions of the medial talar dome. Foot Ankle Int. 1999;20(8):474–80.

74. Tochigi Y, Amendola A, Muir D, Saltzman C. Surgical approach for centrolateral talar osteochondral lesions with an anterolateral osteotomy. Foot Ankle Int. 2002;23(11):1038–9.

75. van Bergen CJ, Tuijthof GJ, Blankevoort L, Maas M, Kerkhoffs GM, van Dijk CN. Computed tomography of the ankle in full plantar flexion: a reliable method for preoperative planning of arthroscopic access to osteochondral defects of the talus. Arthroscopy. 2012;28(7):985–92.

76. van Bergen CJ, Tuijthof GJ, Maas M, Sierevelt IN, van Dijk CN. Arthroscopic accessibility of the talus quantified by computed tomography simulation. Am J Sports Med. 2012;40(10):2318–24.

77. van Dijk CN, Scholten PE, Krips R. A 2-portal endoscopic approach for diagnosis and treatment of posterior ankle pathology. Arthroscopy. 2000;16(8):871–6.

78. Voto SJ, Ewing JW, Fleissner Jr PR, Alfonso M, Kufel M. Ankle arthroscopy: neurovascular and arthroscopic anatomy of standard and trans-achilles tendon portal placement. Arthroscopy. 1989;5(1):41–6.

79. Wang L, Gui J, Gao F, Yu Z, Jiang Y, Xu Y, et al. Modified posterior portals for hindfoot arthroscopy. Arthroscopy. 2007;23(10):1116–23.

80. Willits K, Sonneveld H, Amendola A, Giffin JR, Griffin S, Fowler PJ. Outcome of posterior ankle arthroscopy for hindfoot impingement. Arthroscopy. 2008;24(2):196–202.

Approach to Osteochondral Lesions of the Medial Talus

Keir A. Ross, Niall A. Smyth, and John G. Kennedy

Take-Home Points

- *Imaging is an invaluable tool for locating lesions and determining size which should strongly influence preoperative planning.*
- *Approach should be based on the size of the OCL, the preoperative treatment plan, and the location of OCL.*
- *Standard anterior arthroscopy is widely accepted and allows access to at least 50 % of the anterior talar dome.*
- *Posterior arthroscopy via the 2-portal approach is a safe and effective approach when hindfoot access is required.*
- *Arthrotomy may be a feasible alternative to medial malleolar osteotomy but requires further research.*
- *Medial malleolar osteotomy is more transgressive and risky but is a reasonable approach when treatment requires full visualization and access; these techniques require more research on long-term follow-up.*

8.1 Introduction

Osteochondral lesions (OCL) of the talus are a challenge to access due to coverage by the tibial plafond and malleoli. As a result, a variety of approaches have been proposed to gain visualization and/or surgical access to talar lesions. Posteromedial and anterolateral OCLs were classically thought to be the most common location of talar lesions [42]. However, OCLs of the centromedial and centrolateral talus have recently been shown to occur most frequently, with medial lesions occurring more often than lateral lesions [10]. Medial lesions also tend to be larger than lateral lesions [10, 25, 32]. Asymptomatic lesions and lesions seen in pediatric patients may be treated nonoperatively with rest, protected weight bearing, or immobilization [28], but more substantial OCLs typically require surgical intervention. Consequently, this chapter covers surgical approaches to access the OCLs of the medial talus including arthroscopy, arthrotomy, and medial malleolar osteotomy [9].

8.2 Surgical Approaches

8.2.1 Arthroscopic Access to the Medial Talar Dome

Considerable progress has been made in ankle arthroscopy over the past two to three decades. Arthroscopic surgery of the ankle was initially considered technically demanding and had a

K.A. Ross, BS • N.A. Smyth, MD
J.G. Kennedy, MD, MCh, FRCS (Orth) (✉)
Department of Orthopaedic Surgery,
Hospital for Special Surgery,
New York, NY, USA
e-mail: rossk@hss.edu; smythn@hss.edu;
kennedyj@hss.edu

C.N. van Dijk, J.G. Kennedy (eds.), *Talar Osteochondral Defects*,
DOI 10.1007/978-3-642-45097-6_8, © ESSKA 2014

complication rate as high as 26.4 % in 1989 [34]. As both arthroscopic techniques and equipment have become more sophisticated, the average published complication rate of ankle arthroscopy is now 10.3 % [48]. With the technique described by van Dijk and co-workers, the percentage dropped to 3.5 % [48]. The principal treatment modality for OCLs performed arthroscopically is debridement and subchondral stimulation (e.g., microfracture) [47]. While subchondral stimulation has shown successful clinical results at the short and medium term [8], the long-term efficacy of the procedure remains contentious as it results in an infill of fibrocartilage. Some authors have suggested that arthroscopic microfracture is effective for any lesion smaller than 1.5 cm^2 [7, 8, 39]. On the other hand, it has been suggested that this technique is most favorable when lesions are less than 6 mm with minimal damage to the subchondral bone [26]. As a result of this discrepancy, there has been increasing interest in alternative surgical treatment when large lesions are present [28, 47]. Depending on the location of the osteochondral lesion, either arthrotomy or osteotomy may be required to gain access to the joint. However, arthroscopy remains the most common approach to treating talar OCLs and may be performed via either anterior or posterior portals.

8.2.1.1 Patient in Supine Position

Routine anterior arthroscopic examination of the ankle is typically performed with the patient in a supine position and consists of anteromedial and anterolateral portals [40]. The anterolateral portal is created 5 mm below the joint line, lateral to the tertiary peroneal tendon, while being cautious of the superficial peroneal nerve [25, 48]. The anteromedial portal is created 5 mm distal to the joint line, just medial to the anterior tibial tendon. For medial OCL access the surgical instrument will be placed through the medial portal, and the arthroscope is inserted through the lateral portal [25]. Anterior arthroscopy may be performed with or without the use of fixed continuous distraction, but because of reported complication rates with continuous fixed distraction (13.6 %) [39], intermittent soft tissue distraction is more commonly used [48].

Most talar OCLs can be accessed with anterior arthroscopy with the ankle joint plantar flexed (with or without soft tissue distraction) [39], but access becomes more challenging if the lesion is located posterior to the anterior distal tibial rim [35, 36]. For patients with full plantar flexion ability, 48 % of the talar dome can be revealed anterior to the anterior distal tibial rim, meaning OCLs in this region can be accessed through anterior arthroscopic portals without the need for invading the joint [12, 36]. OCLs located posterior to the anterior tibial rim can still be accessed with an arthroscope; however, instrumentation can be difficult to navigate over the talar horizon. A limited plafondplasty, in which the anterior margin of the distal tibia corresponding to the OCD is removed, can be helpful in some cases [3]. In most cases, however, soft tissue joint distraction in the plantar flexed position provides access to the OCD even if it is located posterior to the anterior distal rim. Sometimes a posterolateral working portal is needed. Most talar OCLs can be accessed via arthroscopic portals.

8.2.1.2 Patient in Prone Position

A posterior arthroscopic approach can be used to access OCLs located in the posterior aspect of the talus [40]. Marumoto and Ferkel suggested the use of a posterolateral portal in combination with standard anterior arthroscopy as a method to access the hindfoot [6, 16, 18, 22, 27, 31]. Other approaches include posterolateral and anterolateral portals, two posterolateral portals, and a posterolateral and trans-Achilles portal [11, 13, 16, 22, 44, 45]. Most notably, van Dijk and co-workers proposed a novel posterior 2-portal approach in 2000 that granted arthroscopic access to the hindfoot, posterior ankle, subtalar joints, and extra-articular structures [40].

The original posterior 2-portal approach [40] is the most commonly presented technique for accessing the hindfoot and is used by the senior authors. This technique is performed with the patient in a prone position with the foot and ankle overhanging the end of the table or at the end of the table with a triangular cushion under the distal tibia. With the ankle maintained in a neutral position, a straight line, parallel to the sole of the foot, is drawn between the tips of the lateral and medial malleoli. The posterolateral portal is positioned just proximal to this line and 5 mm anterior to the lateral border of the Achilles tendon. The posteromedial portal is positioned 5 mm anterior to the medial border of the Achilles tendon at the level of the intermalleolar line [33, 38]. Manual dorsiflexion of the ankle is typically sufficient to allow adequate visualization and access of the posterior talus [40]; however, distraction techniques have been described [5].

The chief concern with hindfoot arthroscopy is proximity of the posterolateral portal to the sural nerve and the posteromedial portal to the medial neurovascular bundle [33]. However, the complication rate following hindfoot arthroscopy is low, with a review of 311 cases reporting a complication rate of 2.3 % [48]. It is important to note that this rate is considerably lower than the 24 % complication rate reported following open surgery for the treatment of hindfoot pathology [1].

8.2.2 Open (Non-arthroscopic) Access to the Medial Talar Dome

Large OCLs of the medial talus that require autograft or allograft transplantation may require open access to fully assess the lesions and implant the graft. While autologous chondrocyte implantation (ACI) and minced juvenile cartilage procedures can be performed arthroscopically, many OCLs located in the posteromedial talar dome are best approached with an open procedure [14, 15, 20, 24, 28, 33].

8.2.2.1 Arthrotomy

A simple arthrotomy has been proposed as an alternative to medial malleolar osteotomy [46]. Young and co-workers demonstrated in a cadaver study that a standard anteromedial incision allows access to 50 % of the talus from anterior to posterior and 31 % of the talus from medial to lateral [46]. The novel posteromedial incision, made 3 cm posterior to the medial malleolus, provides access to 33 % of the anterior to posterior length and 36 % of the medial to lateral length. The combination of these two arthrotomies leaves only roughly 20 % of the talus inaccessible. A prior arthrotomy study, using anterolateral, posterolateral, anteromedial, and posteromedial portals, proposed that all but 17 % of the medial talar dome can be revealed [24]. Advantages of this approach over osteotomy include small incisions and minimal transgression of the patient and ankle joint itself [46]. This approach, however, is not commonly used and requires further study.

8.3 Extensile Exposures to the Medial Talar Dome

Medial malleolar osteotomy is an established method for approaching the medial talus and for gaining exposure of the centromedial and posteromedial aspects of the talus [9]. As a large percentage of medial OCLs are located posteriorly [25], a medial malleolar osteotomy is often necessary to visualize an OCL. Furthermore, full visualization with perpendicular access is often necessary for posteromedial OCLs, as they tend to be large lesions [42], requiring osteochondral allograft or autograft transplantation. Disadvantages of this approach include the risk of displacement or migration of the osteotomy, tenderness at osteotomy site, increased immobilization, damage to the long flexors, damage to the articulating surface of the medial tibial plafond, and malunion/nonunion [2, 21, 46].

There are a number of medial malleolar osteotomy techniques including step-cut [2], oblique [37], inverted U [29], crescentic [43], Chevron-type [9, 21], and transverse [30]. Advantages and disadvantages of these techniques vary [37] (Table 8.1), but there is evidence suggesting that the oblique and Chevron-type osteotomies result in good outcomes at follow-up [21, 37]. When performing a medial malleolar osteotomy, the senior authors prefer the use of a Chevron osteotomy.

Table 8.1 Comparison of medial malleolar osteotomy techniques

Osteotomy technique	Exposure/visualization	Advantages	Disadvantages
Transverse	Inadequate	Simple procedure	Talar dome covered by tibial plafond
Inverted U	Inadequate	Simple procedure	Contraindicated for large OCLs, limited range of motion, and narrow joints
Crescentic	No perpendicular access	Conforms to contour of talar dome	Horizontal cut results in no perpendicular access
Step-cut	Excellent	Modified technique provides good access	Difficult to fix the fragment perpendicular to the cut
Oblique	Excellent	Excellent congruity when the cut is made 30° relative to long axis of the tibia	Outcomes vary; fragment migration seen when fixation is not perpendicular to cut; requires precise cut 30° to tibia
Chevron-type	Excellent	Good healing and fixation in short term	May require precise cut 30° to tibia

Amount of exposure, advantages, and disadvantages of medial malleolar osteotomy techniques are outlined for comparison [42]

The Chevron-type medial malleolar osteotomy has been described several times previously [19, 21]. The medial malleolus is exposed using a standard curvilinear medial incision, and a K-wire is then used to establish the apex of the Chevron cut. Under fluoroscopic guidance, the K-wire is advanced to the subchondral plate at the malleolar colliculous (Fig. 8.1). Proper angulation of the guidewire is necessary for exposing the OCL, and angulation can be adjusted based on the location of the lesion but should be around 30° in relation to the long axis of the tibia. Two parallel fixation holes are then drilled in the malleolus for later reduction of the fragment. An oscillating saw is then used to create the osteotomy, with a baby Bennett retractor in place to protect the posterior tibial tendon. Sawing is halted before reaching the articular surface and the osteotomy completed using an osteotome (Fig. 8.2). The procedure is concluded with reduction of the osteotomy fragment. This is achieved by securing predrilled fixation holes using 4.0 mm cannulated screws. A transverse screw is also placed in the malleolus to prevent superior migration (Fig. 8.3).

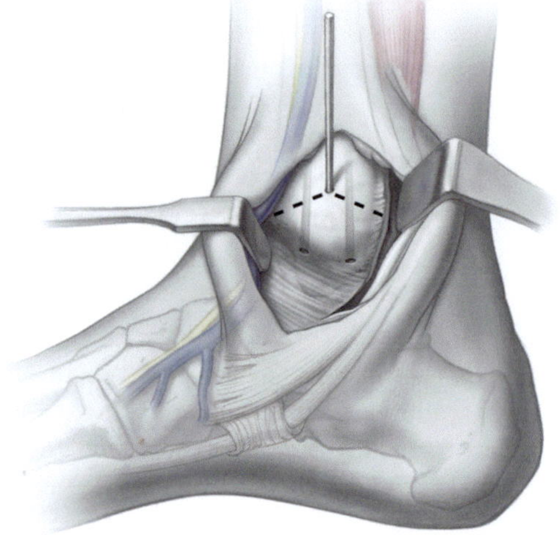

Fig. 8.1 A Chevron cut is made in the medial malleolus after predrilling the fixation holes and placing a guidewire for osteotomy direction (Illustrations copyright of and reproduced with permission from JG Kennedy MD. Reproduction without express written consent is prohibited)

A series of 62 patients undergoing Chevron-type osteotomy demonstrated satisfactory healing and fixation at a median time of 6 weeks.

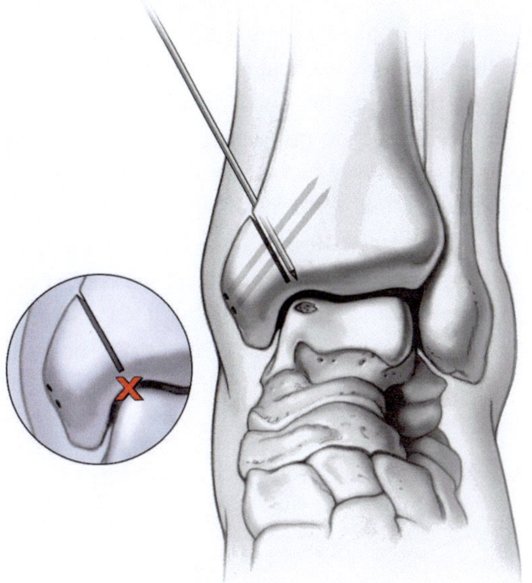

Fig. 8.2 The osteotomy cut is terminated just prior to reaching the subchondral bone and completed with an osteotome (Illustrations copyright of and reproduced with permission from JG Kennedy MD. Reproduction without express written consent is prohibited)

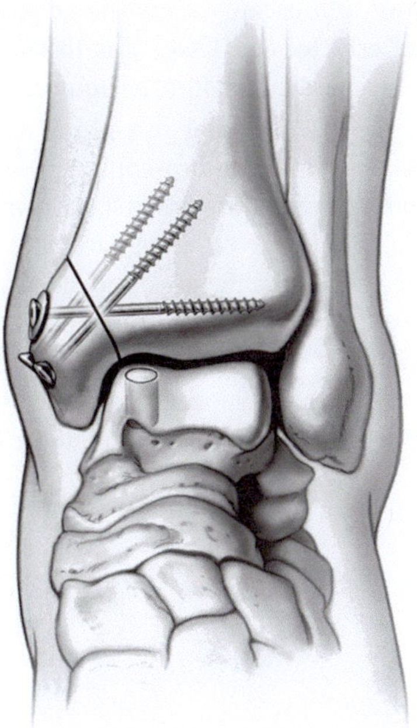

Fig. 8.3 The osteotomy is fixed with two parallel screws and a third transverse screw to prevent superior migration of the osteotomy fragment (Illustrations copyright of and reproduced with permission from JG Kennedy MD. Reproduction without express written consent is prohibited)

Fibrocartilaginous infill was evident in the superficial half of repair tissue at the osteotomy interface, and MRI indicated restored normal tissue in the deep half [21]. In a separate series, 4 of 19 patients had a slight (<2 mm) displacement at the osteotomy site, but this was attributed to technical error [9].

An oblique osteotomy provides adequate visualization of the talus and good congruity when executed properly [21, 37]. Some case series have shown no postoperative complications [27, 31], while others have reported osteoarthritis [17], reduction in plantar flexion [4], reduction in range of motion [4], loss of stability [21, 37], and potential for fragment migration when fixation screws are not applied perpendicular to the osteotomy cut [37]. Failure of the osteotomy to heal in an anatomic position may place higher load on the ankle, potentially leading to arthrosis [25]. Deciding which osteotomy is most appropriate to treat, medial OCLs should be

based on the size and location of the lesion and most importantly on the surgeon's experience with the technique.

Conclusions

Arthroscopic approaches are well established, minimally invasive, and can provide access to most OCLs. Standard anterior arthroscopy can access about 50 % of the talus without invading the joint space, and 75 % of the talus can be accessed with distraction, debridement, and/or arthroscopic invasion of the joint space. This approach is recommended when preoperative imaging indicates an OCL is in an accessible location and does not require full visualization or open treatment [23, 41]. Posterior/hindfoot arthroscopy is a safe and effective approach and should be used when anterior arthroscopy cannot grant access to a posteriorly located OCL. For this approach, careful regard for hindfoot anatomy is required.

A medial malleolar osteotomy should be avoided when an arthroscopic approach can provide access and allow satisfactory treatment of an OCL. However, when the characteristics of a lesion require the use osteochondral transplantation, an open approach with a malleolar osteotomy is a feasible option. Oblique osteotomy requires precision, and adverse outcomes have been reported. In addition, there is a risk of fragment migration when fixation screws are not applied properly [37], and failure of the osteotomy to heal in an anatomic position may place higher load on the ankle, potentially leading to arthrosis [25]. The Chevron-type osteotomy has shown good outcomes but requires long-term follow-up studies.

Ultimately, lesion size and characteristics will impact the treatment of choice and therefore the approach used. OCL location and characteristics must therefore be considered when planning the surgical approach (Fig. 8.4).

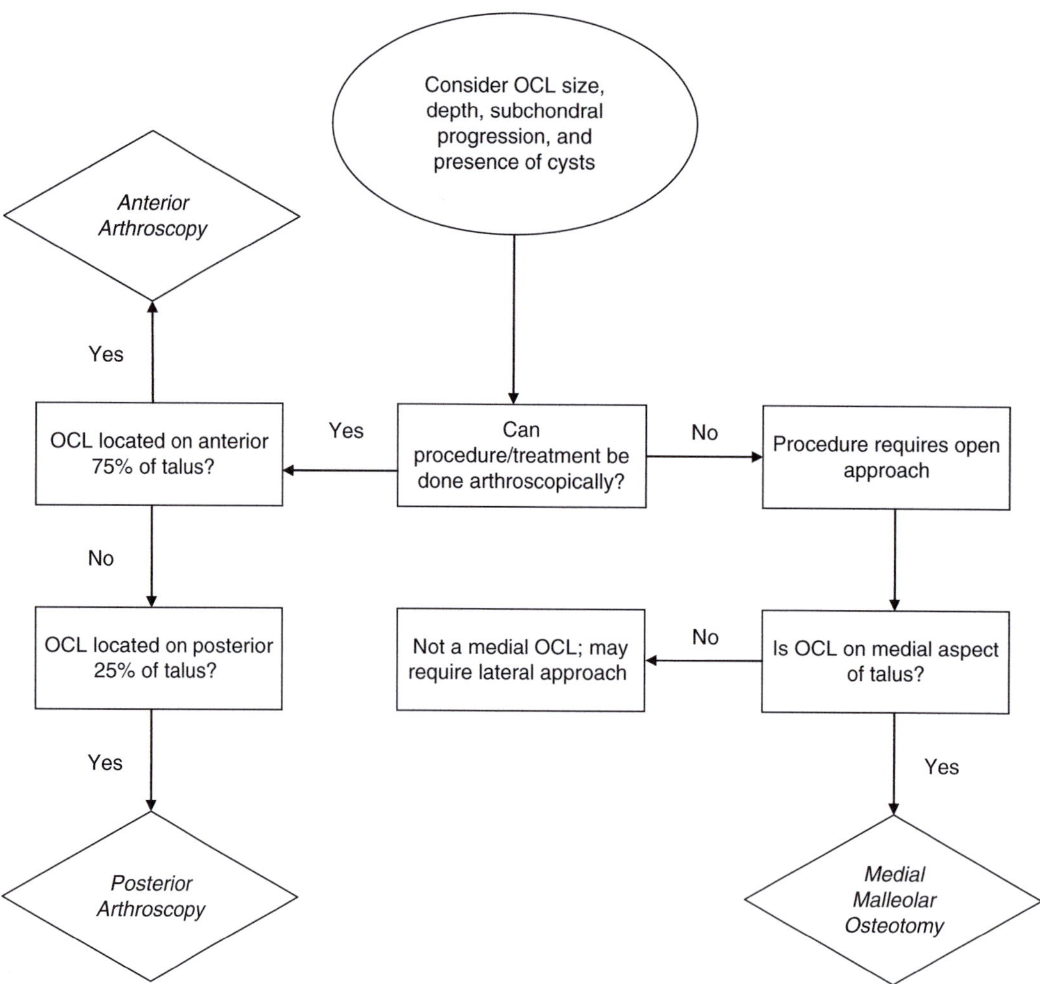

Fig. 8.4 An algorithm for the approach to osteochondral lesions of the medial talar dome. Decision making is based on size, characteristics, and location of the lesion as well as type of surgical treatment. The oval is the starting point, each rectangle is a factor in the decision-making process, and each rhombus is a selected approach and end point

Conflict of Interest The author has no current conflict of interests with the products presented.

References

1. Abramowitz Y, Wollstein R, Barzilay Y, et al. Outcome of resection of a symptomatic os trigonum. J Bone Joint Surg Am. 2003;85-A:1051–7.
2. Alexander IJ, Watson JT. Step-cut osteotomy of the medial malleolus for exposure of the medial ankle joint space. Foot Ankle. 1991;11:242–3.
3. Assenmacher JA, Kelikian AS, Gottlob C, Kodros S. Arthroscopically assisted autologous osteochondral transplantation for osteochondral lesions of the talar dome: an MRI and clinical follow-up study. Foot Ankle Int. 2001;22:544–51.
4. Baltzer AW, Arnold JP. Bone-cartilage transplantation from the ipsilateral knee for chondral lesions of the talus. Arthroscopy. 2005;21:159–66.
5. Beals TC, Junko JT, Amendola A, Nickisch F, Saltzman CL. Minimally invasive distraction technique for prone posterior ankle and subtalar arthroscopy. Foot Ankle Int. 2010;31:316–9.
6. Calder JD, Sexton SA, Pearce CJ. Return to training and playing after posterior ankle arthroscopy for posterior impingement in elite professional soccer. Am J Sports Med. 2010;38:120–4.
7. Choi WJ, Park KK, Kim BS, Lee JW. Osteochondral lesion of the talus: is there a critical defect size for poor outcome? Am J Sports Med. 2009;37:1974–80.
8. Chuckpaiwong B, Berkson EM, Theodore GH. Microfracture for osteochondral lesions of the ankle: outcome analysis and outcome predictors of 105 cases. Arthroscopy. 2008;24:106–12.
9. Cohen BE, Anderson RB. Chevron-type transmalleolar osteotomy: an approach to medial talar dome lesions. Tech Foot Ankle Surg. 2002;1:158–62.
10. Elias I, Zoga AC, Morrison WB, Besser MP, Schweitzer ME, Raikin SM. Osteochondral lesions of the talus: localization and morphologic data from 424 patients using a novel anatomical grid scheme. Foot Ankle Int. 2007;28:154–61.
11. Ferkel RD, Fischer SP. Progress in ankle arthroscopy. Clin Orthop Relat Res. 1989;240:210–20.
12. Ferkel RD, Heath DD, Guhl JF. Neurological complications of ankle arthroscopy. Arthroscopy. 1996;12:200–8.
13. Ferkel RD, Scranton Jr PE. Arthroscopy of the ankle and foot. J Bone Joint Surg Am. 1993;75:1233–42.
14. Hangody L, Rathonyi GK, Duska Z, Vasarhelyi G, Fules P, Modis L. Autologous osteochondral mosaicplasty: surgical technique. J Bone Joint Surg Am. 2004;86:65–72.
15. Hatic SO, Berlet GC. Particulated juvenile articular cartilage graft (DeNovo NT Graft) for treatment of osteochondral lesions of the talus. Foot Ankle Spec. 2010;3:361–4.
16. Horibe S, Kita K, Natsu-ume T, Hamada M, Mae T, Shino K. A novel technique of arthroscopic excision of a symptomatic os trigonum. Arthroscopy. 2008;24:121–4.
17. Jarde O, Trinquier-Lautard JL, Garate F, de Lestang M, Vives P. Osteochondral lesions of the talar dome: surgical treatment in a series of 30 cases. Rev Chir Orthop Reparatrice Appar Mot. 2000;86:608–15.
18. Jerosch J, Fadel M. Endoscopic resection of a symptomatic os trigonum. Knee Surg Sports Traumatol Arthrosc. 2006;14:1188–93.
19. Kennedy JG, Murawski CD. The treatment of osteochondral lesions of the talus with autologous osteochondral transplantation and bone marrow aspirate concentrate: surgical technique. Cartilage. 2011;2:327–36.
20. Kruse DL, Ng A, Paden M, Stone PA. Arthroscopic De Novo NT(®) juvenile allograft cartilage implantation in the talus: a case presentation. J Foot Ankle Surg. 2012;51:218–21.
21. Lamb J, Murawski CD, Deyer TW, Kennedy JG. Chevron-type medial malleolar osteotomy: a functional, radiographic and quantitative T2-mapping MRI analysis. Knee Surg Sports Traumatol Arthrosc. 2013;21:1283–8.
22. Marumoto JM, Ferkel RD. Arthroscopic excision of the os trigonum: a new technique with preliminary clinical results. Foot Ankle Int. 1997;18:777–84.
23. Mintz DN, Tashjian GS, Connell DA, Deland JT, O'Malley M, Potter HG. Osteochondral lesions of the talus: a new magnetic resonance grading system with arthroscopic correlation. Arthroscopy. 2003;19:353–9.
24. Muir D, Saltzman CL, Tochigi Y, Amendola N. Talar dome access for osteochondral lesions. Am J Sports Med. 2006;34:1457–63.
25. Navid DO, Myerson MS. Approach alternatives for treatment of osteochondral lesions of the talus. Foot Ankle Clin. 2002;7:635–49.
26. O'Driscoll SW. The healing and regeneration of articular cartilage. J Bone Joint Surg Am. 1998;80:1795–812.
27. Ogut T, Ayhan E, Irgit K, Sarikaya AI. Endoscopic treatment of posterior ankle pain. Knee Surg Sports Traumatol Arthrosc. 2011;19:1355–61.
28. O'Loughlin PF, Heyworth BE, Kennedy JG. Current concepts in the diagnosis and treatment of osteochondral lesions of the ankle. Am J Sports Med. 2010;38:392–404.
29. Oznur A. Medial malleolar window approach for osteochondral lesions of the talus. Foot Ankle Int. 2001;22:841–2.
30. Ray RB, Coughlin EJ. Osteochondritis dissecans of the talus. J Bone Joint Surg. 1947;29:697–710.
31. Scholten PE, Sierevelt IN, van Dijk CN. Hindfoot endoscopy for posterior ankle impingement. J Bone Joint Surg Am. 2008;90:2665–72.
32. Smyth NA, Fansa AM, Murawski CD, Kennedy JG. Platelet-rich plasma as a biological adjunct to the

surgical treatment of osteochondral lesions of the talus. Tech Foot Ankle Surg. 2012;11:18–25.

33. Smyth NA, Murawski CD, Levine DS, Kennedy JG. Hindfoot arthroscopic surgery for posterior ankle impingement: a systematic surgical approach and case series. Am J Sports Med. 2013;41:1869–76.

34. Sprague NF, Guhl JF, Olson DW. Specific complications: elbow, wrist, hip, and ankle. Complications in arthroscopy. New York: Raven; 1989. p. 99–224.

35. van Bergen CJA, Tujithof GJM, Blankvoort L, Maas M, Kerkoffs GMMJ, van Dijk CN. Computed tomography of the ankle in full plantar flexion: a reliable method for preoperative planning of arthroscopic access to osteochondral defects of the talus. Arthroscopy. 2012;28:985–92.

36. van Bergen CJA, Tujithof GJM, Blankvoort L, Maas M, Sierevelt IN, van Dijk CN. Arthroscopic accessibility of the talus quantified by computed tomography simulation. Am J Sports Med. 2012;40:2318–24.

37. van Bergen CJA, Tuijthof GJM, Sierevelt IN, van Dijk CN. Direction of the oblique medial malleolar osteotomy for exposure of the talus. Arch Orthop Trauma Surg. 2010;131:893–901.

38. van Dijk CN, de Leeuw PA, Scholten PE. Hindfoot endoscopy for posterior ankle impingement. Surgical technique. J Bone Joint Surg Am. 2009;91:287–98.

39. van Dijk CN, van Bergen CJ. Advancements in ankle arthroscopy. J Am Acad Orthop Surg. 2008;16:635–46.

40. van Dijk CN, Scholten PE, Krips R. A 2-portal endoscopic approach for diagnosis and treatment of posterior ankle pathology. Arthroscopy. 2000;16:871–6.

41. Verhagen RA, Maas M, Dijkgraaf MG, Tol JL, Krips R, van Dijk CN. Prospective study on diagnostic strategies in osteochondral lesions of the talus. Is MRI superior to helical CT? J Bone Joint Surg Br. 2005;87:41–6.

42. Verhagen RA, Struijs PA, Bossuyt PM, van Dijk CN. Systematic review of treatment strategies for osteochondral defects of the talar dome. Foot Ankle Clin. 2003;8:233–42.

43. Wallen EA, Fallat LM. Crescentic transmalleolar osteotomy for optimal exposure of the medial talar dome. J Foot Surg. 1989;28:389–94.

44. Willits K, Sonneveld H, Amendola A, Giffin JR, Griffin S, Fowler PJ. Outcome of posterior ankle arthroscopy for hindfoot impingement. Arthroscopy. 2008;24:196–202.

45. Yilmaz C, Eskandari MM. Arthroscopic excision of the talar Stieda's process. Arthroscopy. 2006;22:225.

46. Young KW, Deland JT, Lee KT, Lee YK. Medial approaches to osteochondral lesion of the talus without medial malleolar osteotomy. Knee Surg Sports Traumatol Arthrosc. 2010;18:634–7.

47. Zengerink M, Struijs PA, Tol JL, van Dijk CN. Treatment of osteochondral lesions of the talus: a systematic review. Knee Surg Sports Traumatol Arthrosc. 2010;18:238–46.

48. Zengerink M, van Dijk CN. Complications in ankle arthroscopy. Knee Surg Sports Traumatol Arthrosc. 2012;20:1420–31.

Approach to Osteochondral Lesions of the Tibial Plafond

Steven M. Raikin

Take-Home Points

Osteochondral lesions of the tibial plafond are:

- *Rare as compared to osteochondral lesions of the talar dome (3.7 %)*
- *Do not occur in any predictable location or zone within the plafond*
- *May be associated with periarticular cysts requiring bone grafting*
- *Treated with arthroscopic debridement and microfracture/marrow stimulation*
- *Not as predictable as seen with arthroscopic management of talar dome lesions*

9.1 Introduction

Osteochondral lesions were first described by König in the distal femoral condyles of the knee in 1888 [11]. It was only in 1922 that Kappis described similar lesions in the ankle, involving the articular surface of the talar dome [10]. In 1959 Berndt and Harty classified these lesions and reported that the majority were secondary to trauma and were due in fact to transchondral fractures of the talar dome [1]. There are, however,

S.M. Raikin, MD
Department of Orthopaedic Surgery,
Rothman Institute, Jefferson Medical College,
Thomas Jefferson University Hospital,
Philadelphia, PA, USA
e-mail: steven.raikin@rothmaninstitute.com

numerous underlying etiological factors which can cause osteochondral lesions in the talus. Examples of this are vascular insults (local osteonecrosis) of various causes, hormonal dysfunction, and hereditary genetic factors with a strong intra-family association and a relatively high bilateral rate (10–25 %). As such Ferkel proposed changing the name from OCD to osteochondral lesions of the talus, or OLT [9].

Involvement of the distal tibial plafond was even more recently defined when in 1985 Parisian described finding distal tibial lesion in two of 15 ankles treated arthroscopically for osteochondral lesions [14]. In reviewing the literature, there is no predominant underlying etiology causing lesions within the tibial plafond, with traumatic and nontraumatic history having statistically equal incidence.

9.2 Incidence

Approximately 4 % of all osteochondral lesions developing in the joints of the body occur in the ankle joint [11]. Most of these are found in the talar dome. Two large studies evaluating a combined 1,640 ankles with osteochondral lesions found 61 (3.7 %) within the distal tibial plafond (OLTP) [6, 13]. The average age of patients with OLTP was 38 years old, with no specific gender and side predominance. Bilateral lesions have only been reported in one case report [17].

OLTP can occur concomitantly with OLT. This is found in an average of 18.75 % of cases

C.N. van Dijk, J.G. Kennedy (eds.), *Talar Osteochondral Defects*,
DOI 10.1007/978-3-642-45097-6_9, © ESSKA 2014

where OLTP are seen [6, 13]. The majority of these are within different geographical zones of the ankle, with less than 20 % of these being "kissing" or matching lesions on opposite sides of the ankle joint [3, 5, 6, 13].

There are very few published papers on OLTP with a total of only 88 lesions described in the English literature, for which 74 came from three studies [5, 6, 13]. This makes scientific analysis of most aspects of these lesions very difficult, being a significant limitation of this chapter.

9.3   Location Within the Plafond

Osteochondral lesion of the talus occurs most frequently within the equatorial zone of the medial talar dome (53 %), followed by the equatorial zone of the lateral talus (26 %) [7]. Due to the relative rarity of OLTP, defining the distribution of lesions geographically has been more difficult. The author previously described a 9-zone grid system of locations of OLTP, similar to that described in the talar dome. Plotting the distribution of 38 OLTP (the largest published study on OLTP) demonstrated a non-statistically significant distribution of these lesions geographically within the grid. There was, however, a tendency for lesions to be more frequently located within the medial central to medial posterior quadrant of the distal tibial plafond [6].

9.4   Diagnosis

Most patients with OLTP present with nonspecific history of gradually developing deep ankle pain [20]. History of prior trauma may be present in some cases. Patients usually complain of pain in the ankle which is activity related. The pain is often generalized to the ankle joint and nonspecific in nature. Functional ankle instability may be an associated complaint due to a pain reflex emanating from the subchondral bone.

Clinical evaluation and examination again is very nonspecific. The ankle may or may not have an effusion. Most patients have tenderness at the ankle joint line anteriorly, but this is usually poorly defined and located. It is not infrequent that the side of the tenderness or pain complaint is not concomitant with the site of the actual lesion once diagnosed. The ankle should be evaluated for all generalized causes of ankle pain.

Evaluatory radiographs should be performed with weight bearing and should include an anteroposterior view, mortise view, and lateral view. In many cases the radiographs appear normal, but careful scrutiny for abnormal shadows or cysts within the distal tibial plafond region should be performed (Fig. 9.1).

Diagnosis is usually made on a CT scan or magnetic resonance imaging (MRI) [2, 6]. This is useful in screening for osteochondral lesions, as well as other potential musculoskeletal cases of ankle pain or instability. The MRI is used to diagnose the lesion, as well as access the biological activity of the lesion. This is seen as signal change consistent with bone marrow edema within the subchondral bone adjacent to the lesion (Fig. 9.2). Absence of bone marrow edema may suggest that a lesion seen within the distal tibia may be inactive and an incidental finding not responsible for the patients pain. This may additionally be evaluated on a 3-phase technetium-labeled bone scan.

The MRI is not however very accurate in determining the true size and depth of the lesion, nor the presence of subtle associated subchondral cysts, which are all better evaluated on CT scans (Fig. 9.3). For preoperative planning CT scan is the preferred option [21].

9.5   Nonoperative Treatment

Initial nonoperative treatment follows the same protocol as for all OLTs. This includes initial rest, immobilization, and unloading protocol, in either a fracture boot or cast. The duration of nonoperative treatment is not well defined and should include input from the patient.

The natural history of OLTP and the success rate of nonoperative treatment are currently

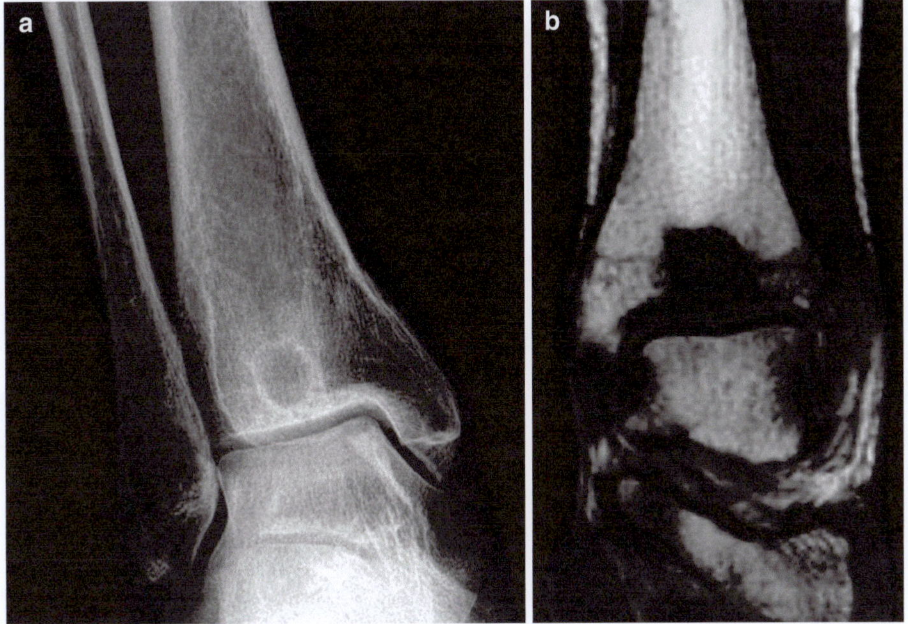

Fig. 9.1 Anteroposterior radiograph (**a**) and MRI (**b**) demonstrating an osteochondral defect in the tibial plafond (OLTP) with a large overlying periarticular cyst

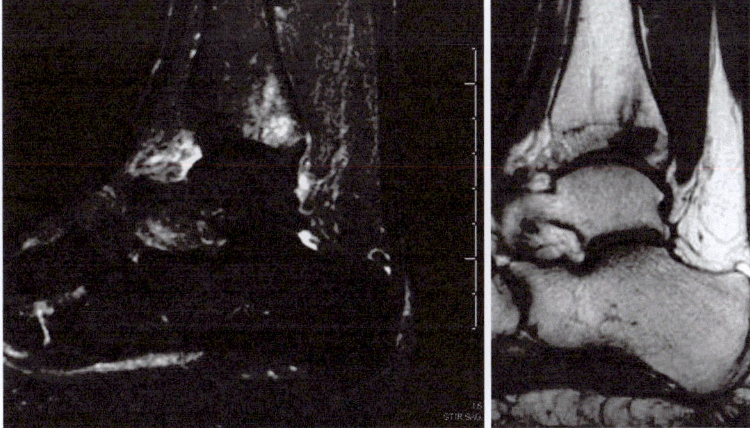

Fig. 9.2 Sagittal T2 and T2 MRI images demonstrating a posterior OLTP with active bone marrow edema

unknown. Shearer described 54 % good and excellent results with nonoperative treatment of OLT [16], while the author of this chapter reviewed sequential MRI studies of patients with diagnosed OLTs and showed that 45 % had MRI evidence of improvement (although 55 % did get worse or stayed the same) [8]. It is unclear whether these results translate to lesions in the tibial plafond.

Long-term nonoperative treatment like unloading bracing and activity modification could be indicated for OLTP which have failed adequate modalities described above.

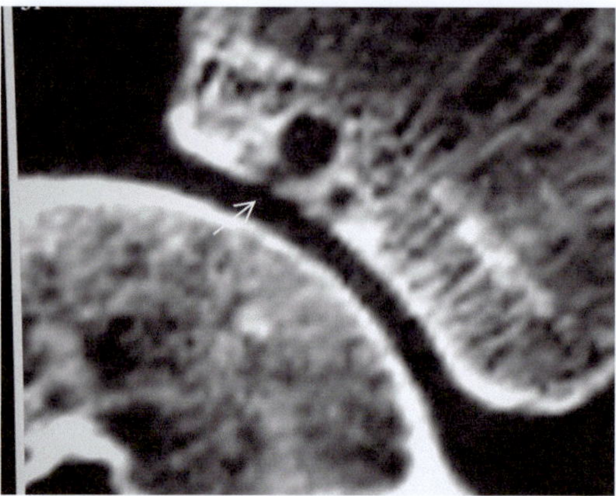

Fig. 9.3 Sagittal cut CT scan demonstrating a small anterior periarticular cyst associated with an OLTP. *White arrow* indicates the intra-articular extension of the cyst demonstrating osteochondral involvement

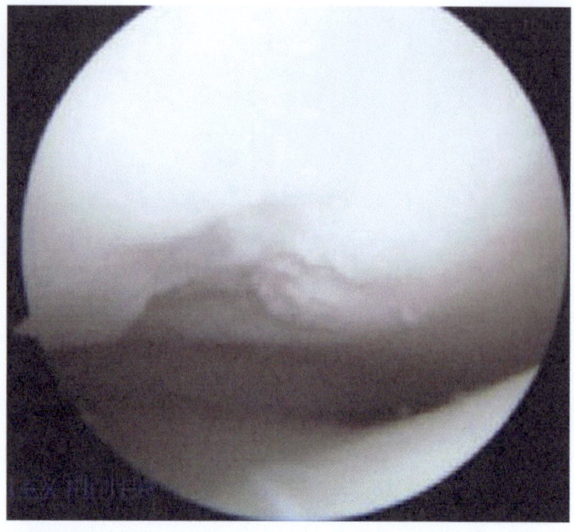

Fig. 9.4 Arthroscopic view of OLTP in the central plafond

9.6 Operative Treatment

Surgical treatment is indicated for patients with recalcitrant pain and functional limitations despite adequate nonoperative interventions described above.

Most OLTP can be surgically managed arthroscopically. Utilizing standard anteromedial and anterolateral portals, a diagnostic evaluation should be performed as described by Ferkel to evaluate for associated pathologies [9]. Very posterior lesions can be addressed via a posterior arthroscopic approach described by Van Dijk with the patient positioned prone [19].

Once identified (Fig. 9.4), the OLTP is managed by debriding nonviable or damaged cartilage and bone, curetting the rim and base of the lesion to ensure a stable cartilaginous rim and a vascularized bone base (Fig. 9.5).

Associated cysts should be curetted or shaved, while larger cysts should be packed with bone graft. Bone grafting is usually performed in an antegrade manner. The debrided lesion is located arthroscopically with the ball tip of a microvector guide. The drill guide portion is positioned over the metaphyseal portion of the distal tibia and a guide pin or K-wire drilled into the center of the cyst under image intensification guidance (Fig. 9.6). Sequential cannulated

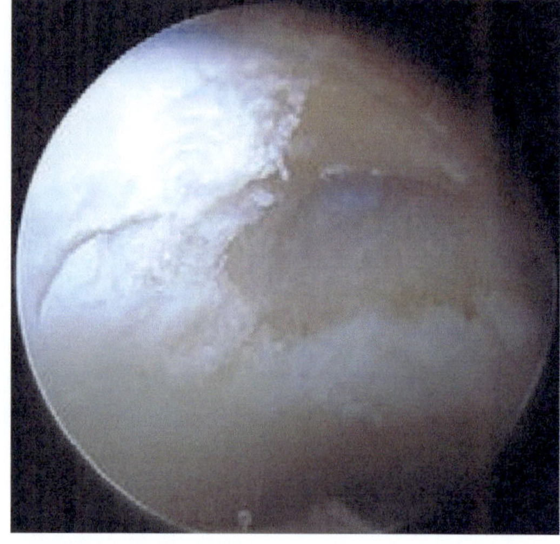

Fig. 9.5 OLTP post debridement of unstable cartilage

drill bits are drilled over the wire creating an access channel to the cyst large enough to insert a curette (Fig. 9.7). The curette is used to scrape and remove the membranous cystic lining of the cyst (Fig. 9.8) and any sclerotic bone bordering the cyst, leaving bleeding cancellous bone at the cyst's borders. Following irrigation, the arthroscope can be inserted down the bone tunnel to confirm the cyst has been adequately debrided and prepared under direct visualization. Bone graft (autologous, allograft, or synthetic) is then inserted down the bone tunnel and impacted

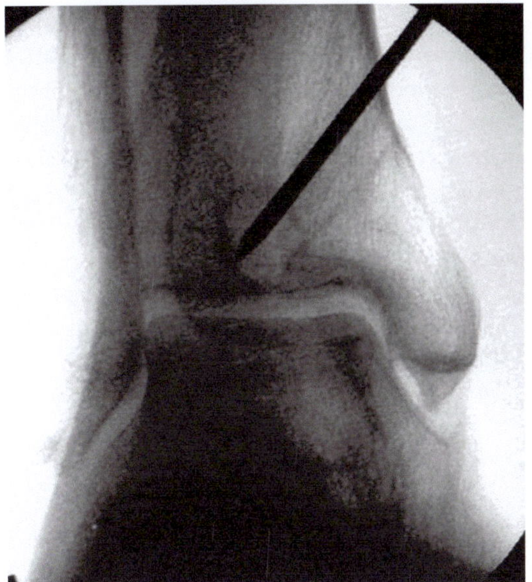

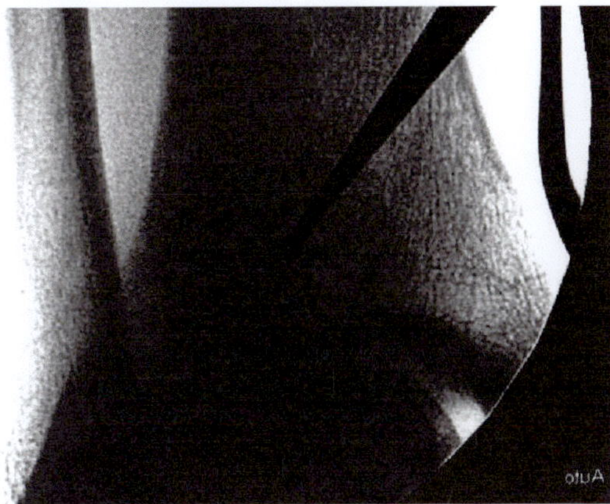

Fig. 9.8 Intraoperative image intensification image demonstrating curette debriding the walls of the cyst prior to grafting

Fig. 9.6 Intraoperative image intensification image demonstrating placement of guide pin within the center of the distal tibial cyst

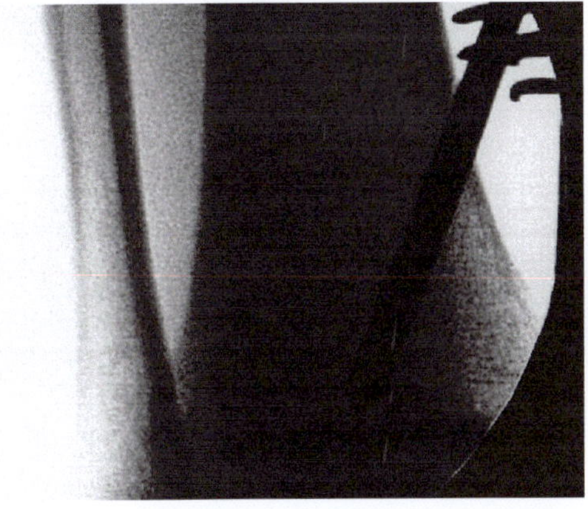

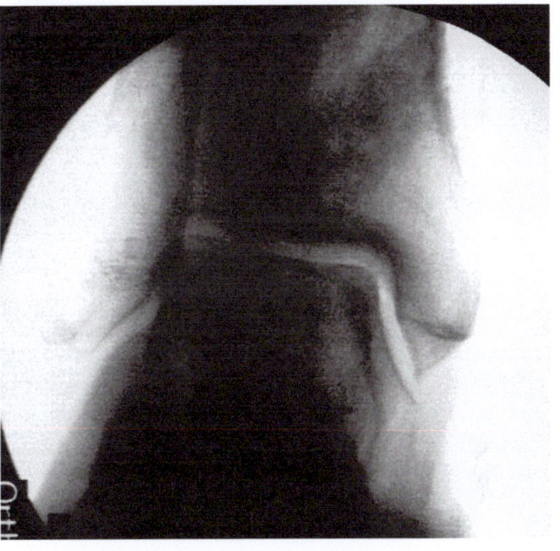

Fig. 9.9 Intraoperative image intensification image demonstrating antegrade packing of bone graft material filling the cyst and access channel

Fig. 9.7 Intraoperative image intensification image demonstrating reamer drilling into the cyst to enlarge the access channel

into the cyst utilizing a bone tamp. Complete fill of the cyst can usually be seen under image intensification (Fig. 9.9). Adequate packing of the cyst is important to prevent synovial fluid entering through the joint into the cyst which may result in resorption of the graft or reformation of the cyst. This is assessed arthroscopically through the ankle joint while probing the communicating OLTP.

Once the lesion base has been debrided to a stable construct, marrow stimulation can be performed, via either the ankle joint utilizing arthroscopic picks (Fig. 9.10) {author's preference} or antegrade utilizing a drill bit or K-wire through the microvector guide. Once the "microfracture" holes have been created, the tourniquet is deflated and/or the arthroscopic pump is turned off and the area is monitored for aggressive bleeding or extravasation of bone marrow cells from the lesion base (Fig. 9.11).

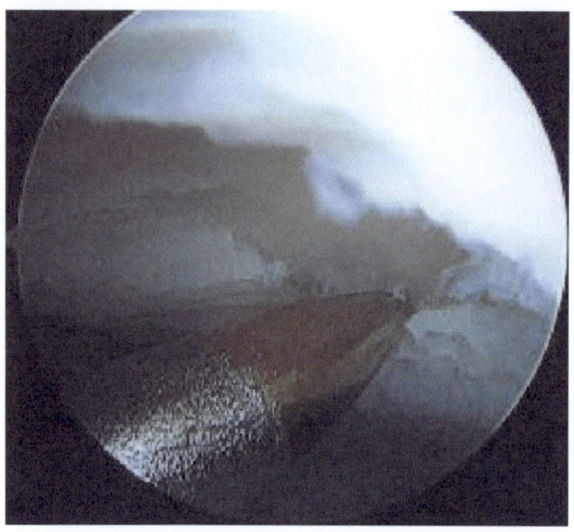

Fig. 9.10 Arthroscopic view of a microfracture pick prior to penetration into the base of a debrided OLTP

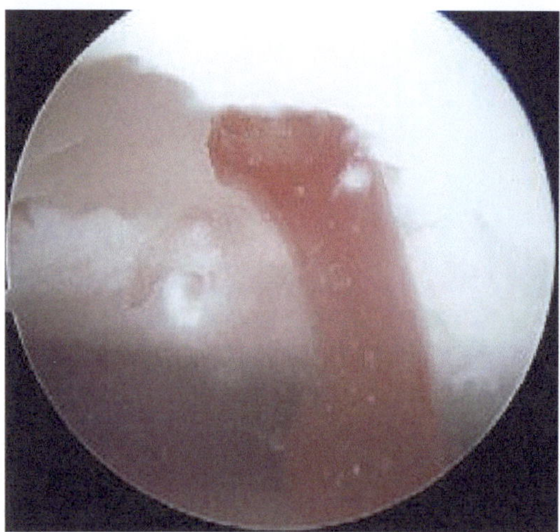

Fig. 9.11 Arthroscopic view demonstrating adequate bleeding from microfracture pick hole at the base of the OLTP allowing marrow-stimulated healing of the lesion

9.6.1 Postoperative Management

Postoperative management of arthroscopically treated osteochondral lesions of the ankle remains controversial as far as how long to keep the patient non-weight bearing and/or protected (braced) following surgery. No clear protocols exist following arthroscopic marrow stimulation of OLTP, but the author keeps his patients non-weight bearing for 6 weeks after surgery. A bulky dressing is applied for the first week; patients are encouraged to move the ankle out of their protective boot as soon as they can tolerate this. Active range of motion is encouraged very early in the postoperative period with the theoretical advantage of encouraging the inflow of synovial fluid for cartilage nutrition.

After 6 weeks, patients are allowed to begin weight bearing as tolerated, initially in a protective boot which is weaned as comfort allows. This protocol is similar to that described by Cuttica and co-workers in their patients [5].

9.6.2 Results of Surgical Treatment

Only two case series of arthroscopically treated OLTP have been published [5, 12]. The first included 23 patients, but only 17 were available for follow-up at 44 months. Additionally there was a broad spectrum of different treatment modalities used with ten patients receiving only an abrasion chondroplasty and seven receiving marrow stimulation (five antegrade drilling, two microfracture picking). Two cases (12 %) additionally had iliac crest bone grafting of large associated cysts. The authors did demonstrate a significant improvement in AOFAS-AH score with 14 of 17 describing their results as good or excellent. There were two poor results. Both of these were complex cases, one of which had an associated cyst requiring bone grafting and the other having both an OLTP and an OLT within the same joint. Due to the small numbers in the study, no difference could be found between different treatment modalities used [13]. The second study evaluated 13 patients managed arthroscopically over a 6-year time period. All underwent debridement and microfracture of the tibial lesion. An underlying cyst was present in three cases (23 %), and these cases additionally underwent bone grafting of the cysts. Patients were followed for an average of 38 months postoperatively. The results of this study demonstrated a 43 % improvement on AOFAS-AH scores as compared to preoperative levels, which was a significant improvement. Despite this there were only seven (54 %) good results, with four (31 %) patients evaluated as having a poor result – three requiring revision surgery and one being on disability for chronic pain. They concluded that surgical management of OLTP can lead to improved outcomes, but caution that treatment predictability and outcomes are less than that seen with management of OLTs [5].

In the authors personal experience (currently unpublished) of 25 cases (7 % of arthroscopically treated osteochondral lesions of the ankle), there were four (16 %) patients with associated subchondral cysts requiring concomitant bone grafting. Results of the data collected to date on 19 patients demonstrate an overall improvement in AOFAS-AH score of 47 % with 15 self rating their results as good or excellent, two as fair, and two as poor. Both patients with poor results were posttraumatic cases with degenerative changes seen more diffusely at the time of arthroscopy that had been predicted on preoperative evaluation.

9.7 New Horizons

Larger lesions, recurrent lesions, and some cystic lesions may not be amenable to arthroscopic debridement and marrow stimulation.

Osteochondral autograft plugs have been described in a case report to treat these lesions [18]. The osteochondral autograft transfer system (OATS) has been recently modified with a "switch tube" (Fig. 9.12) allowing osteochondral plugs harvested from the knee joint to be inserted in an antegrade manner once the OLTP has been cored or drilled out.

Additionally there are case reports of utilizing synthetic osteochondral plugs [15] and osteochondral allografts [4] to treat these difficult lesions.

Conclusion

Osteochondral lesions of the distal tibial plafond (OLTP) represent only 3.7 % of osteochondral lesions within the ankle joint, with the remaining lesions occurring in the talar dome. Relatively small studies on these rare lesions demonstrated that approximately 17 % of these will have a large overlying communicating cyst, and 20 % will have an associated osteochondral lesion of the talus – most in a different zone to the tibial lesion.

Lesions recalcitrant to nonoperative treatment can be managed with arthroscopic debridement and microfracture, with additional bone grafting of the overlying cyst as needed. This protocol results in improved outcomes and function with 73 % of patients reporting excellent or good results. The results however are not as good or predictable as those seen with isolated lesion involving the talar dome, with a greater proportion of poor results.

Conflict of Interest The author has no current conflict of interests with the products presented.

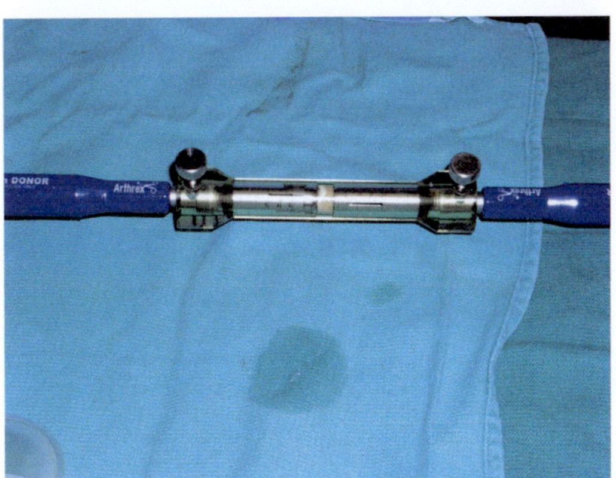

Fig. 9.12 "Switch stick" utilized for reversing a harvested osteochondral plug prior to antegrade insertion for management of a large OLTP (Courtesy of Pierce Scranton, M.D.)

References

1. Berndt AL, Harty M. Transchondral fractures (osteochondritis dissecans) of the talus. J Bone Joint Surg. 1959;41(A):988–1929.
2. Bui-Mansfield LT, Kline M, Chew FS, Rogers LF, Lenchik L. Osteochondritis dissecans of the tibial plafond: imaging characteristics and a review of the literature. AJR Am J Roentgenol. 2000;175(5):1305–8.
3. Canosa J. Mirror image osteochondral defects of the talus and distal tibia. Int Orthop. 1994;18(6):395–6.
4. Chapman CB, Mann JA. Distal tibial osteochondral lesion treated with osteochondral allografting: a case report. Foot Ankle Int. 2005;26(11):997–1000.
5. Cuttica DJ, Smith WB, Hyer CF, Philbin TM, Berlet GC. Arthroscopic treatment of osteochondral lesions of the tibial plafond. Foot Ankle Int. 2012;33(8):662–8.

6. Elias I, Raikin SM, Schweitzer ME, Besser MP, Morrison WB, Zoga AC. Osteochondral lesions of the distal tibial plafond: localization and morphologic characteristics with an anatomical grid. Foot Ankle Int. 2009;6:524–9.

7. Elias I, Zoga AC, Morrison WB, Besser MP, Schweitzer ME, Raikin SM. Osteochondral lesions of the talus: localization and morphologic data from 424 patients using a novel anatomical grid scheme. Foot Ankle Int. 2007;28(2):154–61.

8. Elias I, Jung JW, Raikin SM, Schweitzer MW, Carrino JA, Morrison WB. Osteochondral lesions of the talus: change in MRI findings over time in talar lesions without operative intervention and implications for staging systems. Foot Ankle Int. 2006;27(3):157–66.

9. Ferkel RD. Arthroscopic surgery: the foot & ankle. Philadelphia: Lippincott-Raven; 1996.

10. Kappis M. Weitere beitrage zur traumatisch-mechanischen entstehung der "spontanen" knorpela biosungen. Deutsche Zeitschrift Chirurgie. 1922; 171:13–29.

11. König F. Uber Freie Jorper in der Gelenken. Deutsche Zeitschrift Chirurgie. 1888;27:90–109.

12. Lindholm TS, Osterman K, Vankka E. Osteochondritis dissecans of elbow, ankle and hip: a comparison survey. Clin Orthop Relat Res. 1980;148:245–53.

13. Mologne TS, Ferkel RD. Arthroscopic treatment of osteochondral lesions of the distal tibia. Foot Ankle Int. 2007;28(8):865–72.

14. Parisien JS, Vangsness T. Operative arthroscopy of the ankle. Three years' experience. Clin Orthop Relat Res. 1985;199:46–53.

15. Pearce CJ, Lutz MJ, Mitchell A, Calder JD. Treatment of a distal tibial osteochondral lesion with a synthetic osteochondral plug: a case report. Foot Ankle Int. 2009;30(9):900–3.

16. Shearer C, Loomer R, Clement D. Nonoperatively managed stage 5 osteochondral talar lesions. Foot Ankle Int. 2002;23(7):651–4.

17. Sopov V, Liberson A, Groshar D. Bilateral distal tibial osteochondral lesion: a case report. Foot Ankle Int. 2001;22(11):901–4.

18. Ueblacker P, Burkart A, Imhoff AB. Retrograde cartilage transplantation on the proximal and distal tibia. Arthroscopy. 2004;20(1):73–8.

19. van Dijk CN, Scholten PE, Krips R. A 2-portal endoscopic approach for diagnosis and treatment of posterior ankle pathology. Arthroscopy. 2000;16(8): 871–6.

20. van Dijk CN, Reilingh ML, Zengerink M, van Bergen CJ. Osteochondral defects in the ankle: why painful? Knee Surg Sports Traumatol Arthrosc. 2010; 18(5):570–80.

21. Verhagen RA, Maas M, Dijkgraaf MG, Tol JL, Krips R, van Dijk CN. Prospective study on diagnostic strategies in osteochondral lesions of the talus. Is MRI superior to helical CT? J Bone Joint Surg Br. 2005; 87(1):41–6.

Maartje Zengerink and C. Niek van Dijk

M. Zengerink, MD, PhD (✉)
Department of Orthopaedic Surgery,
Orthopaedic Research Centre Amsterdam,
Academic Medical Center, University of Amsterdam,
Amsterdam, The Netherlands
e-mail: m.zengerink@amc.uva.nl

C.N. van Dijk, MD, PhD
Department of Orthopaedic Surgery
and Traumatology, Academic Medical Center,
University of Amsterdam, Amsterdam,
The Netherlands
e-mail: c.n.vandijk@amc.uva.nl

> **Take-Home Points**
> - *Recommended treatment for asymptomatic/low symptomatic lesions is conservative.*
> - *Recommended treatment for symptomatic lesions ≤15 mm is excision, curettage, and BMS.*
> - *For symptomatic lesions ≥15 mm, consider fixation (for posttraumatic cases and juveniles), or bone marrow stimulation, or OATS.*
> - *For large talar cystic lesions, consider antegrade or retrograde drilling with or without a bone transplant or OATS.*
> - *For secondary lesions, consider OATS or ACI.*

10.1 Introduction

Treatment strategies for osteochondral lesions (OCL) of the ankle vary widely. Moreover, they have substantially increased over the past two decades, due to technical progress. In the case of a patient with a symptomatic OCL, it can be a challenge for the surgeon to choose from this wide pallet of treatment strategies. Publications are numerous, but often involve only one technique and therefore lack comparison. Stages of OCL vary between the studies, as do patient characteristics, surgical experience, and follow-up. Pooling the data of these studies can provide new information useful in decision making.

The various nonsurgical and surgical techniques for treatment of symptomatic OCL include rest or cast immobilization, excision of the lesion, excision and curettage, excision combined with curettage and drilling/microfracturing (i.e., bone marrow stimulation – BMS), placement of an autogenous (cancellous) bone graft, antegrade (transmalleolar) drilling (TMD), retrograde drilling, fixation and newer techniques like osteochondral transplantation (osteochondral autograft transfer system – OATS), and autologous chondrocyte implantation (ACI). The last two techniques focus at replacement and regeneration of hyaline cartilage, respectively.

Publications on the effectiveness of these treatment strategies vary. The goal of these treatment strategies is always to diminish symptoms like pain and swelling and to improve function. In most cases of OCL of the talus, several treat-

C.N. van Dijk, J.G. Kennedy (eds.), *Talar Osteochondral Defects*,
DOI 10.1007/978-3-642-45097-6_10, © ESSKA 2014

ment options are viable. The choice of treatment is based on the type and size of the lesion and on preferences of the treating clinician [12, 13]. A meta-analysis provides information that is not available from these separate publications. It summarizes the effectiveness of different treatment strategies to result in a more accurate outcome. A statistical reanalysis on basis of source data makes the outcome more reliable.

For talar OCL, three systematic reviews were undertaken in the past [56, 62, 69], of which the second was an update of the first. The last review involved new data but also followed a different research protocol. The most important difference was that only a series of ten patients and more were included, instead of "extended case series" of two patients and more. Another important difference was that it involved a quality assessment of the included studies. We will discuss the last review, published in 2010, since it includes the newer techniques like OATS and ACI [69]. Based on the results of this review, we will provide a guideline concerning the best treatment for the different stages of OCL of the ankle.

10.2 Materials and Methods

10.2.1 Data Sources

Electronic databases MEDLINE, EMBASE, CENTRAL, and DARE (January 1966– December 2006) were screened. As main keywords "Therapy; Treat*; Talus; Talar; Ankle; Cartilage*; Osteochondritis Dissecans; Chondral; Osteochondral; and Transchondral" were used. The search strategy for MEDLINE was (therapy or treat$) and (talar or talus or ankle) and (cartilag$ or osteochondritis dissecans or talar or chondral or osteochondral or transchondral). No language limitations were imposed. Reference lists of the selected studies were searched for additional articles.

10.2.2 Study Selection, Inclusion, and Exclusion Criteria

The published studies were independently assessed for inclusion by two investigators. Specifically developed forms were used for the

review. Agreement was needed for inclusion. In case of disagreement, the opinion of a third independent investigator was decisive. The manuscripts were blinded to the author and institute to prevent investigator bias. Included were all RCTs or quasi-experimental research that evaluated the effectiveness of treatment strategies for osteochondral lesions of the talus. This included case series. Studies were included if treatment for OCL of the talus was properly described and the outcome was well defined. Published studies describing the results of the following treatment strategies were included: nonoperative treatment – rest, nonoperative treatment – cast, excision of the fragment, excision and curettage, excision and curettage and drilling/microfracturing, placement of a cancellous bone graft, antegrade (transmalleolar) drilling, OATS, ACI, retrograde drilling, and fixation of the lesion.

Exclusion criteria for studies and/or patients were the evaluation of a combination of diagnoses without separately describing the results for talar OCL, follow-up less than 6 months, inadequately described therapy, age under 18 years, studies in which less than ten patients were included (excluding single case reports), the lesser extensive of a double publication, studies with no well-defined outcome, and if there was a combination of therapies described and results were not described per therapy. In case of double publications, only the most elaborate publication was selected.

10.2.3 Data Extraction

Successful treatment was defined as an excellent or good result at follow-up. This had to be defined by an accepted scoring system, like the AOFAS Ankle/Hindfoot scale [28] and the Hannover scoring system [59]. If success rate was not labeled by the author, but the results were well described, they were fitted into the widely accepted score of Thompson and Loomer [61]. The proportion of the patient population with successful treatment was noted and percentages were calculated. For each treatment strategy, study size weighted success rates were calculated. The primary outcomes were the effects of treatment on symptoms, measured by scoring systems concerning the ankle (mainly the AOFAS Ankle/Hindfoot scale).

10.2.4 Quality Assessment

A quality assessment of the included studies was performed, using the Newcastle-Ottawa Scale (NOS) [67] adjusted for case series. It was originally developed as an instrument to provide an easy and convenient tool for quality assessment of nonrandomized studies, i.e., case-control and cohort studies, to be used in a systematic review. It uses a "star" rating system to judge quality based on three aspects of the study: selection of study groups, comparability of study groups, and ascertainment of either the exposure or outcome of interest (dependent on assessment of case-control or cohort study, respectively). The maximum number of stars a study may receive in each of these three categories is 4, 2, and 3, respectively, for a total of 9 possible stars. The validity of the scale has been previously established. In orthopedic literature, the vast majority of publications involve case series. We adjusted the NOS for case series to perform a quality assessment of the included case series. Studies were scored for study design (0–2 stars), selection (0–1 star), and assessment of outcome (0–2 stars) (Appendix 1).

10.3 Results

10.3.1 Description of Studies

Over 2,000 articles were identified by the search strategy. One-hundred-eighty-three publications describing the results of treatment of talar OCL could be identified. Since only one randomized clinical trial was found [20], the conventional measures of summarizing estimates of effectiveness could not be used. Pooling of the estimates of the outcome in individual studies was used instead.

A total of 131 studies were excluded due to one or more exclusion criteria, being combination of diagnoses ($n = 14$), inappropriate duration of follow-up ($n = 14$), improper description of therapy ($n = 8$), age under 18 years ($n = 17$), case report ($n = 33$), double publication ($n = 17$), non-interpretable results ($n = 37$), less than ten patients ($n = 37$), and a combination of therapies ($n = 25$) (Table 10.1). This left 52 studies describing the results of 65 treatment groups. Three described the results of nonoperative treatment – rest, 4 of

Table 10.1 Criteria that were used

Exclusion criterion	No.
Combination of diagnoses	14
Follow-up <6 months	14
Therapy inadequately described	8
<18 years old	17
Single case report	33
Double publication	17
No well-defined outcome	37
<10 patients	37
Combination of therapies	25
Total no. of excluded studies	**202**

nonoperative treatment – cast, 4 of excision, 13 of excision and curettage, 18 of excision and curettage and BMS, 3 of retrograde drilling, 4 of ACI, 9 of OATS, 1 of fixation with bone pegs, 4 of cancellous bone grafting, and 2 of antegrade (transmalleolar) drilling.

10.3.2 Population Characteristics

In the 52 eligible studies, the total number of included patients with an OCL of the talus was 1,361. Average age was 31 years (18–75), and 63 % were male and 37 % female. The right ankle was involved in 57 % and the left in 43 %. Lesions were medial in 62 %, lateral in 36 %, central in 1 %, and medial and lateral in 1 %. A history of ankle trauma was reported in 86 % of cases. There was a primary defect in 84 %. For about half of the patients, the Berndt and Harty stage was mentioned. In 13 % it considered a Berndt and Harty stage 1 lesion, in 22 % a stage 2 lesion, in 40 % a stage 3 lesion, and in 25 % a stage 4 lesion. For evaluation of the result of therapy, the AOFAS Ankle/Hindfoot scale was most used [28] (Table 10.2).

10.3.3 Treatment Strategies

10.3.3.1 Nonoperative Treatment: Rest

This may be rest and/or restriction of (sporting) activities with or without treatment of nonsteroidal anti-inflammatory drugs (NSAIDs). The aim is to unload the damaged cartilage so edema can resolve and necrosis is prevented. Another objective could be healing of a (partly) detached fragment to the surrounding bone. Eighty-six patients,

Table 10.2 Scoring systems used for treatment of talar osteochondral lesions in the included studies. Some studies used more than one scoring system

Scoring system	No. of studies
AOFAS Ankle/Hindfoot scale	16
Scoring system developed by the authors	18
Hannover score	5
Patient satisfaction score	5
Criteria proposed by Berndt and Harty	5
Visual analog scale	3
Martin score	3
Alexander and Lichtman	3
Ogilvie-Harris score	2
MODEMS	2
Karlsson scoring scale	2
Tegner score	1
Evaluation proposed by Loomer	1
Mazur score	1
Freiburg ankle score	1
SANE	1
According to Thompson and Loomer	1
McCullough score	1

divided over three studies, were treated with rest for OCD [6, 49, 55]. The rationale to choose nonoperative treatment was not always clearly described. Stage of the lesion was not described. Two studies date back from 1953 [49] and 1975 [6]. At the time these studies were published, surgical treatment of talar OCL wasn't as common as it is today. The duration of symptoms prior to institution of nonoperative treatment was either unreported or ranged from subacute to acute (<6 weeks) to chronic (>6 weeks). In the most recent study, patients were given the choice between operative and nonoperative treatment and chose nonoperative treatment [55]. Conservative treatment consisted of weightbearing as tolerated. In 39 of 86 patients (45 %), conservative treatment reported to be successful (range 20–54 %).

10.3.3.2 Nonoperative Treatment: Cast

Unloading the damaged cartilage is the aim of cast treatment. Duration of cast immobilization is between 3 weeks and 4 months. Four studies reported the results of this treatment [6, 9, 26, 45], and they date back at least two decades. In most cases, it involved a Berndt and Harty stage II or III lesion. In 44 of the 83 patients (53 %), the treatment was reported to be successful (range 29–69 %).

10.3.3.3 Excision

This involves excision of the partially detached fragment, without treating the defect that is left. Four studies reported the results of excision [14, 27, 41, 45]. In two studies excision was performed for superficial cartilaginous lesions, with mainly intact underlying subchondral bone. It could also involve a loose intra-articular fragment. In one study the lesions showed bony necrosis underneath. In 32 of 59 patients, the result was reported to be successful (54 %). Success rates varied from 30 to 88 %.

10.3.3.4 Excision and Curettage

After excision of the loose body, the surrounding necrotic subchondral tissue is curetted using either an open or arthroscopic technique. Most patients had a Berndt and Harty stage III or IV lesion, although also stage II lesions occurred. Thirteen studies, a total of 259 patients, reported the results of OCD treatment by excision and curettage [6, 9, 14, 20, 26, 27, 36, 37, 39, 42, 43, 46, 48]. In 199 of 259 patients, a successful result was reported (77 %). The success rate varied from 56 to 94 %.

10.3.3.5 Excision, Curettage, and BMS

Bone marrow stimulation involves creating multiple connections with the subchondral bone. It follows excision and curettage. The connections to the subchondral bone can be accomplished by drilling or microfracturing. The aim is to partially destroy the calcified zone that is most often present and to create multiple openings into the subchondral bone. Intra-osseous blood vessels are disrupted, and the release of growth factors leads to the formation of a fibrin clot. The formation of local new blood vessels is stimulated, bone marrow cells are introduced in the OCL, and fibrocartilaginous tissue is formed. Most patients had a Berndt and Harty stage III or IV lesion, but stage I and II lesions also occurred. Lesions were usually not larger than 1.5 cm in diameter. A total of 18 studies, including 388 patients, described the results of BMS [1, 3, 5, 7, 11, 16, 17, 20–22, 25, 38, 40, 41, 52, 57, 60, 63]. In 329 of 386 patients, treatment was reported to be successful (85 %). The success rate varied from 46 to 100 %.

10.3.3.6 Excision, Curettage, and Autogenous Bone Graft

In this technique, the defect that remains after excision and curettage is filled with autogenous cancellous bone. The objective is to restore the weightbearing properties of the talus. Indications for treatment were large, often medial lesions, exceeding 1.5 cm in diameter. Four publications reported the results of this technique, for 74 patients [8, 16, 29, 31]. In 45 of 74 patients, the result was successful (61 %). Success rates varied from 41 to 93 %.

10.3.3.7 Antegrade (Transmalleolar) Drilling

An OCL that is hard to reach because of its location on the talar dome can be drilled through the malleolus. A K-wire is inserted about 3 cm proximal to the tip of the medial malleolus and directed across the medial malleolus into the lesion through the intact cartilage. Two publications described the results of this technique, for 41 patients [30, 48]. In 26 patients, the result was reported to be successful (63 %, range 32–100 %).

10.3.3.8 Osteochondral Transplantation/OATS® (Arthrex)

These are the alternative to allografts for the treatment of OCL. Two related procedures have been developed: mosaicplasty and osteochondral autograft transfer system. Both are reconstructive bone grafting techniques that use one or more cylindrical osteochondral grafts from the less weightbearing periphery of the ipsilateral knee. The transplants are then placed into the prepared defect site on the talus. The objective is to reproduce the mechanical, structural, and biochemical properties of the original hyaline articular cartilage which has become damaged. It is performed either by an open approach or by an arthroscopic procedure. Indications involve large, often medial lesions, sometimes with a cyst underneath. Sometimes it is used as a secondary treatment, after failed primary (surgical) treatment. Nine studies described the results of 243 patients treated with OATS [2, 18, 20, 23, 32, 35, 51, 53, 54]. Good/excellent results were obtained in 212 patients (87 %). Success rates varied from 74 to 100 %. Morbidity of the donor knee joint was seen in 12 % of patients (0–37 %). Three studies did not discuss the possibility of postoperative knee pain [23, 32, 51].

10.3.3.9 Autologous Chondrocyte Implantation/ACI

The aim of ACI is to regenerate tissue with a high percentage of hyaline-like cartilage. First, a region of healthy articular cartilage is arthroscopically identified and a biopsy is taken. The tissue is minced and enzymatically digested. Chondrocytes are separated by filtration, and the isolated chondrocytes are cultivated in culture medium for 11–21 days. In a second stage, an arthrotomy is performed, and the chondral lesion is excised up to the healthy surrounding cartilage. A periosteal flap is removed from the tibia and sutured to the surrounding rim of normal cartilage. The cultured chondrocytes are then injected beneath the periosteal flap. Lesions larger than 1 cm^2, in the absence of generalized osteoarthritic changes, are suitable for this technique. Four studies, describing 59 patients, were included [4, 19, 44, 68]. In 45 of 59 patients (76 %), a successful result was reported. The success rate varied from 70 to 92 %.

10.3.3.10 Retrograde Drilling

In case of a primary OCL with more or less intact cartilage with a large subchondral cyst, or in case a defect is hard to reach via the usual anterolateral and anteromedial portals, retrograde drilling is suitable. For medial lesions, arthroscopic drilling can take place through the sinus tarsi. For lateral lesions, the cyst is approached from anteromedial. Revascularisation is induced in the subchondral bone, and subsequently the forma-

Table 10.3 Results per treatment strategy

Treatment strategy	No. of studies	No. of patients	No. of patients good/excellent result	Success percentage (%)	Range (%)
Nonoperative, rest	3	86	39	45	20–54
Nonoperative, cast	4	83	44	53	29–69
Excision	4	59	32	54	30–88
Excision and curettage	13	259	199	77	56–94
Excision, curettage, and BMS	18	388	329	85	46–100
Autogenous bone graft	4	74	45	61	41–93
TMD	2	41	26	63	32–100
OATS	9	243	212	87	74–100
ACI	4	59	45	76	70–92
Retrograde drilling	3	42	37	88	81–100
Fixation, bone pegs	1	27	24	89	–
Total	**65**	**1,361**	**1,032**	76	20–100

Described are the number of included studies per treatment strategy as mentioned in the first column, the cumulative number of patients per treatment strategy, the number of patients with a good or excellent result at follow-up, the success percentage per treatment strategy, and finally the range of the success percentages

BMS bone marrow stimulation, *ACI* autologous chondrocyte implantation, *OATS* osteochondral autograft transfer system, *TMD* transmalleolar drilling

tion of new bone is stimulated. A cancellous graft may be placed to fill the gap. Three publications, comprising 42 patients, were included [30, 50, 58]. It mainly involved medial lesions. Size of the lesions was not described. Postoperatively immediate range-of-motion exercises were commenced in all studies. After 2 [50], 4 [30], or 6 [58] weeks postoperatively, partial weightbearing was started. In 37 of 42 patients, this treatment was reported to be successful (88 %, range 81–100 %).

10.3.3.11 Fixation

Large loose fragments can be secured to the underlying bone using either a screw, pin, rod, or fibrin glue. One publication, for a total of 27 patients, met our inclusion criteria [33]. In this study, stage II–IV lesions were elevated, the bed was curetted and drilled, and after alignment of the fragment, it was reattached with at least two bone pegs from the distal tibia. Results were reported to be successful in 24 patients (89 %).

Results are summarized in Table 10.3.

10.3.4 Quality Assessment of Included Studies

On "study design," together 52 studies scored a total of 28 stars, out of a possible 104. On "selection," 48 out of 52 possible stars were scored. On "outcome," 34 out of 104 stars were scored.

10.4 Discussion

The most important finding of the review we discuss was that bone marrow stimulation (BMS), osteochondral transplantation (OATS) and autologous chondrocyte implantation (ACI) could be identified as the three most effective treatment options.

The review summarizes 65 study groups in 52 studies which describe treatment strategies for osteochondral talar lesions. There was a great diversity in trials concerning patient characteristics, staging of the defect, duration of follow-up, and outcome measures. A relatively large number of studies were dedicated to treatment by excision

Table 10.4 Success percentages (patients with a good/excellent result at follow-up after treatment of an osteochondral talar lesion) of a previous review by Verhagen et al. [66] compared to the current review

Treatment strategy	Verhagen et al., studies published up to 2000 (%)	Current review, studies published up to 2006 (%)
Nonoperative treatment – rest	45	45
Nonoperative treatment – cast	–	53
Excision	38	54
Excision and curettage	76	77
Excision, curettage, and BMS	86	85
Autogenous bone graft	85	61
TMD	–	63
OATS	94	87
ACI	–	76
Retrograde drilling	81	88
Fixation	73	89
Total		**76**

and curettage, excision and curettage and BMS, and OATS. The number of patients in other categories, mainly retrograde drilling, fixation, and transmalleolar drilling, was too limited for a reliable interpretation of the results. Therefore, no definitive conclusions could be drawn. Recommendations concerning these techniques must be judged accordingly. Some techniques do not apply to all Berndt and Harty OCL stages or are only suitable in the acute phase (<6 weeks). Retrograde drilling is usually reserved for large OCL with intact overlying cartilage, as confirmed by arthroscopy. It is the treatment of choice when there is a large subchondral cyst with overlying healthy cartilage. The studies concerning retrograde drilling did not describe size of the lesions [30, 50, 58]. Fixation is indicated for large fragments that can be reattached. It is applied especially in (sub)acute cases and in adolescents and children. Transmalleolar drilling is performed when a defect is hard to reach because of its location on the talar surface. A disadvantage is that healthy tibial cartilage is damaged. The reported results do not support the use of this technique [30, 48]. Besides, most talar lesions can be reached by means of the standard anterior or posterior arthroscopic approach, using intermittent distraction and a 90° microfracture probe [64, 65, 70].

The results of nonoperative treatment were poor compared to operative treatment. In spite of this, and especially in acute cases, nonoperative treatment should always be the first treatment to be considered.

Today, most publications on treatment of OCL of the talus involve arthroscopic excision, curettage and bone marrow stimulation, and ACI and OATS. They scored success percentages of 85 %, 76 %, and 87 %, respectively. ACI is a relatively expensive technique, and OATS gives morbidity from knee complaints in a relevant number of patients – up to 36 % [2, 18, 34, 47]. Therefore, we recommend arthroscopic excision, curettage, and BMS to be the first treatment of choice for primary OCL. It is relatively inexpensive, and there is low morbidity, a quick recovery, and a high success rate.

The results of the last review differ slightly from the results described in the previous review of Verhagen and co-workers [66]. Results of both reviews are listed in Table 10.4. The success percentage for BMS has changed very little. Verhagen included 21 studies and 227 patients; this review included 18 studies and 388 patients. The success rate went from 86 to 85 %. For OATS, the success rate changed from 94 to 87 %. Verhagen found one study with 36 patients treated with this technique. The last review identified nine eligible studies comprising 243 patients. The ACI technique was not included in the previous review by Verhagen et al. The last review identified four studies, comprising 59 patients, describing the results of ACI, leading to a success percentage of 76 %. The exclusion criteria of the last review were stricter than the previous review. Considering the number of patients, Verhagen and co-workers excluded single case reports but included a series of two patients and more. To be included in the last review, each study group had to involve ten patients or more. This excluded the "extended case reports" and only allowed true case series to be evaluated. The initial goal was to only include study groups of 20 patients or more. This protocol however excluded too many studies, and the criterion was stretched to ten patients. In comparison to Tol [62], this eliminated 13 studies (and 18 treatment groups) and in comparison to Verhagen [66] 30 studies.

The highest level of evidence is formed by randomized clinical trials. It would have been preferable if the review included more RCTs. However, only one RCT was identified, describing the results of chondroplasty (excision and curettage), microfracturing, and osteochondral transplantation [20]. Looking at the setup and inclusion of this study, one can debate whether this study was a truly randomized trial, as is also stated by the authors of the article. No case-control studies were identified.

Assessment of quality by the adjusted NOS showed that studies scored low on study design. Seven out of 52 studies were prospective in design. Most case series were retrospectively executed, however, and in nine studies the pro- or retrospective nature of the study was not even described. Twenty-one studies accounted for the protocol they had followed, but the majority of studies didn't mention a protocol or did not describe it properly. Nearly all studies reported on a representative patient group. Studies scored

Table 10.5 Recommended treatments for different types of osteochondral lesions

Type	Treatment
Asymptomatic/low symptomatic lesions	Conservative
Symptomatic lesions ≤15 mm	Excision, curettage, and BMS
Symptomatic lesions ≥15 mm	Consider fixation[a]/BMS/OATS
Large talar cystic lesion	Consider antegrade/retrograde drilling ± bone transplant/OATS
Secondary lesions	Consider OATS/ACI

[a]Posttraumatic cases, juveniles

moderately concerning "outcome": no blind assessment was described. Often it was not clear whether patients were scored by someone else than the author. Loss to follow-up exceeded 5 % in many cases. Scoring low on the items described above leads to a higher chance of introducing bias.

The eleven treatment strategies we discuss can be assigned to one of four treatment methods they are based on: (1) conservative treatment (i.e., nonoperative treatment with rest or cast), (2) debridement with or without bone marrow stimulation (i.e., excision, excision and curettage, excision and curettage with BMS, excision and curettage with autogenous bone graft and antegrade (transmalleolar) drilling), (3) replacement of the defect with cartilage (i.e., OATS and ACI), and (4) securing the lesion to the talar dome (i.e., retrograde drilling and fixation).

The current treatment options, OATS, ACI, and BMS, show similar results, although ACI scores somewhat lower. Since OATS leads to co-morbidity in up to 36 %, and ACI has a high cost, the best available treatment option for symptomatic lesions up to 15 mm is excision, curettage, and BMS. For other lesions we recommend treatment as described in Table 10.5, supported by the ISAKOS consensus [10].

Recently, two other systematic reviews concerning OCL of the talus have been published

[15, 24]. The first concerns outcome data of only arthroscopic debridement and microfracture as the primary treatment for OCL of the talus [15]. The review finds a good to excellent score in 80.2 % of patients. Microfracture wasn't compared to other treatments. The result is consistent with the success rate we have found. The other systematic review concerning OCL of the talus performed a descriptive analysis of outcome data [24]. The authors concluded that there were gross inconsistencies and an underreporting of data between studies, so that comparing is not possible. We agree that the reporting of outcome data needs to be improved. However, in their study postoperative outcome data were scored well. Despite the fact that the reporting of patient and outcome data needs to be improved, a systematic review of the currently published studies remains the best available evidence.

Conclusion

Based on the current best available evidence, at present, treatment by means of debridement and bone marrow stimulation is the most effective treatment strategy for symptomatic OCL of the talus. To draw definitive conclusions, sufficiently powered, randomized clinical trials with uniform methodology and validated outcome measures should be initiated.

Conflict of Interest The author has no current conflict of interests with the products presented.

Appendix 1: Newcastle-Ottawa Quality Assessment Scale

Adjusted for Case Series
Study Design
1. Type of study
   (a) Prospective*
   (b) Retrospective
   (c) Other
   (d) Not described

2. Setup
   (a) According to protocol*
   (b) Without protocol
   (c) No protocol described
Selection
3. Representativeness of included patients
   (a) Truly representative of the average talar OCD patient in the community*
   (b) Somewhat representative of the average talar OCD patient in the community*
   (c) Selected group of patients by surgeon
   (d) No description of the derivation of the patient group
Outcome
4. Assessment of outcome
   (a) Independent blind assessment*
   (b) Record linkage*
   (c) Self-report
   (d) No description
5. Adequacy of follow-up of series
   (a) Complete follow-up – all subjects accounted for*
   (b) Subjects lost to follow-up unlikely to introduce bias – small number lost (<5 %)*
   (c) Follow-up rate <95 % and no description of those lost
   (d) No statement

Number of Assigned Stars

Study design (5)	Selection (6)	Outcome (7)

*Every included study was separately assessed for quality using an adjusted version of the Newcastle-Ottawa Scale, as described above. It was performed by scoring each study for study design (0–2 stars), selection of patients (0–1 star), and outcome (0–2 stars). The designs that earned a star are marked with a *. For each study, the total number of stars is noted in the box above.*

References

1. Alexander AH, Lichtman DM. Surgical treatment of transchondral talar-dome fractures (osteochondritis dissecans). Long-term follow-up. J Bone Joint Surg Am. 1980;62(4):646–52.
2. Al-Shaikh RA, Chou LB, Mann JA, Dreeben SM, Prieskorn D. Autologous osteochondral grafting for talar cartilage defects. Foot Ankle Int. 2002;23(5):381–9.
3. Baker Jr CL, Morales RW. Arthroscopic treatment of transchondral talar dome fractures: a long-term follow-up study. Arthroscopy. 1999;15(2):197–202.
4. Baums MH, Heidrich G, Schultz W, Steckel H, Kahl E, Klinger HM. Autologous chondrocyte transplantation for treating cartilage defects of the talus. J Bone Joint Surg Am. 2006;88(2):303–8.
5. Becher C, Thermann H. Results of microfracture in the treatment of articular cartilage defects of the talus. Foot Ankle Int. 2005;26(8):583–9.
6. Blom JM, Strijk SP. Lesions of the trochlea tali. Osteochondral fractures and osteochondritis dissecans of the trochlea tali. Radiol Clin (Basel). 1975;44(5):387–96.
7. Bonnin M, Bouysset M. Arthroscopy of the ankle: analysis of results and indications on a series of 75 cases. Foot Ankle Int. 1999;20(11):744–51.
8. Bruns J. Osteochondrosis dissecans tali. Results of surgical therapy. Unfallchirurg. 1993;96(2):75–81.
9. Canale ST, Belding RH. Osteochondral lesions of the talus. J Bone Joint Surg Am. 1980;62(1):97–102.
10. Chan KM, Karlsson J. ISAKOS-FIMS world consensus conference on ankle instability, Hollywood, Florida. 2005
11. Chin TW, Mitra AK, Lim GH, Tan SK, Tay BK. Arthroscopic treatment of osteochondral lesion of the talus. Ann Acad Med Singapore. 1996;25(2):236–40.
12. Choi WJ, Park KK, Kim BS, Lee JW. Osteochondral lesion of the talus: is there a critical defect size for poor outcome? Am J Sports Med. 2009;37(10):1974–80.
13. Chuckpaiwong B, Berkson EM, Theodore GH. Microfracture for osteochondral lesions of the ankle: outcome analysis and outcome predictors of 105 cases. Arthroscopy. 2008;24(1):106–12.
14. Demaziere A, Ogilvie-Harris DJ. Operative arthroscopy of the ankle. 107 cases. Rev Rhum Mal Osteoartic. 1991;58(2):93–7.
15. Donnenwerth MP, Roukis TS. Outcome of arthroscopic debridement and microfracture as the primary treatment for osteochondral lesions of the talar dome. Arthroscopy. 2012;28(12):1902–7.
16. Draper SD, Fallat LM. Autogenous bone grafting for the treatment of talar dome lesions. J Foot Ankle Surg. 2000;39(1):15–23.
17. Flick AB, Gould N. Osteochondritis dissecans of the talus (transchondral fractures of the talus): review of the literature and new surgical approach for medial dome lesions. Foot Ankle. 1985;5(4):165–85.
18. Gautier E, Kolker D, Jakob RP. Treatment of cartilage defects of the talus by autologous osteochondral grafts. J Bone Joint Surg Br. 2002;84(2):237–44.
19. Giannini S, Buda R, Grigolo B, Vannini F, De Franceschi L, Facchini A. The detached osteochondral fragment as a source of cells for autologous chondrocyte implantation (ACI) in the ankle joint. Osteoarthritis Cartilage. 2005;13(7):601–7.
20. Gobbi A, Francisco RA, Lubowitz JH, Allegra F, Canata G. Osteochondral lesions of the talus: randomized controlled trial comparing chondroplasty, microfracture, and osteochondral autograft transplantation. Arthroscopy. 2006;22(10):1085–92.
21. Guido G, Azzone S, Gianotti S, Donati L. Posttraumatic osteochondral lesions of the arthroscopically treated ankle. Chirurgia del Piede. 2005;29:61–6.
22. Hakimzadeh A, Munzinger U. 8. Osteochondrosis dissecans: results after 10 or more years. c). Osteochondrosis dissecans of the ankle joint: long-term study. Orthopade. 1979;8(2):135–40.
23. Hangody L, Fules P. Autologous osteochondral mosaicplasty for the treatment of full-thickness defects of weight-bearing joints: ten years of experimental and clinical experience. J Bone Joint Surg Am. 2003;85-A Suppl 2:25–32.
24. Hannon CP, Murawski CD, Fansa AM, Smyth NA, Do H, Kennedy JG. Microfracture for osteochondral lesions of the talus: a systematic review of reporting of outcome data. Am J Sports Med. 2013;41(3):689–95.
25. Hunt SA, Sherman O. Arthroscopic treatment of osteochondral lesions of the talus with correlation of outcome scoring systems. Arthroscopy. 2003;19(4):360–7.
26. Huylebroek JF, Martens M, Simon JP. Transchondral talar dome fracture. Arch Orthop Trauma Surg. 1985;104(4):238–41.
27. Kelberine F, Frank A. Arthroscopic treatment of osteochondral lesions of the talar dome: a retrospective study of 48 cases. Arthroscopy. 1999;15(1):77–84.
28. Kitaoka HB, Alexander IJ, Adelaar RS, Nunley JA, Myerson MS, Sanders M. Clinical rating systems for the ankle-hindfoot, midfoot, hallux, and lesser toes. Foot Ankle Int. 1994;15(7):349–53.
29. Kolker D, Murray M, Wilson M. Osteochondral defects of the talus treated with autologous bone grafting. J Bone Joint Surg Br. 2004;86(4):521–6.
30. Kono M, Takao M, Naito K, Uchio Y, Ochi M. Retrograde drilling for osteochondral lesions of the talar dome. Am J Sports Med. 2006;34(9):1450–6.
31. Kouvalchouk JF, Schneider-Maunoury G, Rodineau J, Paszkowski A, Watin-Augouard L. Osteochondral lesions of the dome of the talus with partial necrosis. Surgical treatment by curettage and filling. Rev Chir Orthop Reparatrice Appar Mot. 1990;76(7):480–9.
32. Kreuz PC, Steinwachs M, Erggelet C, Lahm A, Henle P, Niemeyer P. Mosaicplasty with autogenous talar autograft for osteochondral lesions of the talus after failed primary arthroscopic management: a prospective study with a 4-year follow-up. Am J Sports Med. 2006;34(1):55–63.
33. Kumai T, Takakura Y, Kitada C, Tanaka Y, Hayashi K. Fixation of osteochondral lesions of the talus using

cortical bone pegs. J Bone Joint Surg Br. 2002;84(3): 369–74.

34. LaPrade RF, Botker JC. Donor-site morbidity after osteochondral autograft transfer procedures. Arthroscopy. 2004;20(7):e69–73.

35. Lee CH, Chao KH, Huang GS, Wu SS. Osteochondral autografts for osteochondritis dissecans of the talus. Foot Ankle Int. 2003;24(11):815–22.

36. Lundeen RO, Stienstra JJ. Arthroscopic treatment of transchondral lesions of the talar dome. J Am Podiatr Med Assoc. 1987;77(8):456–61.

37. Martin DF, Baker CL, Curl WW, Andrews JR, Robie DB, Haas AF. Operative ankle arthroscopy. Long-term followup. Am J Sports Med. 1989;17(1):16–23; discussion 23.

38. Mendicino RW, Lee MS, Grossman JP, Shromoff PJ. Oblique medial malleolar osteotomy for the management of talar dome lesions. J Foot Ankle Surg. 1998; 37(6):516–23.

39. Ming SH, Tay Keng Jin D, Amit Kanta M. Arthroscopic treatment of osteochondritis dissecans of the talus. Foot Ankle Surg. 2004;10:181–6.

40. Munoz M, Aznar P, Utrilla L. Lesiones osteocondrales mediales de astrágalo. valoración del abordaje quirúrgico transmaleolar. Rev Ortop Traumatol. 2002; 46:510–4.

41. O'Farrell TA, Costello BG. Osteochondritis dissecans of the talus. The late results of surgical treatment. J Bone Joint Surg Br. 1982;64(4):494–7.

42. Ogilvie-Harris DJ, Sarrosa EA. Arthroscopic treatment of osteochondritis dissecans of the talus. Arthroscopy. 1999;15(8):805–8.

43. Parisien JS. Arthroscopic treatment of osteochondral lesions of the talus. Am J Sports Med. 1986; 14(3):211–7.

44. Petersen L, Brittberg M, Lindahl A. Autologous chondrocyte transplantation of the ankle. Foot Ankle Clin. 2003;8(2):291–303.

45. Pettine KA, Morrey BF. Osteochondral fractures of the talus. A long-term follow-up. J Bone Joint Surg Br. 1987;69(1):89–92.

46. Pritsch M, Horoshovski H, Farine I. Arthroscopic treatment of osteochondral lesions of the talus. J Bone Joint Surg Am. 1986;68(6):862–5.

47. Reddy S, Pedowitz DI, Parekh SG, Sennett BJ, Okereke E. The morbidity associated with osteochondral harvest from asymptomatic knees for the treatment of osteochondral lesions of the talus. Am J Sports Med. 2007;35(1):80–5.

48. Robinson DE, Winson IG, Harries WJ, Kelly AJ. Arthroscopic treatment of osteochondral lesions of the talus. J Bone Joint Surg Br. 2003;85(7):989–93.

49. Roden S, Tillegard P, Unanderscharin L. Osteochondritis dissecans and similar lesions of the talus: report of fifty-five cases with special reference to etiology and treatment. Acta Orthop Scand. 1953;23(1):51–66.

50. Rosenberger RE, Fink C, Bale RJ, El Attal R, Muhlbacher R, Hoser C. Computer-assisted minimally invasive treatment of osteochondrosis disse-cans of the talus. Oper Orthop Traumatol. 2006;18(4): 300–16.

51. Sammarco GJ, Makwana NK. Treatment of talar osteochondral lesions using local osteochondral graft. Foot Ankle Int. 2002;23(8):693–8.

52. Schuman L, Struijs PA, van Dijk CN. Arthroscopic treatment for osteochondral defects of the talus. Results at follow-up at 2 to 11 years. J Bone Joint Surg Br. 2002;84(3):364–8.

53. Scranton Jr PE, Frey CC, Feder KS. Outcome of osteochondral autograft transplantation for type-V cystic osteochondral lesions of the talus. J Bone Joint Surg Br. 2006;88(5):614–9.

54. Scranton Jr PE, McDermott JE. Treatment of type V osteochondral lesions of the talus with ipsilateral knee osteochondral autografts. Foot Ankle Int. 2001;22(5): 380–4.

55. Shearer C, Loomer R, Clement D. Nonoperatively managed stage 5 osteochondral talar lesions. Foot Ankle Int. 2002;23(7):651–4.

56. Struijs PA, Tol JL, Bossuyt PM, Schuman L, van Dijk CN. Treatment strategies in osteochondral lesions of the talus. Review of the literature. Orthopade. 2001;30(1):28–36.

57. Takao M, Uchio Y, Kakimaru H, Kumahashi N, Ochi M. Arthroscopic drilling with debridement of remaining cartilage for osteochondral lesions of the talar dome in unstable ankles. Am J Sports Med. 2004; 32(2):332–6.

58. Taranow WS, Bisignani GA, Towers JD, Conti SF. Retrograde drilling of osteochondral lesions of the medial talar dome. Foot Ankle Int. 1999;20(8):474–80.

59. Thermann H. Treatment of osteochondritis dissecans of the talus: a long term follow-up. Sports Med Arthrosc Rev. 1994;284–8.

60. Thermann H, Becher C. Microfracture technique for treatment of osteochondral and degenerative chondral lesions of the talus. 2-year results of a prospective study. Unfallchirurg. 2004;107(1):27–32.

61. Thompson JP, Loomer RL. Osteochondral lesions of the talus in a sports medicine clinic. A new radiographic technique and surgical approach. Am J Sports Med. 1984;12(6):460–3.

62. Tol JL, Struijs PA, Bossuyt PM, Verhagen RA, van Dijk CN. Treatment strategies in osteochondral defects of the talar dome: a systematic review. Foot Ankle Int. 2000;21(2):119–26.

63. Van Buecken K, Barrack RL, Alexander AH, Ertl JP. Arthroscopic treatment of transchondral talar dome fractures. Am J Sports Med. 1989;17(3):350–5; discussion 355–6.

64. Van Dijk CN. Hindfoot endoscopy for posterior ankle pain. Instr Course Lect. 2006;55:545–54.

65. Van Dijk CN, Verhagen RA, Tol HJ. Technical note: resterilizable noninvasive ankle distraction device. Arthroscopy. 2001;17(3):E12.

66. Verhagen RA, Struijs PA, Bossuyt PM, van Dijk CN. Systematic review of treatment strategies for osteochondral defects of the talar dome. Foot Ankle Clin. 2003;8(2):233–42, viii–ix.

67. Wells G, Shea B, O'Connell D. The newcastle-ottawa scale for assessing the quality of nonrandomized studies in meta-analyses. In: Proceedings of the 3rd symposium on systematic reviews. Beyond the basics: improving quality and impact. Oxford; 2000.
68. Whittaker JP, Smith G, Makwana N, et al. Early results of autologous chondrocyte implantation in the talus. J Bone Joint Surg Br. 2005;87(2):179–83.
69. Zengerink M, Struijs PA, Tol JL, van Dijk CN. Treatment of osteochondral lesions of the talus: a systematic review. Knee Surg Sports Traumatol Arthrosc. 2010;18(2):238–46.
70. Zengerink M, Szerb I, Hangody L, Dopirak RM, Ferkel RD, van Dijk CN. Current concepts: treatment of osteochondral ankle defects. Foot Ankle Clin. 2006;11(2):331–59, vi.

Outcome Scores

11

Inger N. Sierevelt, Christiaan J.A. van Bergen,
Karin Grävare Silbernagel, Daniel Haverkamp,
and Jón Karlsson

The art and science of asking questions is the source of all knowledge.

Thomas Berger

Take-Home Points
- *The AOFAS is a frequently used outcome measure for talar OCD, but some concerns of the score are discussed.*
- *The FAOS and the FAAM are functional patient-reported outcome scores that are useful in the clinical assessment of patients with talar OCD.*
- *The 11-point NRS is a suitable, valid, and practical scale to assess pain intensity.*
- *Postoperative imaging can be used for objective assessment of surgical repair.*

11.1 Introduction

Outcome assessment is critical in evaluating the efficacy of orthopedic procedures. Questionnaires are used to assess the patient's perspective on the degree of impairment, pain, disability, and quality of life. Many outcome scores have been developed to assess the effect of orthopedic interventions for various ankle disorders. Scoring systems that have been used in the evaluation of talar osteochondral defects (OCDs) are presented in a systematic review [52]. The selection of the appropriate outcome measure is dependent not only on the patient population but to a greater extent on the outcome of interest.

To be able to evaluate treatment effect, the outcome measure should be reliable, valid, and sensitive to changes over time [41]. Additional information on minimal clinically important changes for the outcome measures in this specific patient population may be important to evaluate treatment results in the day-by-day clinical practice.

Frequently used outcome scores are discussed in this chapter (Table 11.1). In addition to these clinical outcome measures, the authors discuss scoring systems based on postoperative imaging after the treatment of talar OCDs (Table 11.2).

I.N. Sierevelt, PT, MSc (✉)
C.J.A. van Bergen, MD, PhD
Orthopaedic Research Centre Amsterdam,
Department of Orthopaedic Surgery,
Academic Medical Center, University
of Amsterdam, Amsterdam, The Netherlands
e-mail: i.sierevelt@gmail.com;
c.j.vanbergen@amc.uva.nl

K.G. Silbernagel, PT, ATC, PhD
Department of Physical Therapy, Samson College
of Health Sciences, University of the Sciences
in Philadelphia, Philadelphia, PA, USA

D. Haverkamp, MD, PhD
Department of Orthopaedic Surgery,
Slotervaart Hospital, Amsterdam, The Netherlands
e-mail: daniel@drhaverkamp.com

J. Karlsson, MD, PhD
Department of Orthopaedics, Sahlgrenska
University Hospital, Gothenburg University,
Gothenburg, Sweden
e-mail: jon.karlsson@telia.com

C.N. van Dijk, J.G. Kennedy (eds.), *Talar Osteochondral Defects*,
DOI 10.1007/978-3-642-45097-6_11, © ESSKA 2014

Table 11.1 Overview of clinical and functional outcome scores for foot and ankle

Foot and Ankle Outcome Score [32]	Foot and Ankle Ability Measure [26]
Symptoms	*Foot and Ankle Ability Measure (FAAM)*
Do you have swelling in your foot/ankle?	Standing
Do you feel grinding, hear clicking, or any other type of noise when your foot/ankle moves?	Walking on even ground
	Walking on even ground without shoes
Does your foot/ankle catch or hang up when moving?	Walking up hills
Can you straighten your foot/ankle fully?	Walking down hills
Can you bend your foot/ankle fully?	Going up stairs
How severe is your foot/ankle stiffness after first wakening in the morning?	Going down stairs
	Walking on uneven ground
How severe is your foot/ankle stiffness after sitting, lying, or resting later in the day?	Stepping up and down curbs
	Squatting
Pain	Coming up on your toes
How often do you experience foot/ankle pain?	Walking initially
Twisting/pivoting on your foot/ankle	Walking 5 min or less
Straightening foot/ankle fully	Walking approximately 10 min
Bending foot/ankle fully	Walking 15 min or greater
Walking on flat surface	Home responsibilities
Going up or down stairs	Activities of daily living
At night while in bed	Personal care
Sitting or lying	Light to moderate work (standing, walking)
Standing upright	Heavy work (push/pulling, climbing, carrying)
Function, daily living	Recreational activities
Descending stairs	*FAAM sports scale*
Ascending stairs	Running
Rising from sitting	Jumping
Standing	Landing
Bending to floor/pick up an object	Starting and stopping quickly
Walking on flat surface	Cutting/lateral movements
Getting in/out of car	Low impact activities
Going shopping	Ability to perform activity with your normal technique
Putting on socks/stockings	Ability to participate in your desired sport as long as you would like
Rising from bed	
Taking off socks/stockings	**Hannover questionnaire** [42]
Lying in bed (turning over, maintaining foot/ankle position)	*Symptoms severity scale*
	How severe is your pain in the evening?
Getting in/out of bath	How often did you have pain within the past 2 weeks?
Sitting	Do you feel any pain during the day?
Getting on/off toilet	How often do you feel pain during the day?
Heavy domestic duties (moving heavy boxes, scrubbing floors, etc.)	How long does your pain last during the day?
	Do you have swelling around your ankle and/or foot in the evening?
Light domestic duties (cooking, dusting, etc.)	
Function, sports and recreational activities	How often did you have swelling around your ankle and/or foot during the past 2 weeks in the evening?
Squatting	
Running	How often do you have swelling of your ankle and/or foot during the day?
Jumping	
Twisting/pivoting on your injured foot/ankle	Do you feel any stiffness in your foot or ankle?

Table 11.1 (continued)

Kneeling	Does the stiffness bother you?
Quality of life	*Questionnaire functional status*
How often are you aware of your foot/ankle problem?	Do you have difficulties to climb stairs?
Have you modified your lifestyle to avoid potentially damaging activities to your foot/ankle?	Do you have difficulties driving a car (brake, clutch, gas pedal)?
How much are you troubled with lack of confidence in your foot/ankle?	Do you have difficulties to walk on uneven or slippery ground?
In general, how much difficulty do you have with your foot/ankle?	Are you able to walk fast or do jogging?
	Are you able to jump (small ditch or puddle)?
AOFAS ankle-hindfoot score [16]	You have difficulties with single leg stance?
Pain	How long does it take for your leg to get fatigued?
Function	Do you feel your operated leg is more weak than the uninjured one?
Activity limitations, support requirement	
Maximum walking distance	How you would describe your gait?
Walking surfaces	Do you have problems wearing conventional shoes?
Gait abnormality	**Ogilvie-Harris score** [30]
Sagittal motion (flexion plus extension)	Pain
Hindfoot motion (inversion plus eversion)	Swelling
Ankle-hindfoot stability (anteroposterior, varus-valgus)	Stiffness
Alignment	Limping
	Activity

Table 11.2 Overview of several radiographic (Van Dijk, modified Takakura, modified Kellgren-Lawrence) and MRI (MOCART) scoring systems for the ankle joint

Van Dijk scale [49]	Magnetic resonance observation of cartilage repair tissue [24]
Van Dijk scale [49]	**Magnetic resonance observation of cartilage repair tissue** [24]
(0) Normal joint or subchondral sclerosis	
(I) Osteophytes without joint space narrowing	Degree of defect repair and filling of the defect
(II) Joint space narrowing with or without osteophytes	Complete (on a level with adjacent cartilage)
(III) (Sub)total disappearance or deformation of the joint space	Hypertrophy (over the level of the adjacent cartilage)
	Incomplete (under the level of the adjacent cartilage; underfilling)
Modified Takakura scale [40]	> 50 % of the adjacent cartilage
(1) No joint space narrowing but early sclerosis and osteophyte formation	< 50 % of the adjacent cartilage Subchondral bone exposed (complete delamination or dislocation and/or loose body)
(2) Narrowing of the joint space medially	
(3a) Obliteration of the joint space limited to the facet of medial malleolus with subchondral bone contact	Integration to border zone Complete (complete integration with adjacent cartilage)
(3b) Obliteration of the joint space advanced to the roof of the talar dome with subchondral bone contact	Incomplete (incomplete integration with adjacent cartilage)
Modified Kellgren-Lawrence scale [15]	Demarcating border visible (split-like)
(0) No radiographic findings of osteoarthritis	Defect visible
(1) Minute osteophytes of doubtful clinical significance	< 50 % of the length of the repair tissue
(2) Definite osteophytes with unimpaired joint space	> 50 % of the length of the repair tissue
(3) Definite osteophytes with moderate joint space narrowing	Surface of the repair tissue Surface intact (lamina splendens intact)

(continued)

Table 11.2 (continued)

(4) Definite osteophytes with severe joint space narrowing and subchondral sclerosis	Surface damaged (fibrillations, fissures, and ulcerations)
	< 50 % of repair tissue depth
	> 50 % of repair tissue depth or total degeneration
	Structure of the repair tissue
	Homogenous
	Inhomogeneous or cleft formation
	Signal intensity of the repair tissue
	Dual T2-FSE
	Isointense
	Moderately hyperintense
	Markedly hyperintense
	3D-GE-FS
	Isointense
	Moderately hypointense
	Markedly hypointense
	Subchondral lamina
	Intact
	Not intact
	Subchondral bone
	Intact
	Non-intact (edema, granulation tissue, cysts, sclerosis)
	Adhesions
	No
	Yes
	Effusion
	No
	Yes

11.2 Clinical and Functional Outcome Measures

11.2.1 The American Orthopaedic Foot & Ankle Society: Ankle-Hindfoot Score

The American Orthopaedic Foot & Ankle Society (AOFAS) has developed four rating systems, in which the clinical status of the ankle and foot is reported [16]. In the original publication, the AOFAS ankle-hindfoot score was described to be used for ankle replacement, ankle arthrodesis, ankle instability operations, subtalar arthrodesis, subtalar instability operations, talonavicular arthrodesis, calcaneocuboid arthrodesis, calcaneal osteotomy, calcaneus fracture, talus fracture, and ankle fractures [16]. This scale incorporates both subjective and objective factors with a maximal score of 100, indicating no symptoms or impairments. The scale includes nine items that can be divided into three subscales (pain, function, and alignment). Pain consists of one item with a maximal score of 40, indicating no pain. Function consists of seven items with a maximal score of 50, indicating full function. Alignment consists of one item with a maximal score of 10, indicating good alignment.

The AOFAS ankle-hindfoot score, as a complete score, has been shown to be valid [22, 37, 51]. The score has shown good responsiveness over time in two studies, with reported effect sizes of 1.69 [22] and 1.12 [38]. The subjective portion of the scale has been shown to be valid and reliable [12]. The objective portion of the scale has not been evaluated for reliability. This is one of the main criticisms of the AOFAS score. The second major concern of the AOFAS score is the weighting and calculations of the items; for example, high scores are obtained relatively easily (i.e., ceiling effect). Furthermore, the subscale pain is heavily weighted (40 points), and there is a 20-point difference between rating pain as severe (almost always present) and moderate (daily). To establish reliability, validity, and responsiveness, the scale has been evaluated related to a wide spectrum of diagnoses, such as general ankle-hindfoot complaints [37], pending ankle or foot surgery [12], surgically treated calcaneal fractures [51], and end-stage ankle arthritis [22]. However, there is no study that has evaluated the psychometric properties in patients with talar OCD.

11.2.2 The Foot and Ankle Outcome Score

The Foot and Ankle Outcome Score (FAOS) [32] is a patient-reported score, which evaluates symptoms and functional limitations related to the foot and ankle (www.koos.nu). It includes five different subscales: pain (nine items), other symptoms (stiffness, swelling, and range of motion; seven items), activities of daily living (17 items), sports and recreational activities (five items), and foot-and-ankle-related quality of life (four items). The items are scored on a 0–4-point scale and then normalized, resulting in a subscale score of 0–100. A score of 100 equals no symptoms or difficulty with activities. The FAOS is based on the Knee injury and Osteoarthritis Outcome Score (KOOS) and has been shown to have good validity and reliability in patients with ankle injury [32]. When used as an outcome measure for patients with Achilles tendinopathy, it has been shown to be responsive to changes over time [17, 33]. No study has evaluated the minimal clinically important difference, nor has the reliability or validity been investigated specifically for talar OCD. The FAOS is available in numerous languages (www.koos.nu), enabling its use in international multicenter studies.

11.2.3 The Hannover Ankle Score

The Hannover ankle score was developed by the Medizinische Hochschule Hannover; therefore, it can also be found as the Medizinische Hochschule Hannover ankle score or MHH score.

The Hannover ankle score consists of 20 questions with five graded response options that are filled out by the patient. The score consists of three domains: pain (five questions), swelling (five questions), and function (10 questions). These questions result in a score between 0 and 100.

The score was developed and first mentioned in a study by Thermann and co-workers [42]. It is based on the scales for the measurement of severity of symptoms and functional status by Levine and co-workers, which was designed for carpal tunnel syndrome [19]. The English version can be found in the initial publication. However, the questionnaire used in these patients was a German version. No translation protocols were mentioned. Thus, this questionnaire has not been designed according to the methodological guidelines, nor has it been properly validated. Only a test-retest reliability coefficient of 0.91 was reported [43].

11.2.4 The Foot and Ankle Ability Measure

The Foot and Ankle Ability Measure (FAAM) is a patient-reported questionnaire and was designed at the University of Pittsburgh. Martin and co-workers in 2005 thoroughly described the design and validation process [26]. The score was designed to evaluate changes in self-reported physical function in individuals with leg, ankle, and foot musculoskeletal disorders. The questionnaire was constructed by using the following four steps to develop a self-reported evaluative instrument: (1) generation of potential items, (2) initial item reduction, (3) final item reduction, and (4) acquisition of validity evidence to support interpretation of the score [26].

The FAAM comprises two separately scored subscales: the activities of daily living (ADL) subscale (21 items) and the sports subscale (eight items). Each item is scored on a five-point Likert scale from 4 to 0, with 4 being "no difficulty" and 0 being "unable to do." Items without a response are marked as not applicable and are not counted. The total number of items with a response is multiplied by four to get the highest potential score. The total item score is divided by the highest potential score and then multiplied by 100 to produce the FAAM score that ranges between 0 and 100. A higher score represents a higher level of physical function for both the ADL and sports subscales. The minimal clinically important differences for the FAAM are 8 and 9 points for the ADL and sports subscales, respectively.

Since its introduction, the construct validity, reliability, and responsiveness have been tested for several indications. In all these indications, the FAAM has been shown to be a valid subjective measurement tool [6, 9, 25]. There is, however, no specific information in the literature on psychometric properties for talar OCD. The FAAM has been translated and validated into several languages [4, 27, 29].

In conclusion, the FAAM is a well-validated questionnaire suitable for several foot and ankle pathologies.

11.2.5 The Ogilvie-Harris and Berndt and Harty Scores

Both the Ogilvie-Harris and Berndt and Harty scores are simple scoring systems to evaluate the effect of treatment. They are specifically useful to provide a success rate rather than a score.

The Ogilvie-Harris score consists of five items, including pain, swelling, stiffness, limping, and activity [30]. Either the patient or the examiner rates each item as excellent, good, fair, or poor. The lowest grade of each of the five items determines the final score.

The Berndt and Harty outcome question was specifically introduced for ankle OCDs. It is a single question with three possible answers, which allows patients to categorize their ankles into good, fair, or poor [3]. The score was slightly modified in 2003 because the original language was confusing [11]. In this modified score, patients with a "good" outcome have no symptoms of pain, swelling, or instability or experience slightly annoying, but not disabling, symptoms; patients with a "fair" outcome report that the symptoms are somewhat improved, although some disability problems persist; a "poor" outcome indicates that the overall symptoms remain unchanged [11].

Both the Ogilvie-Harris and the Berndt and Harty scores have been used in various studies on the treatment of osteochondral ankle defects [11, 35, 48], which makes it possible to compare the results of different studies. However, neither score has been validated. The Berndt and Harty outcome question has been shown to have a good correlation with both the single assessment numeric evaluation ($r = 0.81$) and the Martin outcome system ($r = 0.69$) [11].

11.3 Pain Assessment

Measurement of pain intensity is a quantitative estimate of the subjective interpretation of the severity of the pain experienced by the patient. The most frequently used methods to assess pain intensity are (1) the visual analog scale (VAS), (2) the numeric rating scale (NRS), and (3) the verbal rating scale (VRS). All pain rating scales have been extensively studied in several different populations, and validity and reliability have been demonstrated [10]. However, there is high variation in pain descriptors of the scales, time frames used to assess pain intensity (e.g., last week, last month), and specific situations for which pain intensity has to be assessed (e.g., rest, activity).

11.3.1 Visual Analog Scale

The VAS is a 100 mm line that represents the severity of the pain; the ends of the scale are anchored by two extremes of pain, such as "no pain" on one side and "worst imaginable pain" on the other side. The patient is asked to mark the line to indicate the pain intensity.

Various minimal clinically important differences are proposed for the VAS for musculoskeletal conditions. A minimal clinically important difference of 15 mm was proposed for low back pain (30 % from baseline) [31], 20 mm for knee osteoarthritis (41 % from baseline), and 15 for hip osteoarthritis (32 % from baseline) [44].

11.3.2 Numeric Rating Scale

The NRS is an 11-, 21-, or 101-point scale where the end points often are the extremes "no pain" and "worst imaginable pain" or "unbearable pain." The NRS measures pain severity by asking the patient to select a number that represents the severity of the pain. The NRS can be administered graphically (NRS) or verbally (VNRS). The 11-point (V)NRS (0–10) is used most frequently [10].

The minimal clinically important difference of the 11-point NRS is two points, reported for both low back pain [31] and chronic musculoskeletal pain (rheumatoid arthritis; knee, hip, and hand osteoarthritis; and ankylosing spondylitis) [34], both implying a change from baseline of approximately 30 %.

11.3.3 Verbal Rating Scale

The VRS consists of a list of adjectives that are commonly used to describe increasing pain intensity. It should comprise the extremes of the scale, such as "no pain" and "worst imaginable pain." The amount of response options can vary but has to be sufficient to capture the gradations of pain intensities experienced by the patient. Rank numbers are assigned to response options, with highest numbers indicating most pain.

In summary, all three scales perform generally well, although specific studies on reliability, validity, and minimal clinically important difference for patients with talar OCD are lacking. All scales are sensitive to changes over time [5, 21, 36]. The VRS, however, is slightly less sensitive than the NRS and the VAS [5, 8, 21], possibly due to the limited amount of response options. The NRS and the VRS are both easy to administer with good compliance. The VAS scale appears to be more complicated than NRS and VRS [10]. Despite the fact that the scales are highly correlated, they cannot be used interchangeably [20, 36].

Since the psychometric properties of the pain scales are sufficient, the choice for the type of scale can be based on practical considerations, such as ease of administration and type of population. The authors prefer the NRS because of its ease and compliance.

11.4 Postoperative Imaging

11.4.1 Radiography

Radiographs are frequently obtained in the postoperative assessment of talar OCDs, especially to evaluate degenerative changes in the joint. Several radiographic grading systems have been developed for the osteoarthritic ankle joint [14, 39, 49]. The scales focus on the presence of osteophytes and joint space narrowing. The Kellgren and Lawrence system was not designed specifically for the ankle [14]. The Takakura system focuses mainly on the medial joint space [39]. The van Dijk OA classification evaluates the complete talocrural joint and has been used for the evaluation of talar OCD [35, 48].

Moon and co-workers compared the van Dijk scale [49], the modified Kellgren-Lawrence scale [15], and modified Takakura [40] scales and concluded that all these scales were reliable and valid [28]. Interobserver and intraobserver comparisons (weighted kappa) of each scale were found to be satisfactory (Kellgren and Lawrence, 0.51–0.81; Takakura, 0.65–0.88; van Dijk, 0.64–0.89). However, the predictability of the scales for cartilage damage, as observed by arthroscopy, was only moderate (intraclass correlation coefficients, 0.42–0.51) [28].

11.4.2 Computed Tomography

To objectively assess the bone repair, multislice helical computed tomography (CT) scans can be obtained [45]. CT has been shown to be accurate in the follow-up of talar OCDs [53]. The scanning protocol involves "ultra high-resolution" axial slices with an increment of 0.3 mm and a thickness of 0.6 mm and multi-planar coronal and sagittal 1-mm reconstructions [46]. One can measure the completeness, thickness, and level of the subchondral plate (i.e., flush, depressed, or proud), as well as bone volume filling of the defect and postoperative loose bony particles [45, 47]. However, to our knowledge, a postoperative grading system based on CT is unavailable.

11.4.3 Magnetic Resonance Imaging

Magnetic resonance imaging (MRI) evaluation of OCD repair tissue has gained popularity in recent years. The scanning protocol incorporates proton density and fast spin-echo acquisitions for cartilage evaluation [24]. Some investigators have quantified MRI results by self-developed criteria [2, 13], but a more objective, well-known, and frequently used method is the magnetic resonance observation of cartilage repair tissue (MOCART) [23, 24]. Nine variables describe the morphology and signal intensity of the repair tissue compared with the adjacent native cartilage, the degree of filling of the defect, the integration to the border zone, the description of the surface and structure, the signal intensity, the status of the subchondral lamina and subchondral bone, the appearance of adhesions, and the presence of synovitis [24]. This system has good interobserver reliability, with intraclass correlation coefficients of >0.81 in eight of nine variables [23]. However, the association of the MOCART with the clinical situation is not exactly clear. In a study by Aurich and co-workers, there was no relation between the MOCART and clinical outcome after matrix-associated chondrocyte implantation of the talus [1]. In another study, three out of five variables of the modified MOCART showed good correlation with second-look arthroscopy after autologous chondrocyte implantation in the ankle, while two out of five variables showed poor correlation [18].

> **Conclusions**
>
> Valid and reliable outcome measures are available for several ankle conditions. However, none of the clinical and functional outcome scores have been psychometrically investigated for the specific patient population with talar

OCD. The AOFAS has been used most frequently in studies on the treatment of talar OCD [52] but has some serious concerns. Both the FAAM and the FAOS are suitable questionnaires for patients with various ankle conditions. However, minimal clinically important differences of these scales are desirable for proper evaluation of outcomes of OCD treatment.

Pain assessment for patients with talar OCD is important since pain is the predominant symptom. Although the described pain scales have been properly validated, they lack information on the minimal clinically important difference for this patient group. Most important in a clinical or research setting is the use of standardized pain descriptors, clear time frames, and unambiguous description concerning the context of pain assessment. The 11-point NRS has, in our opinion, some advantages and would be the most practical and valid choice for the use of pain assessment.

In addition to specific ankle scores, the authors recommend to use a general quality-of-life score in clinical studies, such as the short form-36 or the EuroQoL [7, 50].

Postoperative imaging can be a useful adjunct to clinical outcome scoring.

Conflict of Interest The author has no current conflict of interests with the products presented.

References

1. Aurich M, Bedi HS, Smith PJ, Rolauffs B, Muckley T, Clayton J, Blackney M. Arthroscopic treatment of osteochondral lesions of the ankle with matrix-associated chondrocyte implantation: early clinical and magnetic resonance imaging results. Am J Sports Med. 2011;39:311–9.
2. Becher C, Driessen A, Hess T, Longo UG, Maffulli N, Thermann H. Microfracture for chondral defects of the talus: maintenance of early results at midterm follow-up. Knee Surg Sports Traumatol Arthrosc. 2010;18:656–63.
3. Berndt AL, Harty M. Transchondral fractures (osteochondritis dissecans) of the talus. J Bone Joint Surg Am. 1959;41:988–1020.
4. Borloz S, Crevoisier X, Deriaz O, Ballabeni P, Martin RL, Luthi F. Evidence for validity and reliability of a French version of the FAAM. BMC Musculoskelet Disord. 2011;12:40.

5. Breivik EK, Bjornsson GA, Skovlund E. A comparison of pain rating scales by sampling from clinical trial data. Clin J Pain. 2000;16:22–8.

6. Carcia CR, Martin RL, Drouin JM. Validity of the Foot and Ankle Ability Measure in athletes with chronic ankle instability. J Athl Train. 2008;43:179–83.

7. EuroQol Group. EuroQol–a new facility for the measurement of health-related quality of life. Health Policy. 1990;16:199–208.

8. Ferreira-Valente MA, Pais-Ribeiro JL, Jensen MP. Validity of four pain intensity rating scales. Pain. 2011;152:2399–404.

9. Goldstein CL, Schemitsch E, Bhandari M, Mathew G, Petrisor BA. Comparison of different outcome instruments following foot and ankle trauma. Foot Ankle Int. 2010;31:1075–80.

10. Hjermstad MJ, Fayers PM, Haugen DF, Caraceni A, Hanks GW, Loge JH, Fainsinger R, Aass N, Kaasa S. Studies comparing Numerical Rating Scales, Verbal Rating Scales, and Visual Analogue Scales for assessment of pain intensity in adults: a systematic literature review. J Pain Symptom Manage. 2011;41:1073–93.

11. Hunt SA, Sherman O. Arthroscopic treatment of osteochondral lesions of the talus with correlation of outcome scoring systems. Arthroscopy. 2003;19:360–7.

12. Ibrahim T, Beiri A, Azzabi M, Best AJ, Taylor GJ, Menon DK. Reliability and validity of the subjective component of the American Orthopaedic Foot and Ankle Society clinical rating scales. J Foot Ankle Surg. 2007;46:65–74.

13. Imhoff AB, Paul J, Ottinger B, Wortler K, Lammle L, Spang J, Hinterwimmer S. Osteochondral transplantation of the talus: long-term clinical and magnetic resonance imaging evaluation. Am J Sports Med. 2011;39:1487–93.

14. Kelgrenn JH, Lawrence JS. Radiological assessment of osteo-arthrosis. Ann Rheum Dis. 1957;16:494–502.

15. Kijowski R, Blankenbaker D, Stanton P, Fine J, De SA. Arthroscopic validation of radiographic grading scales of osteoarthritis of the tibiofemoral joint. AJR Am J Roentgenol. 2006;187:794–9.

16. Kitaoka HB, Alexander IJ, Adelaar RS, Nunley JA, Myerson MS, Sanders M. Clinical rating systems for the ankle-hindfoot, midfoot, hallux, and lesser toes. Foot Ankle Int. 1994;15:349–53.

17. Knobloch K, Schreibmueller L, Longo UG, Vogt PM. Eccentric exercises for the management of tendinopathy of the main body of the Achilles tendon with or without an AirHeel Brace. A randomized controlled trial. B: effects of compliance. Disabil Rehabil. 2008;30:1692–6.

18. Lee KT, Choi YS, Lee YK, Cha SD, Koo HM. Comparison of MRI and arthroscopy in modified MOCART scoring system after autologous chondrocyte implantation for osteochondral lesion of the talus. Orthopedics. 2011;34:e356–62.

19. Levine DW, Simmons BP, Koris MJ, Daltroy LH, Hohl GG, Fossel AH, Katz JN. A self-administered questionnaire for the assessment of severity of symptoms and functional status in carpal tunnel syndrome. J Bone Joint Surg Am. 1993;75:1585–92.

20. Lund I, Lundeberg T, Sandberg L, Budh CN, Kowalski J, Svensson E. Lack of interchangeability between visual analogue and verbal rating pain scales: a cross sectional description of pain etiology groups. BMC Med Res Methodol. 2005;5:31.

21. Lundeberg T, Lund I, Dahlin L, Borg E, Gustafsson C, Sandin L, Rosen A, Kowalski J, Eriksson SV. Reliability and responsiveness of three different pain assessments. J Rehabil Med. 2001;33:279–83.

22. Madeley NJ, Wing KJ, Topliss C, Penner MJ, Glazebrook MA, Younger AS. Responsiveness and validity of the SF-36, Ankle Osteoarthritis Scale, AOFAS Ankle Hindfoot Score, and Foot Function Index in end stage ankle arthritis. Foot Ankle Int. 2012;33:57–63.

23. Marlovits S, Singer P, Zeller P, Mandl I, Haller J, Trattnig S. Magnetic resonance observation of cartilage repair tissue (MOCART) for the evaluation of autologous chondrocyte transplantation: determination of interobserver variability and correlation to clinical outcome after 2 years. Eur J Radiol. 2006;57:16–23.

24. Marlovits S, Striessnig G, Resinger CT, Aldrian SM, Vecsei V, Imhof H, Trattnig S. Definition of pertinent parameters for the evaluation of articular cartilage repair tissue with high-resolution magnetic resonance imaging. Eur J Radiol. 2004;52:310–9.

25. Martin RL, Hutt DM, Wukich DK. Validity of the Foot and Ankle Ability Measure (FAAM) in diabetes mellitus. Foot Ankle Int. 2009;30:297–302.

26. Martin RL, Irrgang JJ, Burdett RG, Conti SF, Van Swearingen JM. Evidence of validity for the Foot and Ankle Ability Measure (FAAM). Foot Ankle Int. 2005;26:968–83.

27. Mazaheri M, Salavati M, Negahban H, Sohani SM, Taghizadeh F, Feizi A, Karimi A, Parnianpour M. Reliability and validity of the Persian version of Foot and Ankle Ability Measure (FAAM) to measure functional limitations in patients with foot and ankle disorders. Osteoarthritis Cartilage. 2010;18:755–9.

28. Moon JS, Shim JC, Suh JS, Lee WC. Radiographic predictability of cartilage damage in medial ankle osteoarthritis. Clin Orthop Relat Res. 2010;468:2188–97.

29. Nauck T, Lohrer H. Translation, cross-cultural adaption and validation of the German version of the Foot and Ankle Ability Measure for patients with chronic ankle instability. Br J Sports Med. 2011;45:785–90.

30. Ogilvie-Harris DJ, Mahomed N, Demaziere A. Anterior impingement of the ankle treated by arthroscopic removal of bony spurs. J Bone Joint Surg Br. 1993;75:437–40.

31. Ostelo RW, de Vet HC. Clinically important outcomes in low back pain. Best Pract Res Clin Rheumatol. 2005;19:593–607.

32. Roos EM, Brandsson S, Karlsson J. Validation of the foot and ankle outcome score for ankle ligament reconstruction. Foot Ankle Int. 2001;22:788–94.

33. Roos EM, Engstrom M, Lagerquist A, Soderberg B. Clinical improvement after 6 weeks of eccentric exercise in patients with mid-portion Achilles tendinopathy – a randomized trial with 1-year follow-up. Scand J Med Sci Sports. 2004;14:286–95.

34. Salaffi F, Stancati A, Silvestri CA, Ciapetti A, Grassi W. Minimal clinically important changes in chronic musculoskeletal pain intensity measured on a numerical rating scale. Eur J Pain. 2004;8:283–91.
35. Schuman L, Struijs PA, van Dijk CN. Arthroscopic treatment for osteochondral defects of the talus. Results at follow-up at 2 to 11 years. J Bone Joint Surg Br. 2002;84:364–8.
36. Sindhu BS, Shechtman O, Tuckey L. Validity, reliability, and responsiveness of a digital version of the visual analog scale. J Hand Ther. 2011;24:356–63.
37. SooHoo NF, Shuler M, Fleming LL. Evaluation of the validity of the AOFAS Clinical Rating Systems by correlation to the SF-36. Foot Ankle Int. 2003; 24:50–5.
38. SooHoo NF, Vyas R, Samimi D. Responsiveness of the foot function index, AOFAS clinical rating systems, and SF-36 after foot and ankle surgery. Foot Ankle Int. 2006;27:930–4.
39. Takakura Y, Tanaka Y, Kumai T, Tamai S. Low tibial osteotomy for osteoarthritis of the ankle. Results of a new operation in 18 patients. J Bone Joint Surg Br. 1995;77:50–4.
40. Tanaka Y, Takakura Y, Hayashi K, Taniguchi A, Kumai T, Sugimoto K. Low tibial osteotomy for varus-type osteoarthritis of the ankle. J Bone Joint Surg Br. 2006;88:909–13.
41. Terwee CB, Bot SD, de Boer MR, van der Windt DA, Knol DL, Dekker J, Bouter LM, de Vet HC. Quality criteria were proposed for measurement properties of health status questionnaires. J Clin Epidemiol. 2007;60:34–42.
42. Thermann H. Treatment of osteochondritis dissecans of the talus. Sports Med Arthrosc. 1994;2:284–8.
43. Thermann H, Hufner T, Schratt E, Held C, von GS, Tscherne H. Long-term results of subtalar fusions after operative versus nonoperative treatment of os calcis fractures. Foot Ankle Int. 1999;20:408–16.
44. Tubach F, Ravaud P, Baron G, Falissard B, Logeart I, Bellamy N, Bombardier C, Felson D, Hochberg M, van der Heijde D, et al. Evaluation of clinically relevant changes in patient reported outcomes in knee and hip osteoarthritis: the minimal clinically important improvement. Ann Rheum Dis. 2005;64:29–33.
45. van Bergen CJ, Blankevoort L, de Haan RJ, Sierevelt IN, Meuffels DE, d'Hooghe PR, Krips R, van DG, van Dijk CN. Pulsed electromagnetic fields after arthroscopic treatment for osteochondral defects of the talus: double-blind randomized controlled multicenter trial. BMC Musculoskelet Disord. 2009;10:83.
46. van Bergen CJ, de Leeuw PA, van Dijk CN. Treatment of osteochondral defects of the talus. Rev Chir Orthop Reparatrice Appar Mot. 2008;94:398–408.
47. van Bergen CJ, de Leeuw PA, van Dijk CN. Potential pitfall in the microfracturing technique during the arthroscopic treatment of an osteochondral lesion. Knee Surg Sports Traumatol Arthrosc. 2009;17:184–7.
48. van Bergen CJ, Kox LS, Maas M, Sierevelt IN, Kerkhoffs GM, van Dijk CN. Arthroscopic treatment of osteochondral defects of the talus: outcomes at eight to twenty years of follow-up. J Bone Joint Surg Am. 2013;95:519–25.
49. van Dijk CN, Verhagen RA, Tol JL. Arthroscopy for problems after ankle fracture. J Bone Joint Surg Br. 1997;79:280–4.
50. Ware Jr JE, Sherbourne CD. The MOS 36-item short-form health survey (SF-36). I. Conceptual framework and item selection. Med Care. 1992;30:473–83.
51. Westphal T, Piatek S, Halm JP, Schubert S, Winckler S. Outcome of surgically treated intraarticular calcaneus fractures–SF-36 compared with AOFAS and MFS. Acta Orthop Scand. 2004;75:750–5.
52. Zengerink M, Struijs PA, Tol JL, van Dijk CN. Treatment of osteochondral lesions of the talus: a systematic review. Knee Surg Sports Traumatol Arthrosc. 2010;18:238–46.
53. Zinman C, Wolfson N, Reis ND. Osteochondritis dissecans of the dome of the talus. Computed tomography scanning in diagnosis and follow-up. J Bone Joint Surg Am. 1988;70A:1017–9.

Follow-up Imaging for Osteochondral Lesions of the Ankle

Keir A. Ross, Niall A. Smyth, Francesca Vannini, and John G. Kennedy

Take-Home Points

- *Standard radiography is an imaging method historically used most, but it is unable to evaluate cartilage. It is used for assessing bone healing postoperatively if an osteotomy is required during the surgical procedure.*
- *Technological advancements have increased the utility of CT, and it remains practical for assessing subchondral injury and preoperative planning.*
- *MRI is the cartilage imaging modality of choice and is becoming increasingly well established. Technological advancements allow for improved assessment of cartilage structure and biology, but it requires expertise and knowledge of cartilage repair procedures.*
- *Second-look arthroscopy allows excellent assessment of cartilage but should not be performed solely for follow-up purposes as MRI provides equal, if not more, information about the articular surface through to the cartilage-bone interface.*

12.1 Introduction

Imaging methods for assessing osteochondral lesions (OCL) at follow-up include standard radiographs (x-ray), computed tomography (CT), magnetic resonance imaging (MRI), and second-look arthroscopy. These modalities have been correlated with clinical outcome measures and have been used simultaneously in order to compare their relative sensitivity and specificity for assessment of OCLs [16, 17, 20, 22, 24, 35, 36, 38]. Standard radiographs are simple and well established but are unable to assess articular cartilage. Second-look arthroscopy has the advantage of direct visualization, and it has the obvious disadvantage of requiring an additional invasive procedure at follow-up. MRI and CT have the advantage of being noninvasive. Furthermore, technological advancements have increased cartilage assessment efficacy. A standard should be set with respect to which modality and what time points should be chosen for follow-up imaging.

K.A. Ross, BS • N.A. Smyth, MD
J.G. Kennedy, MD, MCh, FRCS (Orth) (✉)
Department of Orthopaedic Surgery,
Hospital for Special Surgery, New York, NY, USA
e-mail: rossk@hss.edu; smythn@hss.edu;
kennedyj@hss.edu

F. Vannini, MD, PhD
First Clinic of Orthopaedics and Traumatology,
Rizzoli Orthopaedic Institute,
University of Bologna, Bologna, Italy
e-mail: france_vannini@yahoo.it

C.N. van Dijk, J.G. Kennedy (eds.), *Talar Osteochondral Defects*,
DOI 10.1007/978-3-642-45097-6_12, © ESSKA 2014

12.2 Standard Radiography (X-Ray)

Radiography has historically been the most used modality for ankle OCL assessment, with a radiograph-based classification system first established by Berndt and Harty in 1959 [4]. The classification system evaluates the severity of lesions in four stages – stage I, small compression fracture; stage II, incomplete avulsive fracture; stage III, complete avulsion of a fragment without displacement; and stage IV, displaced fragment [4]. This system was augmented in 1989 by Anderson and co-workers [2], but this requires the use of MRI, CT, or scintigraphy. In the augmented system the stages are stage I: subchondral trabecular compression; stage II, incomplete separation of fragment; stage IIA, formation of a subchondral cyst; stage III, unattached, undisplaced fragment; and stage IV, displaced fragment. Although the Berndt and Harty system is simple and commonly used, a prior study has revealed that only 50 % of OCLs could be identified prospectively, and that 66 % could be identified retrospectively [20]. A separate study reported similar findings, with 41 % of OCLs missed upon routine radiological examination [36]. Furthermore, Pritsch and co-workers [31] reported that radiographic findings did not correlate with arthroscopic findings. Due to improved understanding of OCLs, many surgeons now maintain that cartilage assessment/treatment should be based on lesion stability and state of overlying cartilage [22]. This is why most surgeons prefer more advanced techniques for the assessment of articular cartilage. Standard radiographs lack the ability to evaluate the articular surface and are therefore of limited value for routine follow-up imaging or operative outcomes following surgical treatment of OCLs. Radiographs may be useful, however, to assess bone healing if an osteotomy was necessary during the operative procedure (Fig. 12.1).

12.3 Computed Tomography

The technological advancements of high-resolution helical CT and SPECT (single-photon emission computed tomography) have

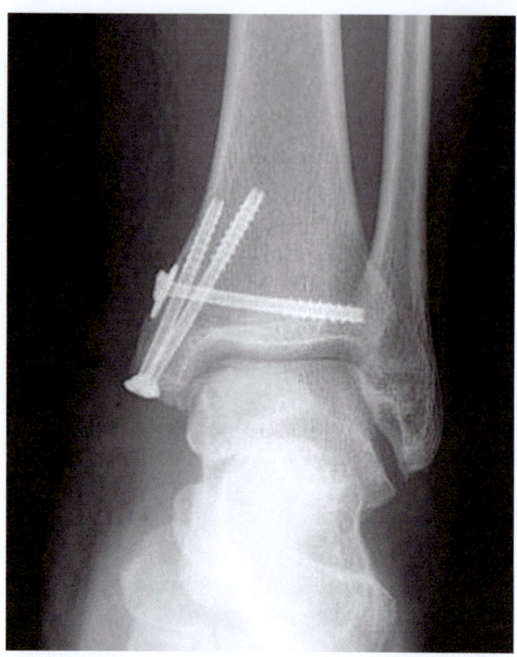

Fig. 12.1 Anterior-posterior x-ray of left ankle following autologous osteochondral transplantation. Healing of the medial malleolar osteotomy required for operative access can be seen. The osteochondral graft has incorporated well and is not seen

improved CT for the purpose of assessing OCLs [19, 36]. Although CT does not have the capability to evaluate articular cartilage, it has been shown to effectively evaluate the size, location, and degree of bony injury in lesions involving subchondral bone [8] (Fig. 12.2). High-resolution helical CT has been compared to both MRI and arthroscopy with results showing that there is no significant difference between modalities in their ability to detect the presence of an OCL. Helical CT was shown to have high specificity (0.99) in accurately grading a lesion and correctly identifies the presence of 81 % of OCLs [36]. Regarding SPECT, it is a three-dimensional scintigraphy bone scan superimposed on a CT scan in order to localize scintigraphic osteoblastic activity and present biological information regarding a lesion [15, 16, 19, 27]. SPECT has also been directly compared to MRI for OCL evaluation and was shown to provide supplemental information that can affect decision making with respect to

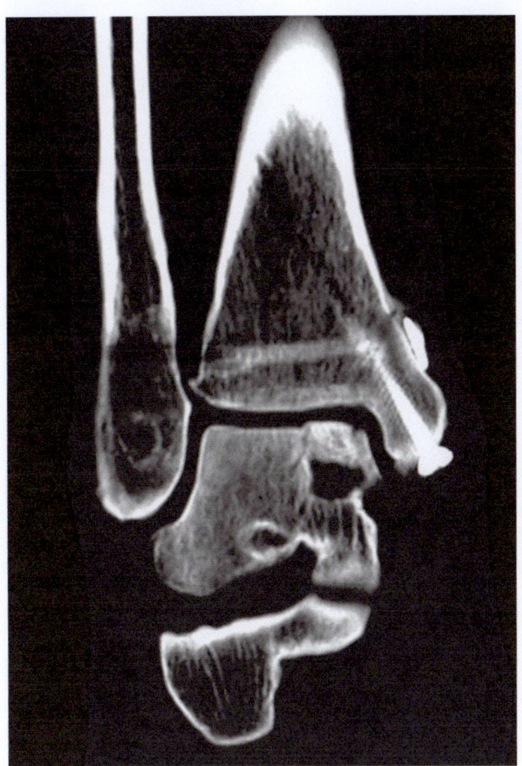

Fig. 12.2 Computed tomography of right ankle in the coronal plane 6 months following autologous osteochondral transplantation. Postoperative cyst formation can be seen

treatment choice. However, poor inter-rater reliability revealed that the techniques are subject to errors in interpretation [19].

MRI signal patterns in the talus resulting from pathologies such as bone edema have been suggested to lead to an overestimation of the extent of bony injury involved in an OCL. Because of this, CT may be a useful addition to MRI at follow up [19, 26, 32]. However, it is important to note that in a comparison study by Verhagen and co-workers assessing MRI, arthroscopy, and helical CT, MRI was noted as the more sensitive modality and identified four OCLs that helical CT did not. Additionally, CT imaging resulted in five false negatives [36]. With regard to follow-up imaging, CT is most pertinent in the presence of subchondral lesions, subchondral cysts, and bone edema, in order to assess the true extent of bone involvement [7].

12.4   Magnetic Resonance Imaging

MRI has been thoroughly studied as a method for evaluating cartilage and has the capacity to distinguish between normal native cartilage, repair cartilage (including fibrocartilage), and synovial tissue [30]. This modality can characterize cartilage morphology, biochemistry, and function and is even sensitive enough to determine collagen orientation and changes associated with degradation [21, 30] (Fig. 12.3). MRI has been used to assess cartilage repair after procedures including bone marrow stimulation techniques, fixation with biodegradable pins, autologous chondrocyte implantation (ACI), and osteochondral autograft and allograft techniques [6, 13]. MRI following these surgical procedures provides evaluation of subchondral bone, three-dimensional geometry of the joint, percent fill of lesion, and signal morphology of repair tissue [13]. Thus, it is an informative objective measure for preoperative diagnosis, surgical planning, and postoperative assessment at follow-up as well as for retrospective and prospective studies [11, 13, 30].

There is also some comparative evidence indicating that MRI is an effective follow-up tool. Magnetic resonance observation of cartilage repair tissue (MOCART) scores have been correlated with American Orthopaedic Foot & Ankle Society (AOFAS) clinical outcome scores at both 5 ± 1 year and 10 years postoperatively following ACI in the talus. MOCART scores were shown to have a direct correlation with AOFAS clinical outcome scores [3, 10]. Additionally, the appearance of cartilage on MRI shows strong correlation with the findings of second-look arthroscopy [16, 18, 24, 38]. Henderson and co-workers compared MRI at 12 months with both second-look arthroscopy and histological evaluation of biopsies in the knee and reported that MRI findings generally agreed with arthroscopic evaluation [14]. The authors concluded that MRI may be as accurate as arthroscopic visual scoring and histological evaluation, when used to assess the state of cartilage [14].

Standard two-dimensional multi-slice turbo or fast spin-echo (FSE) proton density and fat-suppressed proton density sequences acquired in multiple planes are widely accepted as standard

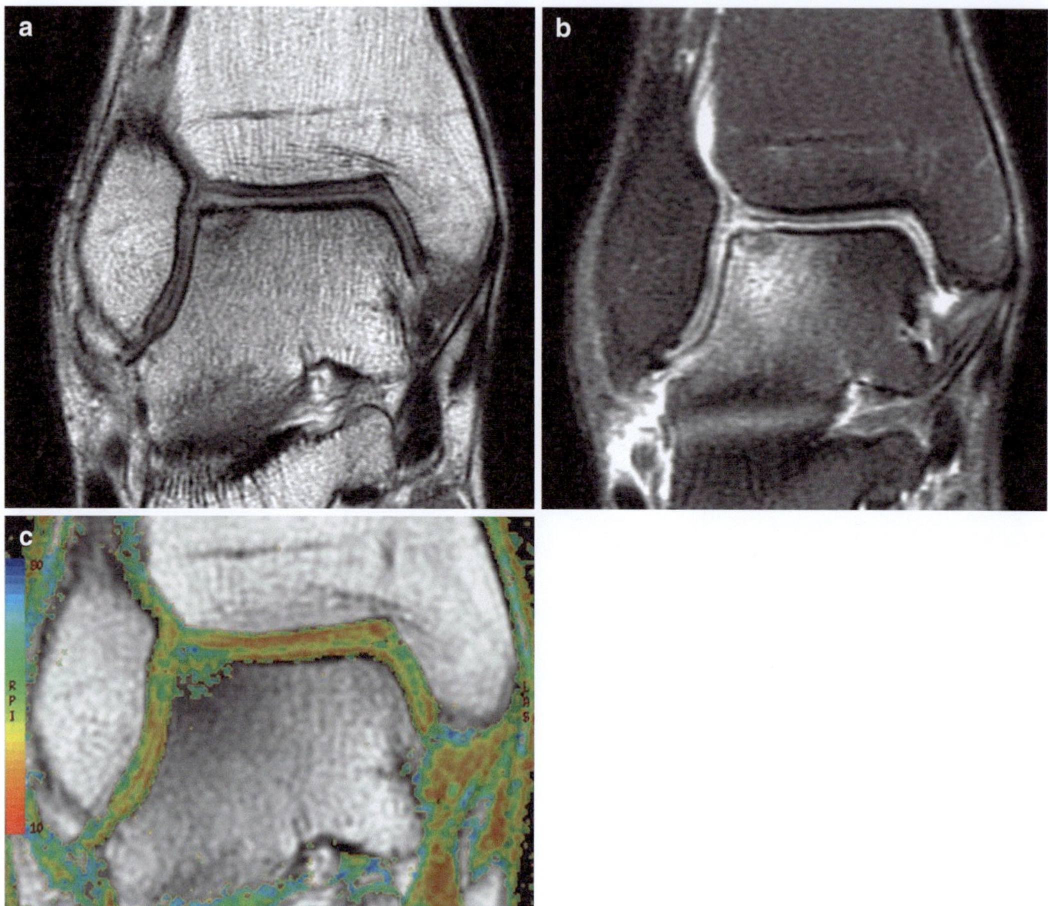

Fig. 12.3 T1 (**a**), T2 weighted (**b**), and T2 mapping (**c**) images of right ankle in the coronal plane. A 6×10 mm full-thickness cartilage defect in the articular cartilage is seen on the lateral talus with extensive adjacent bone marrow edema

MRI cartilage protocol. These are able to evaluate postoperative cartilage healing and morphology. Moreover, technological advancements have produced three-dimensional techniques that can generate models of the joint surface, repair fill, and thickness and volume measurements [28, 29]. Newer, quantitative matrix assessment techniques, including T2 mapping, T1 rho, T1-weighted three-dimensional fat-suppressed fast spoiled gradient echo (FSPGR), and delayed gadolinium-enhanced MRI of cartilage (dGEM-RIC) offer information regarding the histological and biochemical status of repair cartilage [12, 28, 29]. For example, FSPGR MRI is thought to be more sensitive than conventional MRI in detecting talar OCLs and can measure glycosaminoglycan content [12, 26]. T1 rho has been shown to correlate with proteoglycan content [28]. The International Cartilage Repair Society (ICRS) recommends intermediate-weighted FSE and 3D fat-suppressed T1-weighted gradient-echo (GRE) sequences, which are the most commonly used for repair cartilage imaging [6]. With regard to T2 mapping MRI, calculated relaxation times have been related to changes in articular cartilage with respect to collagen presence and orientation [1, 25, 37]. High spatial resolution is another valuable feature that can be attained with 1.5 or 3 Tesla scanners. These scanners allow surface congruity, osseous incorporation, and graft morphology and integration to be evaluated following replacement procedures such as autologous osteochondral transplantation [33]. Specifically, high-resolution MRI is advocated for analysis of articular cartilage defects of the talus because of its ability to reveal clinically relevant features that can impact treatment decisions [7].

It is recommended that MRI follow-up studies take place at 3–6 months after a cartilage repair procedure and again before the end of the first postoperative year [6]. The first follow-up at 3–6 months is for the purpose of evaluating integration of repair tissue and volume of the cartilage. The next round of follow-up imaging, administered within the first year after surgery, allows for assessment of cartilage maturation or graft maturation, in the case of autograft or allograft procedures [33]. Analysis of the imaging requires expertise and familiarity with repair procedures, characteristic MRI features of repair tissue at postoperative intervals, and image acquisition protocols and techniques. The information gained from MRI is vital to patient follow-up after surgical treatment of OCLs for both research and clinical purposes and has become the primary method of noninvasive follow-up imaging.

12.5 Second-Look Arthroscopy

Second-look arthroscopy has the advantage of allowing direct visualization of the articular surface and the ability to probe for softening, ballotability, and fissuring of the cartilage (Fig. 12.4). However, it requires a second operation and invasion of the joint. Therefore, the procedure is rarely performed, and few studies have compared second-look arthroscopy to other cartilage assessment modalities. Arthroscopy is known to provide information that is complimentary to MRI and several scoring systems have been devised on this basis [6]. Ferkel and Cheng proposed a 6-stage arthroscopic grading system that ranges from smooth and intact cartilage to a displaced cartilage fragment [5]. The ICRS has also designed a postoperative arthroscopic assessment system based on the degree to which a defect is filled with repair tissue, the degree of integration of repair tissue with the surrounding cartilage, and the macroscopic appearance of the articular surface [16, 34]. Second-look arthroscopy can be performed using previously created portals, typically

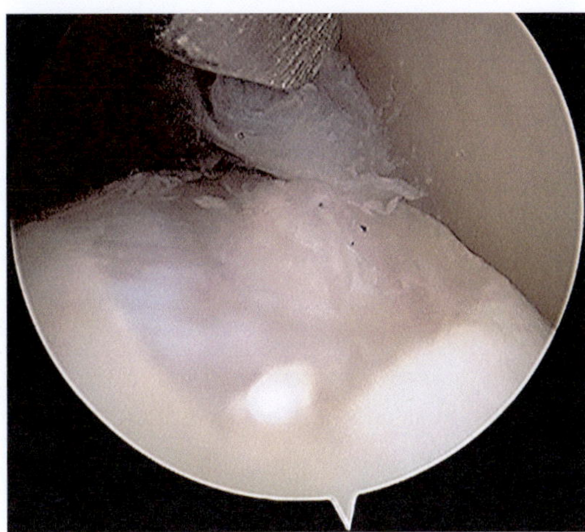

Fig. 12.4 Arthroscopic view of fibrillated cartilage repair. Patient is 2 years postoperative following arthroscopic microfracture of an osteochondral lesion of the medial talar dome

anterolateral, anteromedial, and posterolateral, and is most informative around 1 year postoperatively because cartilage integration and maturation may be assessed [6, 9, 16].

Arthroscopy has been directly compared to other follow-up imaging modalities. Lee and co-workers reported a good correlation between second-look arthroscopy and AOFAS scores 12 months after microfracture treatment, using both the ICRS and Ferkel and Cheng arthroscopic grading systems [16, 23]. With regard to imaging comparison, Lee and co-workers reported that scores for degree of defect repair and filling using second-look arthroscopy and MOCART demonstrated significant agreement and an intraclass correlation coefficient indicating good reliability 1 year following ACI in the talus. However, scores for integration of repair tissue with adjacent cartilage showed poor reliability [17]. A separate study stated that correlations between clinical outcomes, MOCART scores, and second-look arthroscopy were not significantly different, and, thus, second-look arthroscopy was not necessary for follow-up [18]. In another study 12 months following ACI, the paper concluded that due to a moderate correlation between second-look arthroscopy and MRI, MRI seemed to score cartilage maturation less favorably. It was also concluded that surgeon bias may contribute to favor arthroscopic scores, and that MRI may be equally effective as second-look arthroscopy and histology [14].

While arthroscopy allows direct visualization and enables probing of articular cartilage, and arthroscopic scoring has been correlated with clinical outcomes [9], it is invasive and cannot evaluate the subchondral bone. It is therefore not an ideal method for cartilage repair follow-up. If a patient requires a procedure in which the ankle joint must be accessed, whether it be removal of hardware, fracture fixation, or any procedure requiring a portal, arthroscopic inspection of repair cartilage can be performed.

Conclusions

OCL imaging methods for follow-up include standard radiographs, CT, MRI, and second-look arthroscopy. Standard radiography was used historically and the Berndt and Harty scale was the foundation for many cartilage grading systems. While x-ray remains useful for the assessment of acute OCL consolidation, osteotomy alignment and union, arthritis progression, and assessment of hardware, it is unable to evaluate the articular surface at follow-up. CT scans provide comprehensive three-dimensional images and can describe subchondral lesions with high specificity; however, this method is unable to assess articular cartilage and may miss smaller, more superficial OCLs. MRI is the noninvasive cartilage evaluation method of choice and should ideally be done at 3–6 months and approximately 12 months postoperatively. If there is suspicion of bony injury, subchondral cyst formation, or significant bone edema at follow-up, then CT may provide supplemental information. It has been suggested that arthroscopic grading may better predict the extent of articular cartilage repair compared to MRI, but because it is inherently invasive, it should only be done in conjunction with a secondary surgical procedure and not solely for follow-up purposes. Even though MRI does not allow direct visualization, specific protocols allow for a wide array of information to be gathered, including the degree of collagen fiber alignment. Although MRI has been criticized as less forgiving or increasingly sensitive, this modality sets a high standard for cartilage repair and allows for follow-up assessment of both the cartilage and bone for both research and patient care. Much of the literature regarding cartilage imaging focuses on OCL diagnosis rather than postoperative follow-up. Further study and clinical trials comparing imaging modalities at follow-up will help to create an algorithm for modality usage and follow-up imaging timelines.

Conflict of Interest The author has no current conflict of interests with the products presented.

References

1. Alhadlaq HA, Xia Y, Moody JB, Matyas JR. Detecting structural changes in early experimental osteoarthritis of tibial cartilage by microscopic magnetic resonance imaging and polarised light microscopy. Ann Rheum Dis. 2004;63:709–17.
2. Anderson IF, Crichton KJ, Grattan-Smith T, Cooper RA, Brazier D. Osteochondral fractures of the dome of the talus. J Bone Joint Surg Am. 1989;71:1143–52.
3. Battaglia M, Vannini F, Buda R, Cavallo M, Ruffilli A, Monti C, Galletti S, Giannini S. Arthroscopic autologous chondrocyte implantation in osteochondral lesions of the talus: mid-term T2-mapping MRI evaluation. Knee Surg Sports Traumatol Arthrosc. 2011;19:1376–84.
4. Berndt AL, Harty M. Transchondral fractures (osteochondritis dissecans) of the talus. J Bone Joint Surg Am. 1959;41-A:988–1020.
5. Cheng MS, Ferkel RD, Applegate GR. Osteochondral lesions of the talus: a radiologic and surgical comparison. In: Oral presentation presented at: annual meeting of the American Academy of Orthopaedic Surgeons. New Orleans, Feb 1995.
6. Choi YS, Potter HG, Chun TJ. MR imaging of cartilage repair in the knee and ankle. Radiographics. 2008;28:1043–59.
7. Easley ME, Latt LD, Santangelo JR, Merian-Genast M, Nunley 2nd JA. Osteochondral lesions of the talus. J Am Acad Orthop Surg. 2010;18:616–30.
8. Ferkel RD, Flannigan BD, Elkins BS. Magnetic resonance imaging of the foot and ankle: correlation of normal anatomy with pathologic conditions. Foot Ankle. 1991;11:289–305.
9. Ferkel RD, Zanotti RM, Komenda GA, Sgaglione NA, Cheng MS, Applegate GR, Dopirak RM. Arthroscopic treatment of chronic osteochondral lesions of the talus: long-term results. Am J Sports Med. 2008;36:1750–62.

10. Giannini S, Battaglia M, Buda R, Cavallo M, Ruffilli A, Vannini F. Surgical treatment of osteochondral lesions of the talus by open-field autologous chondrocyte implantation: a 10-year follow-up clinical and magnetic resonance imaging T2-mapping evaluation. Am J Sports Med. 2009;37:112S–8.

11. Griffith JF, Lau DT, Yeung DK, Wong MW. High-resolution MR imaging of talar osteochondral lesions with new classification. Skeletal Radiol. 2012;41:387–99.

12. Hao DP, Zhang JZ, Wang ZC, Xu WJ, Liu JH, Yang BT. Osteochondral lesions of the talus: comparison of three-dimensional fat-suppressed fast spoiled gradient-echo magnetic resonance imaging and conventional magnetic resonance imaging. J Am Podiatr Med Assoc. 2010;100:189–94.

13. Hayter C, Potter H. Magnetic resonance imaging of cartilage repair techniques. J Knee Surg. 2011;24:225–40.

14. Henderson IJ, Tuy B, Connell D, Oakes B, Hettwer WH. Prospective clinical study of autologous chondrocyte implantation and correlation with MRI at three and 12 months. J Bone Joint Surg Br. 2003;85:1060–6.

15. Knupp M, Pagenstert GI, Barg A, Bolliger L, Easley ME, Hintermann B. SPECT- CT compared with conventional imaging modalities for the assessment of the varus and valgus malaligned hindfoot. J Orthop Res. 2009;27:1461–6.

16. Lee KB, Bai LB, Yoon TR, Jung ST, Seon JK. Second-look arthroscopic findings and clinical outcomes after microfracture for osteochondral lesions of the talus. Am J Sports Med. 2009;37:63S–70.

17. Lee KT, Choi YS, Lee YK, Cha SD, Koo HM. Comparison of MRI and arthroscopy in modified MOCART scoring system after autologous chondrocyte implantation for osteochondral lesion of the talus. Orthopedics. 2011;34:e356–62.

18. Lee KT, Lee YK, Young KW, Park SY, Kim JS. Factors influencing result of autologous chondrocyte implantation in osteochondral lesion of the talus using second look arthroscopy. Scand J Med Sci Sports. 2012;22:510–5.

19. Leumann A, Valderrabano V, Plaass C, Rasch H, Studler U, Hintermann B, Pagenstert GI. A novel imaging method for osteochondral lesions of the talus comparison of SPECT-CT with MRI. Am J Sports Med. 2011;39:1095–101.

20. Loomer R, Fisher C, Lloyd-Smith R, Sisler J, Cooner T. Osteochondral lesions of the talus. Am J Sports Med. 1993;21:13–9.

21. Maier CF, Tan SG, Hariharan H, Potter HG. T2 quantitation of articular cartilage at 1.5 T. J Magn Reson Imaging. 2003;17:358–64.

22. Mintz DN, Tashjian GS, Connell DA, Deland JT, O'Malley M, Potter HG. Osteochondral lesions of the talus: a new magnetic resonance grading system with arthroscopic correlation. Arthroscopy. 2003;19:353–9.

23. Nam EK, Ferkel RD, Applegate GR. Autologous chondrocyte implantation of the ankle: a 2- to 5-year follow-up. Am J Sports Med. 2009;37:274–84.

24. Nelson DW, DiPaola J, Colville M, Schmidgall J. Osteochondritis dissecans of the talus and knee: prospective comparison of MR and arthroscopic classifications. J Comput Assist Tomogr. 1990;14:804–8.

25. Nieminen MT, Rieppo J, Töyräs J, Hakumäki JM, Silvennoinen J, Hyttinen MM, Helminen HJ, Jurvelin JS. T2 relaxation reveals spatial collagen architecture in articular cartilage: a comparative quantitative MRI and polarized light microscopic study. Magn Reson Med. 2001;46:487–93.

26. O'Loughlin PF, Heyworth BE, Kennedy JG. Current concepts in the diagnosis and treatment of osteochondral lesions of the ankle. Am J Sports Med. 2010;38:392–404.

27. Pagenstert GI, Barg A, Leumann AG, Rasch H, Müller-Brand J, Hintermann B, Valderrabano V. SPECT-CT imaging in degenerative joint disease of the foot and ankle. J Bone Joint Surg Br. 2009;91:1191–6.

28. Potter HG, Black BR, le Chong R. New techniques in articular cartilage imaging. Clin Sports Med. 2009;28:77–94.

29. Potter HG, le Chong R. Magnetic resonance imaging assessment of chondral lesions and repair. J Bone Joint Surg Am. 2009;91:126–31.

30. Potter HG, le Chong R, Sneag DB. Magnetic resonance imaging of cartilage repair. Sports Med Arthrosc. 2008;16:236–45.

31. Pritsch M, Horoshovski H, Farine I. Arthroscopic treatment of osteochondral lesions of the talus. J Bone Joint Surg Am. 1986;68:862–5.

32. Stroud CC, Marks RM. Imaging of osteochondral lesions of the talus. Foot Ankle Clin. 2000;5:119–33.

33. Trattnig S, Millington SA, Szomolanyi P, Marlovits S. MR imaging of osteochondral grafts and autologous chondrocyte implantation. Eur Radiol. 2007;17:103–18.

34. van den Borne MP, Raijmakers NJ, Vanlauwe J, Victor J, de Jong SN, Bellemans J, Saris DB. International Cartilage Repair Society (ICRS) and Oswestry macroscopic cartilage evaluation scores validated for use in autologous chondrocyte implantation (ACI) and microfracture. Osteoarthritis Cartilage. 2007;15:1397–402.

35. Ventura A, Terzaghi C, Legnani C, Borgo E. Treatment of post-traumatic osteochondral lesions of the talus: a four-step approach. Knee Surg Sports Traumatol Arthrosc. 2013;21:1245–50.

36. Verhagen RA, Maas M, Dijkgraaf MG, Tol JL, Krips R, van Dijk CN. Prospective study on diagnostic strategies in osteochondral lesions of the talus. Is MRI superior to helical CT? J Bone Joint Surg Br. 2005;87:41–6.

37. Xia Y. Heterogeneity of cartilage laminae in MR imaging. J Magn Reson Imaging. 2000;11:686–93.

38. Zengerink M, Szerb I, Hangody L, Dopirak RM, Ferkel RD, van Dijk CN. Current concepts: treatment of osteochondral ankle defects. Foot Ankle Clin. 2006;11:331–59.

Return to Sports

Inge C.M. van Eekeren and C. Niek van Dijk

Take-Home Points

- *The time to return to sports depends on the desired level of activity.*
- *Every type of surgery has its specific rehabilitation and guidelines to resume to activity.*

13.1 Introduction

Osteochondral defects (OCD) of the talus often occur after traumatic sprains of the ankle [35]. These lesions can have a severe impact on the quality of life [23, 35]. In case of persisting symptoms, treatment by means of excision and bone marrow stimulation (ECBS) is the gold standard [29]. The primary focus of the rehabilitation after ECBS of an osteochondral defect in the talus is to return to the pre-injury activity level. For athletes, the time in which they can return to pre-injury activity level is also important. The crucial period for return to sports can differ between 3 and 6 months [4, 17, 24]. In case osteochondral autograft transplantation (OATS) is applied, approximately 50–91 % of the patients are able to return to sports [12, 28]. For autologous chondrocyte implantation (ACI), sport activities are allowed after 8–10 months [7, 19, 34]. This chapter focuses on levels of activity and proposes a return to sports algorithm.

13.2 Activity Level

For rehabilitation and return to sports after treatment of an OCD, we propose four levels of activity: *walking, running, noncontact sports,* and *contact sports* [32, 33]. The first and basic level of activity after treatment is return to normal walking, the second is return to running, the third is return to noncontact sport, and the highest level of activity is return to contact sports. These 4 activity levels were originally described for rehabilitation after Achilles tendon ruptures; however, this system can cover the rehabilitation of any ankle injury. It can therefore also be used to monitor the rehabilitation after surgery for talar ODs. Another monitoring method is the ankle activity score as described by Halasi et al. [11]. The authors describe 53 sports, 3 working activities, 4 general activities, and 3 levels within each group. It is therefore a comprehensive scale. Both these methods provide specific scores for ankle joint injuries. For the sake of simplicity we prefer the first method.

I.C.M. van Eekeren, MD, PhD (✉)
Orthopaedic Research Centre Amsterdam,
Department of Orthopaedic Surgery,
Academic Medical Center, University of Amsterdam,
Amsterdam, The Netherlands
e-mail: i.c.vaneekeren@amc.uva.nl

C.N. van Dijk, MD, PhD
Department of Orthopaedic Surgery and
Traumatology, Academic Medical Center, University
of Amsterdam, Amsterdam, The Netherlands
e-mail: c.n.vandijk@amc.uva.nl

C.N. van Dijk, J.G. Kennedy (eds.), *Talar Osteochondral Defects,*
DOI 10.1007/978-3-642-45097-6_13, © ESSKA 2014

13.3 Return to Activity

Level 1: The first phase is return to normal walking. This phase starts on the day of the operation with partial weight-bearing together with training of active range of motion. The most important factor which determines the length of the nonpartial or partial weight-bearing period is the quality and strength of the tissue repair. On the day of the operation, the formation of granulation and thereafter fibrocartilaginous tissue will start. By partially weight-bearing the chondrocytes are nourished by the synovial fluid, and after 6–8 weeks fibrocartilaginous tissue is formed, full weight-bearing is allowed. Weight-bearing stimulates the osteoblasts of bone formation underneath the fibrocartilage. Training of proprioception is started at the end of this phase to regain normal active stability. For ECBS, the length of this first phase with the aim of normal walking is usually between 6 and 8 weeks.

Level 2: The next level of activity is to resume running on even ground. At the start of this activity level, the range of motion should be normal and proprioception should be restored. In order to resume running, it is important to achieve controlled sideways movement and the lower-leg force should be increased to a left/right difference of less than 12 %. This is achieved by training of force, endurance, and technical skills. Pain and swelling that occur after increased activity are signs to slow down the rehabilitation in this phase. Pain and swelling should be gone within 24 h. Return to activity levels is dependent on the type of surgical treatment and will be described in subsequent paragraphs.

Level 3: The third level of activity is return to noncontact sports. At the end of this phase, running on even ground, sprinting, rope jumping, turning, and twisting should be possible. This is achieved by means of further training for speed and endurance.

Level 4: Level 4 is defined as return to contact sports which is the highest level of activity. Training should focus on speed, muscle strength, and endurance which will enable running on uneven ground, generating explosive force, changing direction, and other sports-specific movements.

13.4 Literature Review on Return to Sport After Talar OCD Treatment

13.4.1 Bone Marrow Stimulation

Several authors mention return to sport. Most of them allow return to impact activities at 12 weeks postoperative [20, 24, 25, 29, 35]. Return to non-contact sports is mostly achieved after 4–6 months, depending on muscle strength [5, 8]. Approximately 63–79 % of the patients are able to return to pre-injury sporting level [16, 20]. Even high-demanding sports such as soccer and basketball can be resumed after 4–5 months postoperative [24, 25].

13.4.2 Osteochondral Autograft Transfer (OATS)

Postoperatively, patients are kept non-weight-bearing for 4 weeks, of which the first week in a splint after which range of motion exercises are encouraged. Partial weight-bearing is thereafter allowed for 2 weeks, which can be progressed to full weight-bearing after 6 weeks [15]. Approximately, 50–91 % of the patients are able to return to activity level 3 or 4 [12, 28]. However, there is no mention in the literature as to the time to return to sports.

13.4.3 Allograft Implant

After inserting an allograft, most patients are kept non-weight-bearing in a cast, splint, or walker for 6–12 weeks, depending on the size of the allograft [1, 6, 9, 10, 22, 27]. Meanwhile, active and passive sagittal range of motion exercises are encouraged. The average time for return to normal walking or running is not mentioned in the literature. Depending on the percentage of healing of the allograft into the talus, activity levels were allowed or restricted. Return to full athletic competition is mentioned to be allowed at 1 year after surgery [10].

13.4.4 HemiCAP

After placement of a metal implant by means of an osteotomy of the medial malleolus, patients are kept in a plaster non-weight-bearing cast for 1 or 2 weeks. This is continued with a functional brace for 4–5 weeks. The total period of non-weight-bearing is 6 weeks. After these 6 weeks, patients can progress to full weight-bearing in 1 month [30]. The average time to return to work is 11 weeks (range, 2–25.6). Return to running and sport is generally not the goal of these patients. In our series 75 % wished to go back to running or sports. This was achieved in 25.5 weeks (range 7.1–57.4) by 66.7 % of the patients [31].

13.4.5 Fixation

After fixation of a large osteochondral talar fragment, the rehabilitation depends on the approach used. If an osteotomy of the medial malleolus is needed, a non-weight-bearing cast for 6 weeks is applied [14]. Thereafter, partial weight-bearing is allowed, and by 8–10 weeks patients can progress to full weight-bearing. When the fragment can be fixed by an anterior arthroscopy or anterior arthrotomy, plantarflexion and dorsiflexion are allowed from the first day after the operation. Partial weight-bearing is initiated at 6 weeks and progressed to full weight-bearing at 8 weeks [18]. Progression to activity level 2 can be initiated after 3 months [18] and return to noncontact sports after 4 months [14].

13.4.6 Sliding Calcaneal Osteotomy

Rehabilitation after a sliding calcaneal osteotomy starts with a non-weight-bearing cast for 4 weeks [2, 3, 21, 26]. This is followed by a weight-bearing cast or stabilizing shoe for an additional 4 weeks. The period to return to sports is not described in the literature. In our patients we allow return to running at 12 weeks. Noncontact sports can be resumed at 4 months and contact sports at 5 months.

13.4.7 Autologous Chondrocyte Implantation (ACI)

For autologous chondrocyte implantation a non-weight-bearing or partial weight-bearing period of 6–8 weeks is indicated with active and passive range of motion exercises. After 6 weeks, patients are allowed to progress to full weight-bearing and full range of motion should be achieved after 12 weeks. After 3–4 months, patients can increase the training load and light jogging can be initiated. Higher impact activities and sport-specific training is allowed 8–10 months after surgery [7, 19, 34].

13.4.8 Retrograde Drilling

The rehabilitation after retrograde drilling consists of active range of motion exercises immediately after surgery. Partial weight-bearing is allowed at 2–4 weeks, depending on the size of the defect. Full weight-bearing is normally allowed at 6 weeks postoperative. Advancement to level 3 can be considered after 3 months and to full range of sports at 6 months postoperative [13].

On the basis of the findings described above, we conclude to the timeline as is shown in Fig. 13.1. When an activity level (indicated in blocks with expected time to achieve mentioned above) is achieved, one can progress to the next level.

> **Conclusion**
> The time to return to sports depends on the type of operative repair. To return to contact sports, patients first have to achieve the level of normal walking, followed by running and return to noncontact sports. The specific rehabilitation exercises depend on the desired level

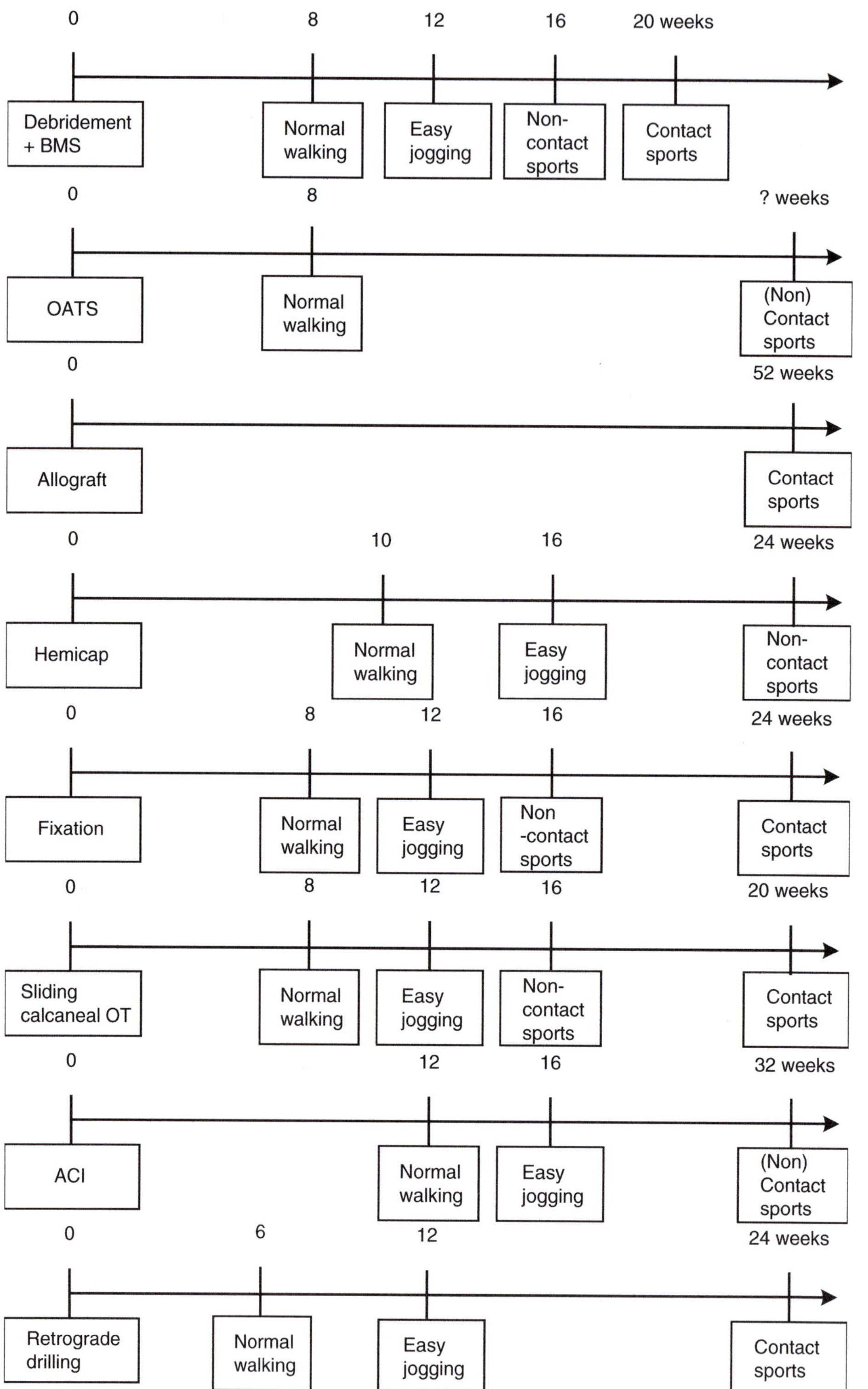

Fig. 13.1 Timeline according to activity levels to return to sports for several treatment options

of activity. A well-motivated, compliant athlete will resume to sports earlier when compared to patients without a strong motivation.

Conflict of Interest The author has no current conflict of interests with the products presented

References

1. Berlet GC, Hyer CF, Philbin TM, Hartman JF, Wright ML. Does fresh osteochondral allograft transplantation of talar osteochondral defects improve function? Clin Orthop Relat Res. 2011;469:2356–66.
2. Catanzariti AR, Lee MS, Mendicino RW. Posterior calcaneal displacement osteotomy for adult acquired flatfoot. J Foot Ankle Surg. 2000;39:2–14.
3. Catanzariti AR, Mendicino RW, King GL, Neerings B. Double calcaneal osteotomy: realignment considerations in eight patients. J Am Podiatr Med Assoc. 2005;95:53–9.
4. Cerynik DL, Lewullis GE, Joves BC, Palmer MP, Tom JA. Outcomes of microfracture in professional basketball players. Knee Surg Sports Traumatol Arthrosc. 2009;17:1135–9.
5. Chuckpaiwong B, Berkson EM, Theodore GH. Microfracture for osteochondral lesions of the ankle: outcome analysis and outcome predictors of 105 cases. Arthroscopy. 2008;24:106–12.
6. El-Rashidy H, Villacis D, Omar I, Kelikian AS. Fresh osteochondral allograft for the treatment of cartilage defects of the talus: a retrospective review. J Bone Joint Surg Am. 2011;93:1634–40.
7. Giannini S, Buda R, Faldini C, Vannini F, Bevoni R, Grandi G, Grigolo B, Berti L. Surgical treatment of osteochondral lesions of the talus in young active patients. J Bone Joint Surg Am. 2005;87 Suppl 2:28–41.
8. Guo QW, Hu YL, Jiao C, Yu CL, Ao YF. Arthroscopic treatment for osteochondral lesions of the talus: analysis of outcome predictors. Chin Med J (Engl). 2010;123:296–300.
9. Haene R, Qamirani E, Story RA, Pinsker E, Daniels TR. Intermediate outcomes of fresh talar osteochondral allografts for treatment of large osteochondral lesions of the talus. J Bone Joint Surg Am. 2012;94:1105–10.
10. Hahn DB, Aanstoos ME, Wilkins RM. Osteochondral lesions of the talus treated with fresh talar allografts. Foot Ankle Int. 2010;31:277–82.
11. Halasi T, Kynsburg A, Tallay A, Berkes I. Development of a new activity score for the evaluation of ankle instability. Am J Sports Med. 2004;32:899–908.
12. Hangody L, Kish G, Modis L, Szerb I, Gaspar L, Dioszegi Z, Kendik Z. Mosaicplasty for the treatment of osteochondritis dissecans of the talus: two to seven year results in 36 patients. Foot Ankle Int. 2001;22:552–8.
13. Kono M, Takao M, Naito K, Uchio Y, Ochi M. Retrograde drilling for osteochondral lesions of the talar dome. Am J Sports Med. 2006;34:1450–6.
14. Kumai T, Takakura Y, Kitada C, Tanaka Y, Hayashi K. Fixation of osteochondral lesions of the talus using cortical bone pegs. J Bone Joint Surg Br. 2002;84:369–74.
15. Lee CH, Chao KH, Huang GS, Wu SS. Osteochondral autografts for osteochondritis dissecans of the talus. Foot Ankle Int. 2003;24:815–22.
16. Lee KB, Bai LB, Chung JY, Seon JK. Arthroscopic microfracture for osteochondral lesions of the talus. Knee Surg Sports Traumatol Arthrosc. 2010;18:247–53.
17. Mithoefer K, Williams III RJ, Warren RF, Wickiewicz TL, Marx RG. High-impact athletics after knee articular cartilage repair: a prospective evaluation of the microfracture technique. Am J Sports Med. 2006;34:1413–8.
18. Nakagawa S, Hara K, Minami G, Arai Y, Kubo T. Arthroscopic fixation technique for osteochondral lesions of the talus. Foot Ankle Int. 2010;31:1025–7.
19. Nam EK, Ferkel RD, Applegate GR. Autologous chondrocyte implantation of the ankle: a 2- to 5-year follow-up. Am J Sports Med. 2009;37:274–84.
20. Ogilvie-Harris DJ, Sarrosa EA. Arthroscopic treatment of osteochondritis dissecans of the talus. Arthroscopy. 1999;15:805–8.
21. Pagenstert GI, Hintermann B, Barg A, Leumann A, Valderrabano V. Realignment surgery as alternative treatment of varus and valgus ankle osteoarthritis. Clin Orthop Relat Res. 2007;462:156–68.
22. Raikin SM. Fresh osteochondral allografts for large-volume cystic osteochondral defects of the talus. J Bone Joint Surg Am. 2009;91:2818–26.
23. Robinson DE, Winson IG, Harries WJ, Kelly AJ. Arthroscopic treatment of osteochondral lesions of the talus. J Bone Joint Surg Br. 2003;85:989–93.
24. Saxena A, Eakin C. Articular talar injuries in athletes: results of microfracture and autogenous bone graft. Am J Sports Med. 2007;35:1680–7.
25. Seijas R, Alvarez P, Ares O, Steinbacher G, Cusco X, Cugat R. Osteocartilaginous lesions of the talus in soccer players. Arch Orthop Trauma Surg. 2010;130:329–33.
26. Stufkens SA, Knupp M, Hintermann B. Medial displacement calcaneal osteotomy. Tech Foot Ankle Surg. 2009;8:85–90.
27. Tasto JP, Ostrander R, Bugbee W, Brage M. The diagnosis and management of osteochondral lesions of the talus: osteochondral allograft update. Arthroscopy. 2003;19 Suppl 1:138–41.
28. Valderrabano V, Leumann A, Rasch H, Egelhof T, Hintermann B, Pagenstert G. Knee-to-ankle mosaicplasty for the treatment of osteochondral lesions of the ankle joint. Am J Sports Med. 2009;37 Suppl 1:105S–11.

29. van Bergen CJ, de Leeuw PA, van Dijk CN. Treatment of osteochondral defects of the talus. Rev Chir Orthop Reparatrice Appar Mot. 2008;94:398–408.
30. van Bergen CJ, Reilingh ML, van Dijk CN. Tertiary osteochondral defect of the talus treated by a novel contoured metal implant. Knee Surg Sports Traumatol Arthrosc. 2011;19:999–1003.
31. van Bergen CJ, van Eekeren IC, Reilingh ML, van Dijk CN. Metal implantation resurfacing for secondary osteochondral defects of the talus. 2013. Ref type: Unpublished work.
32. van Eekeren IC, Reilingh ML, van Dijk CN. Rehabilitation and return-to-sports activity after debridement and bone marrow stimulation of osteochondral talar defects. Sports Med. 2012;42:857–70.
33. van Sterkenburg MN, Donley BG, van Dijk CN. Guidelines for sport resumption. In: van Dijk CN, Karlsson J, Maffuli N, Thermann H, editors. Achilles tendon rupture. Surrey: DJO Publications; 2008. p. 107–16.
34. Whittaker JP, Smith G, Makwana N, Roberts S, Harrison PE, Laing P, Richardson JB. Early results of autologous chondrocyte implantation in the talus. J Bone Joint Surg Br. 2005;87:179–83.
35. Zengerink M, Szerb I, Hangody L, Dopirak RM, Ferkel RD, van Dijk CN. Current concepts: treatment of osteochondral ankle defects. Foot Ankle Clin. 2006;11:331–59, vi.

Inge C.M. van Eekeren, Kyriacos I. Eleftheriou,
Christiaan J.A. van Bergen, and James D.F. Calder

Take-Home Points
- *A single, ideal rehabilitation programme after bone marrow stimulation
  for talar osteochondral defects still does
  not exist.*
- *Further high-quality studies are necessary to provide clinical outcome data to
  support any rehabilitation regimen.*
- *Any protocol may need to be modified
  and individualised for each patient taking into consideration patient and lesion
  factors.*

I.C.M. van Eekeren, MD, PhD (✉)
C.J.A. van Bergen, MD, PhD
Orthopaedic Research Centre Amsterdam,
Department of Orthopaedic Surgery,
Academic Medical Center, University of Amsterdam,
Amsterdam, The Netherlands
e-mail: i.c.vaneekeren@amc.uva.nl;
c.j.vanbergen@amc.uva.nl

K.I. Eleftheriou, MB BS, MD, FRCS (Tr & Orth)
Department of Trauma and Orthopaedics,
Hippocrateon Private Hospital, Nicosia, Cyprus
e-mail: akis@dreleftheriou.com

J.D.F. Calder, MD, FRCS (Tr & Orth), FFSEM
Department of Trauma and Orthopaedics,
Chelsea and Westminster Hospital,
The Fortius Clinic, London, UK
e-mail: j.calder@fortiusclinic.com

14.1 Introduction

The primary treatment of osteochondral defects up
to 15 mm in the talus consists of arthroscopic
debridement (excision and curettage) and bone
marrow stimulation (BMS) [54]. The aim of bone
marrow stimulation is to create multiple connections
with the subchondral bone. This can be accomplished by drilling or by microfracturing. The main
goal after treatment is to return to daily activities
and to the activity level before injury. As yet, there
is no consensus regarding rehabilitation. Reduced
loading and controlled joint motion can stimulate
cartilage repair. Animal studies that compared postoperative continuous passive motion (CPM) and
cast immobilisation showed faster healing with
CPM, as well as thicker and stiffer cartilage with a
greater concentration of proteoglycans [18, 37, 41].
In contrast, prolonged immobilisation and unloading of a joint can deteriorate cartilage, whilst excessive loading can also damage the repaired tissue
[12]. The ideal balance between early versus
delayed weight bearing is difficult to determine.

14.2 Tissue Healing After Arthroscopic BMS

Multiple microfractures disrupt intra-osseous
blood vessels leading to the release of growth
factors and to the formation of a fibrin clot along
with the further release of growth factors and
cytokines which stimulate repair [11, 19]. Within
2 weeks, undifferentiated mesenchymal cells

C.N. van Dijk, J.G. Kennedy (eds.), *Talar Osteochondral Defects*,
DOI 10.1007/978-3-642-45097-6_14, © ESSKA 2014

proliferate and differentiate into chondrocyte-like cells which produce a matrix containing type II collagen and proteoglycans. They also proliferate into osteoblast-like cells which are responsible for new bone formation [20, 22, 35]. At 6–8 weeks, the tissue of the chondral defect contains chondrocyte-like cells in a matrix of proteoglycans, type II collagen (predominantly) and some type I collagen. At 12 weeks, the defects are filled with hyaline-like tissue with mostly type II collagen maturing into a mixture of fibrocartilage and hyaline cartilage [21, 22]. Initially, new woven bone is laid down which is then transformed into lamella bone with the subchondral region modified into a compact bone plate and a reformed tidemark [39].

14.3 Literature on Rehabilitation After Arthroscopic BMS of the Ankle

Debridement of an osteochondral defect has been performed more and more since the 1950s [8]. The use of bone marrow stimulation, by either drilling or microfracturing, combined with debridement was introduced a couple of years later [2, 25]. These surgeries were performed by opening the joint through an arthrotomy with or without an osteotomy of the malleolus [2, 16, 17, 25, 32, 36]. If a malleolar osteotomy was performed, a cast or a postoperative splint was usually recommended for up to 12 weeks [2, 17, 32, 36]. This was often non-weight-bearing for 6–8 weeks, and a varying time to commencement of active and passive range of motion exercises has been described [2, 17, 32, 36]. For cases in which an arthrotomy was performed without an osteotomy, some describe the use of a cast for 1–2 weeks with non-weight-bearing for 8–12 weeks, whereas others begin gentle, active range of motion exercises to 'mould' the new fibrocartilage and then progress to partial weight-bearing over a variable period of time [2, 17, 36].

With the routine introduction of arthroscopic techniques, the standard treatment for osteochondral defects is curettage, debridement and bone marrow stimulation with an overall success rate of 85 % [50, 54]. Despite the good results of the procedure, there is no consensus regarding the postoperative rehabilitation. A period of non-weight-bearing to protect the healing tissue is widely accepted, but the length of this period may vary from 3–5 days to 3 months with no apparent scientific justification being made for the timeframe recommended.

The most conservative approach is to start off with non-weight-bearing for 6–12 weeks with cast, splint or without any support and in some cases including early range of motion exercises [23, 31, 52]. Partial or full weight-bearing is then allowed immediately or within 2 weeks with success rates of 80–90 % [23, 31, 52]. A progressive way is to allow immediate weight-bearing as tolerated or within 2 weeks after surgery, with good to excellent results in 75–100 % of the cases [5, 13–15, 43]. Other articles restricted the weight-bearing to 3–4 weeks or allowed only partial weight-bearing postoperatively [6, 7, 9, 40, 42, 46, 48, 49]. The range of motion can be restricted by cast or posterior splinting [9, 42, 46] or can be progressive with active range of motion exercises or the use of CPM [6, 7, 48].

Most of the studies have good to excellent results on microfracture in 78–100 % of the cases with two exceptions [6, 7, 42, 46, 48]; Bonnin and Bouysset showed only in 66 % of cases a good to excellent result, whilst Robinson et al. found in 52 % a good result. In both studies, the medial lesions were associated with a poor outcome [9, 40]. Regarding rehabilitation, no common factor was found what could explain the difference in outcome compared to the other studies.

In summary, whether weight-bearing should be early or delayed and whether the range of motion should be protected or not is still unclear. A recent study compared the clinical results of early vs. delayed weight-bearing after arthroscopic bone marrow stimulation of the talus [30]. In the early weight-bearing group, partial weight-bearing in a walking boot was allowed after 1 week of posterior splinting. Full weight-bearing was tolerated as soon as possible and active range of motion exercises started within 1 week. After 1 week of a posterior cast, the delayed weight-bearing group was kept on non-weight-bearing and active range of motion exercises with a removable posterior splint for 6 weeks, followed by partial weight-bearing for 2 weeks and thereafter full weight-bearing. They showed no differences in AOFAS, VAS or activity scores at 6, 12 or 37 months follow-up between the early and the delayed weight-bearing group [30]. A potential danger could however be the size of the lesion. Chuckpaiwong et al. showed that larger lesions (>15 mm in diameter) had a worse outcome than smaller lesions (<15 mm in diameter). All these patients were treated with the same rehabilitation protocol, i.e. splinted for 1–2 weeks with partial weight-bearing and advancing to full weight-bearing in a walking boot as soon as tolerated [15]. Recently, Hunt et al. demonstrated that location of peak stress becomes closer to the rim in defect sizes of 10 mm or greater [28]. This threshold is similar to findings in the knee [24] and supported by finite element modelling [38]. This could contribute to clinical failures in larger lesions. It could, therefore, be suggested that in case of larger lesions or anterior lesions, one should prolong the partial weight-bearing period [51].

14.4 Lessons from Knee Microfracture Rehabilitation

Articular cartilage lesions of the knee are common, with arthroscopic findings showing a prevalence of focal chondral and osteochondral defects of 19 % in one study [27] and full-thickness articular lesions of 11 % in another [3]. Since Steadman developed the microfracture technique in the 1980s [44], it has become the most common treatment modality for dealing with such lesions around the knee [10]. Despite the high volume of patients undergoing the procedure [34], there is still some contention on what the postoperative management after knee microfracture should be, and significant variation in practice has been shown between surgeons [47]. This may be because, although it is agreed that protecting the repair at the microfracture site and optimising the environment for hyaline cartilage repair should be central to an appropriate rehabilitation protocol, the experimental and clinical evidence to support a specific regimen is limited [33]. It appears that whilst high shear stresses may lead to failure of the repair at the early postoperative stages, there is evidence that moderate dynamic compression and low shear stresses may be advantageous to the repair tissue and that immobilisation and static compression may have negative effects [4, 26, 29]. Based on such evidence, a detailed rehabilitation regime has been described by Steadman and his group based on the biology of cartilage repair after microfracture [45, 53] and is worthwhile here to review this and look at some of the controversies around this.

Steadman proposed a rehabilitation programme which aims to create an optimal healing environment for the microfracture induced, allowing the latter to mature into a durable repair tissue to replace the underlying defect. The programme entails two protocols: the first for femoral condyle and tibial plateau lesions and the second for patellofemoral lesions. These are detailed below:

14.5 Rehabilitation Protocol for Lesions on the Femoral Condyle or Tibial Plateau

14.5.1 Phase I: 0–8 Weeks

During this first phase of rehabilitation, the aims are to protect the marrow clot, restore range of movement and quadriceps function and decrease swelling. The key components are the use of CPM and only allowing the patient to touch-down weight bear.

Immediately postoperatively the patients are placed on a CPM machine (30–70° at 1 cycle minute^{-1}), which is used for 6–8 h a day for the 8 weeks. Patients who do not tolerate this need to carry out 500 flexion-extension passive range of movement exercise three times a day. At the same time, muscle strengthening exercises are also initiated to restore quadriceps function. No bracing is used during this touch-down weight-bearing phase. At the same time, patellar mobilisations begin, in order to avoid patellar tendon adhesions which can increase joint reaction forces [1];

extensive surgical lysis of adhesions is now routinely incorporated in their treatment protocol [53]. Cryotherapy is also used to control pain and swelling. Deep water running and spinning on a no-resistance bike begins at 2 weeks and progresses as tolerated, aiming for 45 min of continuous spinning by week 8.

14.5.2 Phase II: 9–16 Weeks

Patients are allowed to bear weight with most coming off their crutches after about a week. When patients are able to fully weight bear and have a full range of movement, the rehabilitation then aims to restore normal muscular function and endurance through the use of cardiovascular equipment as well as closed-chain, double leg exercises.

Gradual increases in resistance are added to the bike in order to achieve 45 min of pain-free cycling, but limiting this time accordingly so as not to overload the joint. Treadmill walking on a 7 % incline is also initiated and patients progress through this carefully to limit the impact stress associated with walking (5–10 min only adding 5 min per week as tolerated). Closed-chain exercises continue aiming to build a muscular endurance base.

14.5.3 Phase III: 17–24 Weeks

Once the latter is achieved, rehabilitation then aims to regain muscle strength in the lower limbs. Sports-specific strengthening exercise and lifting techniques are utilised, but patients with significant lesions are progressed more carefully and caution is taken to avoid specific ranges of movement that can impact on the microfracture site.

Running is also initiated, but this is staged and dependent on the severity of the lesion. The goal is for the patient to be able to do 20 min of continuous running after 5 weeks. Exercises to address single-plane agility are also implemented, followed by multi-plane agility exercises.

14.5.4 Phase IV: 25–36 Weeks

Rehabilitation then focuses on allowing the patient to achieve performance abilities specific to their sport. Patients are allowed to return to their sports based on clinical examination, with those that carry out sports that involve cutting, jumping and pivoting advised against return to these until at least 6–9 months after microfracture.

Having considered the evidence from patients undergoing microfracture of knee lesions, which are much more prevalent, it is evident that a clear rehabilitation protocol after microfracture of ankle OCDs may be difficult to suggest at the moment. Some of the issues to consider are the same, however:

1. Any protocol should take into consideration our understanding of articular repair at the ankle, especially with regard to issues such as the times of the different repair phases for the ankle, as well as the effects of motion, loading and shear stresses on the repair.
2. Further high-quality studies are necessary to provide clinical outcome data to support any rehabilitation regimen.
3. Any protocol may need to be modified and individualised for each patient taking into consideration patient and lesion factors.
4. Pain and swelling should be controlled post-operatively to optimise outcomes.
5. Concomitant injuries around the ankle (especially ankle instability) should be addressed.
6. Progression through rehabilitation should be staged taking into consideration all the factors above and the ability of the patient to regain neuromuscular control and thus be able to protect the repair.
7. Patient compliance and psychosocial factors should be considered.

14.6 Proposed Rehabilitation Scheme

From the above, it becomes clear that a single, ideal rehabilitation programme after bone marrow stimulation for talar osteochondral

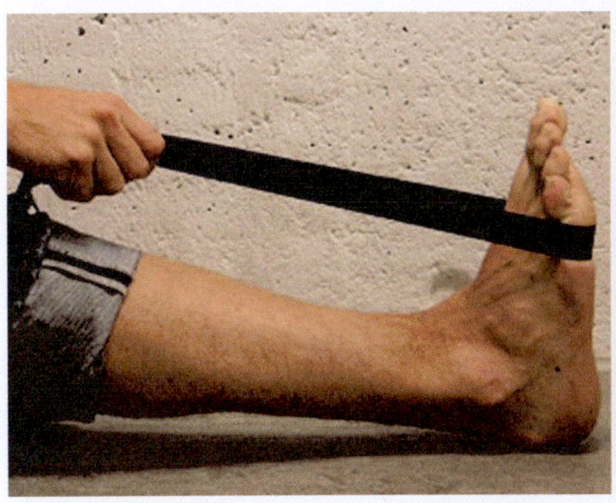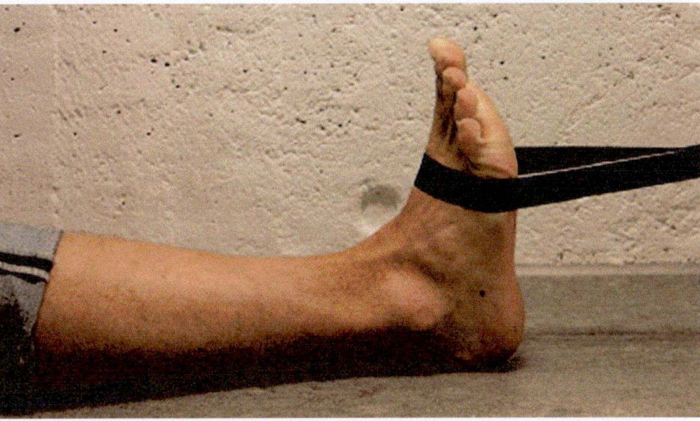

Fig. 14.1 Phase I: extension and flexion exercises against resistance

defects does not exist. Based on the limited literature and an ongoing study, as well as our own experience, the following 6-week rehabilitation scheme is proposed as a guideline [14, 30, 49].

14.6.1 Phase I: 0–2 Weeks

After surgery, the rehabilitation programme is initiated with non-weight-bearing for 2 weeks. In the first week, full non-weight-bearing flexion and extension exercises of the ankle are performed without resistance for 15 min twice a day. During the second week, flexion and extension are performed against resistance (Fig. 14.1).

14.6.2 Phase II: 3–4 Weeks

After these 2 weeks, partial (eggshell) weight-bearing on crutches is allowed, as tolerated. Progression to full weight-bearing is prescribed over a period of 4 weeks. The range of motion exercises against resistance are extended to three to four times a day.

14.6.3 Phase III: 5–6 weeks

During weeks 5 and 6, the patient practises full range of motion against gravity by exercising on a step with both feet simultaneously (Fig. 14.2). After week 6, this exercise can be performed on one leg (Fig. 14.3). The programme can be optionally guided by a physiotherapist.

14.6.4 Phase IV: 7–16 Weeks

Sagittal lunges and exercises can be practised after week 6. Thereafter, patients are allowed to cycle on the home trainer, start walking on the tread mill or use the cross trainer and rowing machine. Balancing and eversion/inversion exercises can be started in this phase. The resumption of sports is detailed in the next chapter 'Return to Sports'. To summarise, a gradual increase to impact activities can be considered after 3–4 months, whilst return to noncontact sports is mostly achieved after 4–6 months.

Additional modalities, such as CPM, cryotherapy or pulsed electromagnetic fields, could possibly be advantageous for an accelerated and improved outcome, but their exact value has to be further investigated. Any protocol may need to be modified and individualised for each patient taking into consideration patient and lesion factors. High-quality future studies will provide further evidence for creating an optimum rehabilitation protocol after microfracture which will be advantageous to patients and the outcome of surgery.

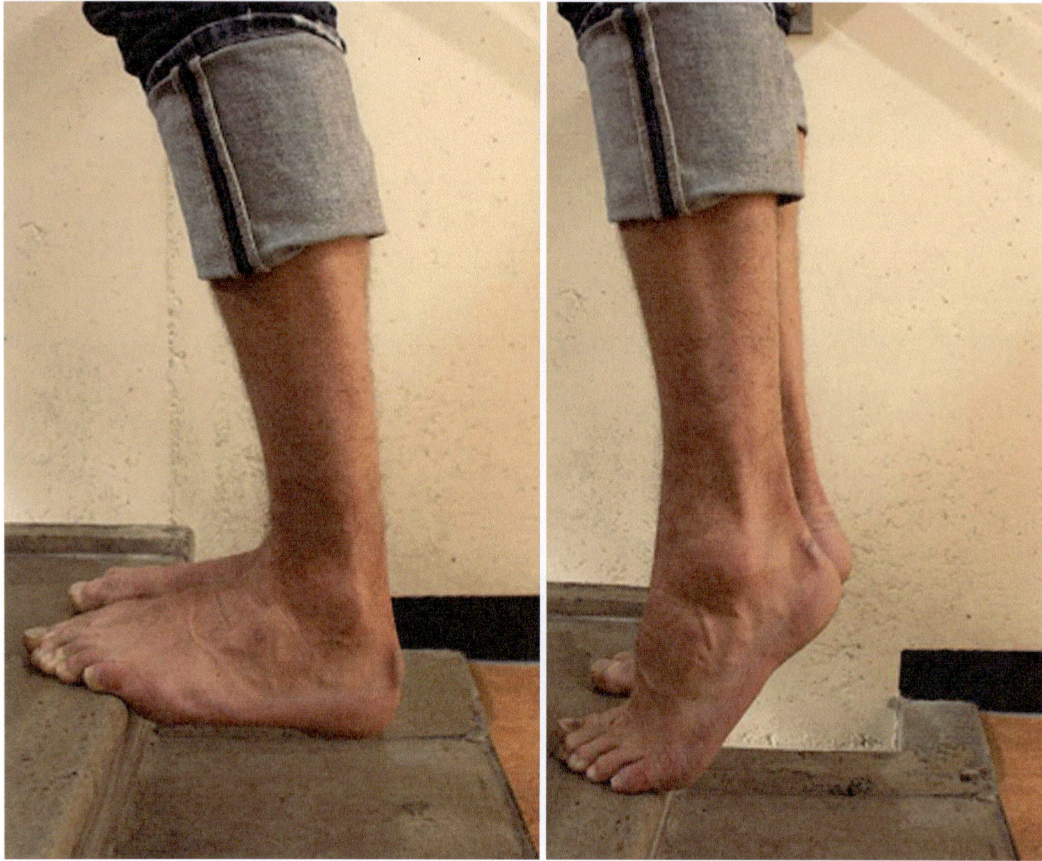

Fig. 14.2 Phase III: full range of motion exercises against gravity on a step on both feet

Conclusion

A single, ideal rehabilitation programme after bone marrow stimulation for talar osteochondral defects still does not exist. It appears that whilst high shear stresses may lead to failure of the repair at the early postoperative stages, there is evidence that moderate dynamic compression and low shear stresses may be advantageous to the repair tissue and that immobilisation and static compression may have negative effects. Rehabilitation with gradual return to weight-bearing after 4 weeks is suggested. Further high-quality studies are necessary to provide clinical outcome data to support any rehabilitation regimen.

Conflict of Interest The author has no current conflict of interests with the products presented

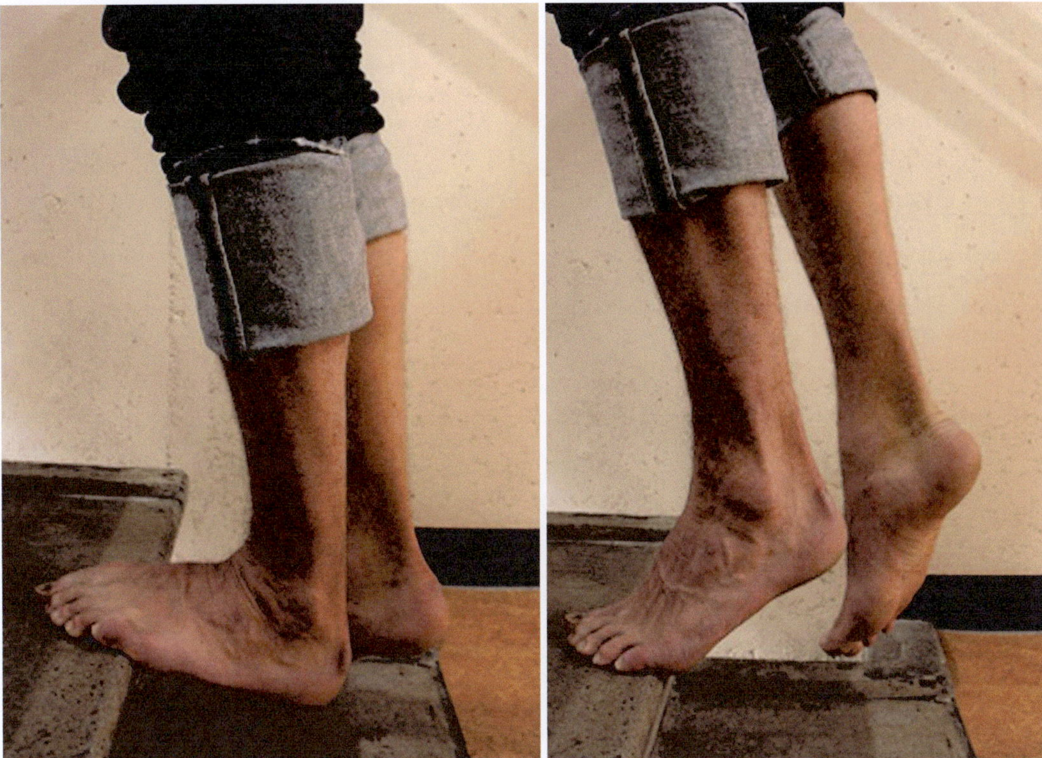

Fig. 14.3 Phase III: full range of motion exercise against gravity on a step on 1 ft

References

1. Ahmad CS, Kwak SD, Ateshian GA, Warden WH, Steadman JR, Mow VC. Effects of patellar tendon adhesion to the anterior tibia on knee mechanics. Am J Sports Med. 1998;26:715–24.
2. Alexander AH, Lichtman DM. Surgical treatment of transchondral talar-dome fractures (osteochondritis dissecans). Long-term follow-up. J Bone Joint Surg Am. 1980;62:646–52.
3. Aroen A, Loken S, Heir S, Alvik E, Ekeland A, Granlund OG, Engebretsen L. Articular cartilage lesions in 993 consecutive knee arthroscopies. Am J Sports Med. 2004;32:211–5.
4. Arokoski JP, Jurvelin JS, Vaatainen U, Helminen HJ. Normal and pathological adaptations of articular cartilage to joint loading. Scand J Med Sci Sports. 2000;10:186–98.
5. Baker Jr CL, Morales RW. Arthroscopic treatment of transchondral talar dome fractures: a long-term follow-up study. Arthroscopy. 1999;15:197–202.
6. Becher C, Driessen A, Hess T, Longo UG, Maffulli N, Thermann H. Microfracture for chondral defects of the talus: maintenance of early results at midterm follow-up. Knee Surg Sports Traumatol Arthrosc. 2010;18:656–63.
7. Becher C, Thermann H. Results of microfracture in the treatment of articular cartilage defects of the talus. Foot Ankle Int. 2005;26:583–9.

8. Berndt AL, Harty M. Transchondral fractures (osteochondritis dissecans) of the talus. J Bone Joint Surg Am. 1959;41-A:988–1020.

9. Bonnin M, Bouysset M. Arthroscopy of the ankle: analysis of results and indications on a series of 75 cases. Foot Ankle Int. 1999;20:744–51.

10. Brophy RH, Rodeo SA, Barnes RP, Powell JW, Warren RF. Knee articular cartilage injuries in the National Football League: epidemiology and treatment approach by team physicians. J Knee Surg. 2009;22:331–8.

11. Buckwalter JA, Mankin HJ. Articular cartilage: degeneration and osteoarthritis, repair, regeneration, and transplantation. Instr Course Lect. 1998;47:487–504.

12. Buckwalter JA, Mow VC, Ratcliffe A. Restoration of injured or degenerated articular cartilage. J Am Acad Orthop Surg. 1994;2:192–201.

13. Chin TW, Mitra AK, Lim GH, Tan SK, Tay BK. Arthroscopic treatment of osteochondral lesion of the talus. Ann Acad Med Singapore. 1996;25:236–40.

14. Choi WJ, Kim BS, Lee JW. Osteochondral lesion of the talus: could age be an indication for arthroscopic treatment? Am J Sports Med. 2012;40:419–24.

15. Chuckpaiwong B, Berkson EM, Theodore GH. Microfracture for osteochondral lesions of the ankle: outcome analysis and outcome predictors of 105 cases. Arthroscopy. 2008;24:106–12.

16. Draper SD, Fallat LM. Autogenous bone grafting for the treatment of talar dome lesions. J Foot Ankle Surg. 2000;39:15–23.

17. Flick AB, Gould N. Osteochondritis dissecans of the talus (transchondral fractures of the talus): review of the literature and new surgical approach for medial dome lesions. Foot Ankle. 1985;5:165–85.

18. French DA, Barber SM, Leach DH, Doige CE. The effect of exercise on the healing of articular cartilage defects in the equine carpus. Vet Surg. 1989;18:312–21.

19. Frenkel SR, Di Cesare PE. Degradation and repair of articular cartilage. Front Biosci. 1999;4:D671–85.

20. Frisbie DD, Oxford JT, Southwood L, Trotter GW, Rodkey WG, Steadman JR, Goodnight JL, McIlwraith CW. Early events in cartilage repair after subchondral bone microfracture. Clin Orthop Relat Res. 2003; 407:215–27.

21. Furukawa T, Eyre DR, Koide S, Glimcher MJ. Biochemical studies on repair cartilage resurfacing experimental defects in the rabbit knee. J Bone Joint Surg Am. 1980;62:79–89.

22. Gill TJ, McCulloch PC, Glasson SS, Blanchet T, Morris EA. Chondral defect repair after the microfracture procedure: a nonhuman primate model. Am J Sports Med. 2005;33:680–5.

23. Gobbi A, Francisco RA, Lubowitz JH, Allegra F, Canata G. Osteochondral lesions of the talus: randomized controlled trial comparing chondroplasty, microfracture, and osteochondral autograft transplantation. Arthroscopy. 2006;22:1085–92.

24. Guettler JH, Demetropoulos CK, Yang KH, Jurist KA. Osteochondral defects in the human knee: influence of defect size on cartilage rim stress and load redistribution to surrounding cartilage. Am J Sports Med. 2004;32:1451–8.

25. Hakimzadeh A, Munzinger U. 8. Osteochondrosis dissecans: results after 10 or more years. c). Osteochondrosis dissecans of the ankle joint: long-term study. Orthopade. 1979;8:135–40.

26. Hinterwimmer S, Krammer M, Krotz M, Glaser C, Baumgart R, Reiser M, Eckstein F. Cartilage atrophy in the knees of patients after seven weeks of partial load bearing. Arthritis Rheum. 2004;50:2516–20.

27. Hjelle K, Solheim E, Strand T, Muri R, Brittberg M. Articular cartilage defects in 1,000 knee arthroscopies. Arthroscopy. 2002;18:730–4.

28. Hunt KJ, Lee AT, Lindsey DP, Slikker III W, Chou LB. Osteochondral lesions of the talus: effect of defect size and plantarflexion angle on ankle joint stresses. Am J Sports Med. 2012;40:895–901.

29. Lane SR, Trindade MC, Ikenoue T, Mohtai M, Das P, Carter DR, Goodman SB, Schurman DJ. Effects of shear stress on articular chondrocyte metabolism. Biorheology. 2000;37:95–107.

30. Lee DH, Lee KB, Jung ST, Seon JK, Kim MS, Sung IH. Comparison of early versus delayed weightbearing outcomes after microfracture for small to mid-sized osteochondral lesions of the talus. Am J Sports Med. 2012;40(9):2023–8.

31. Lee KB, Bai LB, Yoon TR, Jung ST, Seon JK. Second-look arthroscopic findings and clinical outcomes after microfracture for osteochondral lesions of the talus. Am J Sports Med. 2009;37 Suppl 1:63S–70.

32. Mendicino RW, Lee MS, Grossman JP, Shromoff PJ. Oblique medial malleolar osteotomy for the management of talar dome lesions. J Foot Ankle Surg. 1998;37:516–23.

33. Mithoefer K, Hambly K, Logerstedt D, Ricci M, Silvers H, Della VS. Current concepts for rehabilitation and return to sport after knee articular cartilage repair in the athlete. J Orthop Sports Phys Ther. 2012;42:254–73.

34. Negrin L, Kutscha-Lissberg F, Gartlehner G, Vecsei V. Clinical outcome after microfracture of the knee: a meta-analysis of before/after-data of controlled studies. Int Orthop. 2012;36:43–50.

35. O'Driscoll SW. The healing and regeneration of articular cartilage. J Bone Joint Surg Am. 1998;80:1795–812.

36. O'Farrell TA, Costello BG. Osteochondritis dissecans of the talus. The late results of surgical treatment. J Bone Joint Surg Br. 1982;64:494–7.

37. Palmer JL, Bertone AL, Malemud CJ, Carter BG, Papay RS, Mansour J. Site-specific proteoglycan characteristics of third carpal articular cartilage in exercised and nonexercised horses. Am J Vet Res. 1995;56:1570–6.

38. Papaioannou G, Demetropoulos CK, King YH. Predicting the effects of knee focal articular surface injury with a patient-specific finite element model. Knee. 2010;17:61–8.

39. Qiu YS, Shahgaldi BF, Revell WJ, Heatley FW. Observations of subchondral plate advancement

during osteochondral repair: a histomorphometric and mechanical study in the rabbit femoral condyle. Osteoarthritis Cartilage. 2003;11:810–20.

40. Robinson DE, Winson IG, Harries WJ, Kelly AJ. Arthroscopic treatment of osteochondral lesions of the talus. J Bone Joint Surg Br. 2003;85:989–93.

41. Salter RB, Simmonds DF, Malcolm BW, Rumble EJ, MacMichael D, Clements ND. The biological effect of continuous passive motion on the healing of full-thickness defects in articular cartilage. An experimental investigation in the rabbit. J Bone Joint Surg Am. 1980;62:1232–51.

42. Saxena A, Eakin C. Articular talar injuries in athletes: results of microfracture and autogenous bone graft. Am J Sports Med. 2007;35:1680–7.

43. Schuman L, Struijs PA, van Dijk CN. Arthroscopic treatment for osteochondral defects of the talus. Results at follow-up at 2 to 11 years. J Bone Joint Surg Br. 2002;84:364–8.

44. Steadman JR, Rodkey WG, Briggs KK. Microfracture to treat full-thickness chondral defects: surgical technique, rehabilitation, and outcomes. J Knee Surg. 2002;15:170–6.

45. Steadman JR, Rodkey WG, Rodrigo JJ. Microfracture: surgical technique and rehabilitation to treat chondral defects. Clin Orthop Relat Res. 2001;391 Suppl:S362–S369.

46. Takao M, Ochi M, Naito K, Uchio Y, Kono T, Oae K. Arthroscopic drilling for chondral, subchondral, and combined chondral-subchondral lesions of the talar dome. Arthroscopy. 2003;19:524–30.

47. Theodoropoulos J, Dwyer T, Whelan D, Marks P, Hurtig M, Sharma P. Microfracture for knee chondral defects: a survey of surgical practice among Canadian orthopedic surgeons. Knee Surg Sports Traumatol Arthrosc. 2012;20(12):2430–7.

48. Thermann H, Becher C. Microfracture technique for treatment of osteochondral and degenerative chondral lesions of the talus. 2-year results of a prospective study. Unfallchirurg. 2004;107:27–32.

49. van Bergen CJ, Blankevoort L, de Haan RJ, Sierevelt IN, Meuffels DE, d'Hooghe PR, Krips R, van Damme G, van Dijk CN. Pulsed electromagnetic fields after arthroscopic treatment for osteochondral defects of the talus: double-blind randomized controlled multicenter trial. BMC Musculoskelet Disord. 2009;10:83.

50. van Bergen CJ, de Leeuw PA, van Dijk CN. Treatment of osteochondral defects of the talus. Rev Chir Orthop Reparatrice Appar Mot. 2008;94:398–408.

51. van Dijk CN, van Bergen CJ. Advancements in ankle arthroscopy. J Am Acad Orthop Surg. 2008;16:635–46.

52. Van BK, Barrack RL, Alexander AH, Ertl JP. Arthroscopic treatment of transchondral talar dome fractures. Am J Sports Med. 1989;17:350–5.

53. Yen YM, Cascio B, O'Brien L, Stalzer S, Millett PJ, Steadman JR. Treatment of osteoarthritis of the knee with microfracture and rehabilitation. Med Sci Sports Exerc. 2008;40:200–5.

54. Zengerink M, Struijs PA, Tol JL, van Dijk CN. Treatment of osteochondral lesions of the talus: a systematic review. Knee Surg Sports Traumatol Arthrosc. 2010;18:238–46.

Rehabilitation After Replacement Procedures (i.e., OATS, Allograft)

Ágnes Berta, László Hangody, and Mark E. Easley

Take-Home Points

- *The rehabilitation protocol after replacement procedures depends on the size and location (i.e., osteotomy is needed or not) of the osteochondral lesion of the talus and on graft choice (i.e., cylindrical autologous graft/ allograft or structural allograft).*
- *Cylindrical autologous graft/allograft:*
  - *Generally, immediate full ROM is preferred.*
  - *Malleolar osteotomy: typically warrants 4 weeks of non-weight bearing, followed by 2 weeks partial weight bearing.*
  - *Osteotomy was not performed:*
    - *Lesions < 1 cm^2, immediate weight bearing*
    - *Lesions > 1 cm^2, 2 weeks partial loading*
- *Structural allografts: individually, the periods of non-weight bearing, partial weight bearing, and full weight bearing depend on the rate of graft incorporation, which is detected by radiographic imaging techniques. Moreover, graft size and stability at the time of procedure are important, and the fixation of osteotomy must also be considered.*

15.1 Introduction

Autologous osteochondral transplantation techniques, such as osteochondral autologous transfer system (OATS) and mosaicplasty, and osteochondral allograft transplantation aim to repair osteochondral lesions of the talus by providing a hyaline or a hyaline-like gliding surface over the affected area.

The application of autologous osteochondral transplantation techniques to osteochondral lesions of the talus is an extrapolation for similar procedures for the knee, as they were initially developed to treat small- and medium-sized focal chondral and osteochondral defects of the femoral condyles and patellotrochlear surfaces [5–7].

Á. Berta, MD, MSc, MRes (✉)
L. Hangody, MD, PhD, DSc
Department of Orthopaedics and Traumatology,
Uzsoki Hospital, Budapest, Hungary

Department of Traumatology, Semmelweis
University, Budapest, Hungary
e-mail: bertaagnes@hotmail.com;
hangody@t-online.hu

M.E. Easley, MD
Department of Orthopaedic Surgery, Duke University
Medical Center, Durham, NC, USA
e-mail: mark.e.easley@duke.edu

C.N. van Dijk, J.G. Kennedy (eds.), *Talar Osteochondral Defects*,
DOI 10.1007/978-3-642-45097-6_15, © ESSKA 2014

For autologous osteochondral transplantation, single, larger plugs or, for mosaicplasty, multiple smaller cylindrical osteochondral plugs are harvested from the non-articulating or minimally articulating periphery of the patellofemoral area that bears little responsibility in *weight bearing*. These plugs are then inserted into prepared recipient sites in the defective section(s) of cartilage. Grafts harvested from the notch area are less favorable, as they have concave cartilage caps and less elastic underlying bone [10, 25]. Use of multiple smaller grafts instead of one large block may limit donor site morbidity and incongruity at the recipient site. Single plug transfers result in reduced ingrowth of fibrocartilage, and harvesting a single, larger plug may increase the risk of donor site morbidity [15, 26]. Previous experimental trials confirmed the viability of the transplanted hyaline cartilage and fibrocartilage repair of the donor sites [5–7].

Uniquely shaped fresh or fresh frozen structural allografts can be transplanted into osteochondral lesions of the talus in case of massive osteochondral defects.

This chapter discusses the general considerations of rehabilitation and the rehabilitation protocol recommended in the literature after replacement procedures when applied for the treatment of osteochondral lesions of the talus.

15.2 General Considerations

The importance of rehabilitation after cartilage resurfacing procedures is indisputable, and several factors need to be taken into account during the composition of a rehabilitation program to help the patient achieve movement and motion.

It has been proven that immobilization can lead to inadequate nutrition of the cartilage [16]; therefore, immediate full range of movement should be encouraged after all replacement procedures. This observation has been supported by a series of studies investigating the biological concept of continuous passive motion of joints for the postoperative treatment of articular injuries. It was demonstrated that the healing of articular cartilage was enhanced in rabbits by the postoperative use of continuous passive motion [19–22].

Although loading also contributes to proper nutrition, unprotected weight bearing might have a detrimental influence on integration of the bone segment of the transplanted osteochondral graft as seen in an animal study [6]. Mosaicplasty was performed either on the medial, weight bearing or on the trochlear, non-weight-bearing parts of the femoral condyles of two different knees of 18 German shepherd dogs. The dogs were not restricted in movement after surgery. Although survival of the hyaline cartilage could be observed in all cases, significant differences were found between the non-weight-bearing and the weight-bearing areas on radiological and histological examinations. The non-weight-bearing areas had surface congruity in all the cases, with satisfactory bony incorporation and no cartilage degeneration of the grafts. On the contrary, graft subsidence, necrosis of the subchondral bone, and overgrowth with fibrous or fibrocartilaginous tissue were observed in over one third of the weight-bearing cases. Based on these results, at an early stage of autologous osteochondral mosaicplasty, a longer period of postoperative non-weight bearing was recommended. Later it was observed that extended non-weight bearing does not favor tissue regeneration between grafts, and a certain level of loading is necessary for fibrous cartilage formation in the interposed tissue (instead of fibrous repair tissue), which led to shortening the sequence of non-weight bearing and lengthening the sequence of partial weight-bearing period during rehabilitation [1, 7, 11, 14].

The diameter and the number of the grafts also play a role in the determination of the length of the non-weight-bearing period. In a porcine model, single osteochondral grafts, 4.5 and 6.5 mm in diameter, and multiple grafts (3 grafts) 4.5 mm in diameter were transplanted from the trochlea to the weight-bearing area of the lateral femoral condyle [13]. The grafts were pushed in level with the surrounding cartilage surface, and also 3 mm below cartilage level afterward, and the required push-in forces were detected. It was shown that grafts greater in diameter are more stable in absolute values, and multiple grafts may not be as stable as single grafts in the initial period after transplantation. Therefore, restriction of weight bearing is recommended for a certain period of time after replacement procedures to avoid graft subsidence until bony integration occurs.

15.3 Ankle-Specific Considerations

Osteochondral lesions of the talus are difficult to access for replacement procedures, and in most cases, a malleolar osteotomy is needed for proper positioning of the grafts and the instruments. Postoperative management for the osteochondral lesion of the talus must be balanced with the recovery from the required surgical approach. If an osteotomy is necessary to approach the defect, a period of non-weight bearing and partial weight bearing must be incorporated into the rehabilitation protocol. Postoperative regimen for medial malleolar fractures is generally either functional treatment combined with early weight bearing or immobilization in a cast/orthosis for 6 weeks with non-weight bearing [24]. The intraoperative stability of the malleolar fixation also influences the surgeon's confidence in allowing early ROM or weight bearing.

15.4 Recommended Rehabilitation Protocol

After replacement procedures immediate full ROM can be permitted, the length of the non-weight-bearing and partial weight-bearing periods depends on the size of the defect and the stability of the cylindrical osteochondral autologous graft/allograft or the structural allograft and also on the stability of osteotomies or ligament repairs.

15.4.1 Recommended Rehabilitation Protocol Following Cylindrical Osteochondral Autograft and Allograft Transplantation

In case of cylindrical osteochondral autologous graft transplantation, Hangody and co-workers recommend 4 weeks of non-weight bearing, followed by 2 weeks' partial weight bearing with 30–40 kg, if a malleolar osteotomy is performed [8, 9]. When an osteotomy is not required, for example, in case of small (less than 1 cm^2) lesions, immediate weight bearing may be allowed. There are currently no biomechanical data nor level I clinical data supporting this 1-cm^2 size threshold; the recommendation is based on best practice. For larger lesions (greater than 1 cm^2), Hangody and co-workers recommend 2 weeks' partial weight bearing with 30–40 kg postoperatively. They usually allow unprotected weight bearing 4–6 weeks after surgery. Individualized rehabilitation protocols consist of additional active exercises and proprioceptive training. Depending on the clinical and radiological follow-up findings, patients are allowed to return to athletic activities approximately 4–6 months after surgery.

In a retrospective study by Scranton PE Jr and co-workers [23] on the outcome of osteochondral autograft transplantation for type V cystic osteochondral lesions of the talus, the patients remained non-weight bearing in a boot walker for 3 weeks, non-weight bearing without boot walker for the following 3 weeks, and weight bearing in the boot walker for the final 3 weeks and had routine physiotherapy afterward. A malleolar osteotomy for exposure was needed in 26 out of the examined 50 patients, and the rehabilitation protocol was uniform for all subjects.

Emre and co-workers [3] performed open mosaicplasty in osteochondral lesions of the talus with medial malleolar osteotomy in a prospective study on 32 patients, where all patients started range-of-motion exercises immediately after surgery. Weight bearing was allowed 6 weeks after surgery, following radiographic examination of the union of the medial malleolus to ensure satisfactory bone healing.

Imhoff and co-workers [12] analyzed 26 talus OATS procedures in a retrospective long-term clinical and MRI evaluation of osteochondral transplantation of the talus. Malleolar osteotomies were performed in every case when the osteochondral defect could not be reached from the anterior incision, and postoperatively a split lower leg cast was applied for 6 weeks. The postoperative protocol was partial weight bearing for 6 weeks with physiotherapy for both the knee and the ankle. Progression of weight bearing was allowed after 12 weeks when the radiological evidence of union of the osteotomy sites could be detected.

15.4.2 Recommended Rehabilitation Protocol for the Donor Knee Following Autologous Osteochondral Transplantation

Generally, the grafts for autologous osteochondral transplantation are harvested from the asymptomatic, ipsilateral knee of the patient. Macroscopic and histological evaluations of the donor areas showed that the donor sites are filled to the surface with cancellous bone and capped by fibrocartilage by 8–10 weeks, providing an acceptable gliding surface for these less weight-bearing areas [5–7]. Still, the morbidity associated with osteochondral harvest from asymptomatic knees for the treatment of osteochondral lesions of the talus remains a concern.

Hangody and co-workers found [7–9] that patients who had knee surgery only for the harvest of osteochondral plugs rarely had knee complaints. Sixty-three patients who had talar mosaicplasty were evaluated by the Bandi score, and 3 % of the patients had slight donor site disturbances. The knee complaints in 95 % of these patients resolved in 6 weeks, and in 98 % of the patients, the knee complaints resolved completely at 1 year.

Paul and co-workers [17] evaluated 200 patients who had autologous osteochondral graft obtained from an asymptomatic knee for the treatment of osteochondral defects of the talus. The patients were followed for a minimum of 2 years, and the WOMAC (Western Ontario and McMaster Universities Osteoarthritis Index) and the Lysholm score were used to examine the functional outcome. It was shown that the number and the size of the harvested grafts and the age of the patient had no influence on the functional outcome; only a higher body mass index was found to have a potentially negative effect.

To date, there is a paucity of information in the literature on the recommended protocol for the rehabilitation of the donor knee joint to improve knee function and reduce knee symptoms. The focus is on the recipient joint when determining the period of restriction in weight bearing and the start point of full weight bearing.

15.4.3 Recommended Rehabilitation Protocol Following Osteochondral Allograft Transplantation

After transplantation of fresh or fresh frozen structural allografts to osteochondral lesions of the talus, the rehabilitation process should be determined individually, taking the rate of graft incorporation, graft size, and stability at the time of procedure and fixation of osteotomy into consideration.

The intermediate outcomes of fresh talar osteochondral allografts for treatment of large osteochondral lesions of the talus were investigated by Haene and co-workers in 16 patients [4]. All talar lesions had a height ranging between 8 and 13 mm, except for one 20-mm-high lesion, and the surgical approach required a medial malleolar osteotomy in 14 cases, combined fibular and Chaput osteotomies in two ankles, and an arthrotomy in one case. After surgery, in all cases the ankle was immobilized for 10–14 days and placed in a removable walking boot afterward and early range-of-motion exercises were started. Weight bearing was allowed 6–12 weeks after surgery, depending on graft integration.

In a retrospective review, El-Rashidy and co-workers [2] report transfer of fresh osteochondral allografts in 42 patients with focal, contained, unipolar osteochondral lesion of the talus with an average lesion size of 1.5 cm^2. Postoperatively, a non-weight-bearing splint was applied for 2 weeks. After suture removal, a short leg non-weight-bearing cast was used for an additional 2 weeks. A removable short leg splint was applied at 4 weeks, and physical therapy for range of motion was started. The patients remained *non-weight bearing* for 8 weeks, and weight bearing was advanced afterward, usually *to full weight bearing* by 12 weeks.

Large-volume cystic osteochondral lesions of the talus with a mean volume of 6,059 mm^3 were treated with fresh bulk allograft transplantation in 15 patients by Raikin and co-workers [18]. The patients were restrained from weight bearing for 10–12 weeks postoperatively. Active and passive sagittal plane range of motion was allowed after suture removal (2 weeks). Formal physical therapy was started at 6 weeks and progressive protected weight bearing at 10–12 weeks. A fracture boot was used until crosstrabeculation between the graft and host talus could be detected on radiological images, at an average of 18.5 weeks (16–26 weeks) postoperatively.

Conclusions

Replacement procedures intend to restore the articular surface over osteochondral lesions of the talus by the transplantation of cylindrical autologous graft(s)/allograft(s) or structural allograft. The postoperative rehabilitation protocol should start with immediate full ROM exercises, as it promotes nutrition of the transplanted chondrocytes. Restriction in weight bearing and progression to full weight bearing is determined by the size and location of the osteochondral lesion of the talus; the type, size, and stability of the graft; and also the stability of osteotomies or ligament repairs.

Conflict of Interest The author has no current conflict of interests with the products presented

References

1. Bartha L, Vajda A, Duska ZS, Rahmeh H, Hangody L. Autologous osteochondral mosaicplasty grafting. J Orthop Sports Phys Ther. 2006;36(10):739–50.
2. El-Rashidy H, Villacis D, Omar I, Kelikian AS. Fresh osteochondral allograft for the treatment of cartilage defects of the talus: a retrospective review. J Bone Joint Surg Am. 2011;93(17):1634–40.
3. Emre TY, Ege T, Cift HT, Demircioğlu DT, Seyhan B, Uzun M. Open mosaicplasty in osteochondral lesions of the talus: a prospective study. J Foot Ankle Surg. 2012;51(5):556–60.
4. Haene R, Qamirani E, Story RA, Pinsker E, Daniels TR. Intermediate outcomes of fresh talar osteochondral allografts for treatment of large osteochondral lesions of the talus. J Bone Joint Surg Am. 2012;94(12):1105–10.
5. Hangody L, Kárpáti Z. A new surgical treatment of localised cartilaginous defects of the knee. Hung J Orthop Trauma. 1994;37:237–43.
6. Hangody L, Kish G, Kárpáti Z, et al. Autogenous osteochondral graft technique for replacing knee cartilage defects in dogs. Orthop Int Edition. 1997;5(3):175–81.
7. Hangody L, Feczkó P, Kemény D, et al. Autologous osteochondral mosaicplasty for the treatment of full thickness cartilage defects of the knee and ankle. Clin Orthop. 2001;(391 Suppl):328–37.
8. Hangody L, Kish G, Módis L, Szerb I, Gáspár L, Diószegi Z, Kendik Z. Mosaicplasty for the treatment of osteochondritis dissecans of the talus: two to seven year results in 36 patients. Foot Ankle Int. 2001;22(7):552–8.
9. Hangody L. The mosaicplasty technique for osteochondral lesions of the talus. Foot Ankle Clin . 2003;8:259–73.
10. Hangody L, Duska Z, Kárpáti Z. Osteochondral plug transplantation. In: Jackson D, editor. Master techniques in orthopaedics; the knee. Philadelphia: Lippincott Williams & Wilkins; 2008. p. 395–410.
11. Hangody L, Koreny T. Mosaicplasty. In: Cole BJ, Gomoll AH, editors. Biologic joint reconstruction. Thorofare: Slack Inc.; 2009. p. 107–17.
12. Imhoff AB, Paul J, Ottinger B, Wörtler K, Lämmle L, Spang J, Hinterwimmer S. Osteochondral transplantation of the talus long-term clinical and magnetic resonance imaging evaluation. Am J Sports Med. 2011;39(7):1487–93.
13. Kordás G, Szabó JS, Hangody L. Primary stability of osteochondral grafts used in mosaicplasty. Arthroscopy. 2006;22(4):414–21.
14. Kordás G, Szabó JS, Hangody L. The effect of drill-hole length on the primary stability of osteochondral grafts in mosaicplasty. Orthopedics. 2005;28: 401–4.
15. Martin TL, Wilson MG, Robledo J, et al. Early results of autologous bone grafting for large talar osteochondritis dissecans lesions. In: American Orthopaedic Foot and Ankle Society 29th annual meeting, Anaheim; 1999.

16. O'Hara BP, Urban JPG, Maroudas A. Influence of cyclic loading on the nutrition of articular cartilage. Ann Rheum Dis. 1990;49:536–9.
17. Paul J, Sagstetter A, Kriner M, Imhoff AB, Spang J, Hinterwimmer S. Donor-site morbidity after osteochondral autologous transplantation for lesions of the talus. J Bone Joint Surg Am. 2009;91(7):1683–8.
18. Raikin SM. Fresh osteochondral allografts for large-volume cystic osteochondral defects of the talus. J Bone Joint Surg Am. 2009;91(12):2818–26.
19. Salter RB, Ogilvie-Harris DJ. The healing of intra-articular fractures with continuous passive motion. In: Instructional Course Lectures, vol. 28. American Academy of Orthopaedic Surgeons. St. Louis: C. V. Mosby; 1979. p. 102–17.
20. Salter RB, Simmonds DE, Malcolm BW, Rumble EJ, MaclVlichael D, Clements ND. The biological effect of continuous passive motion on the healing of full-thickness defects in articular cartilage. An experimental investigation in the rabbit. J Bone and Joint Surg. 1980;62-A:1232–51.
21. Salter RB, Hamilton HW, Wedge JH, Tile M, Torode IP, O'Driscoll SW, Murnaghan JJ, Saringer JH. Clinical application of basic research on continuous passive motion for disorders and injuries of synovial joints: a preliminary report of a feasibility study. J Orthop Res. 1984;1:325–42.
22. Salter RB. The biologic concept of continuous passive motion of synovial joints. The first 18 years of basic research and its clinical application. Clin Orthop. 1989;242:12–25.
23. Scranton Jr PE, Frey CC, Feder KS. Outcome of osteochondral autograft transplantation for type V cystic osteochondral lesions of the talus. J Bone Joint Surg Br. 2006;88(5):614–9.
24. Simanski CJ, Maegele MG, Lefering R, Lehnen DM, Kawel N, Riess P, Yücel N, Tiling T, Bouillon B. Functional treatment and early weightbearing after an ankle fracture: a prospective study. J Orthop Trauma. 2006;20(2):108–14.
25. Simonian PT, Sussmann PS, Wickiewicz TL, Paletta GA, Warren RF. Contact pressures at osteochondral donor sites in the knee. Am J Sports Med. 1998;26(4):491–4.
26. Speck M, Schweinfurth M, Boerner T. Osteochondral autograft transplantation for traumatic and degenerative lesions of the talus. In: Proceedings of the 4th symposium of the International Cartilage Repair Society, Toronto; 2002.

Rehabilitation After Cartilage Reconstruction

16

Tomasz T. Antkowiak, Richard D. Ferkel,
Martin R. Sullivan, Christopher D. Kreulen, Eric Giza,
and Scott R. Whitlow

Take-Home Points

- *Effective rehabilitation plays an essential role in the success of cartilage restoration procedures. Patients who adhere to a specific rehabilitation program tend to have improved outcomes.*
- *Two primary goals of cartilage reconstruction rehabilitation protocols are local integration of the repair and a return to full strength, range of motion, and function of the joint.*
- *Rehabilitation protocols for cartilage reconstruction must carefully balance protection of the construct with the known tendency for chondrocytes to atrophy when shielded from joint motion and compressive forces.*

- *It takes 12–24 months for cartilage tissue to be fully mature. Progression through the rehabilitation protocols can be tailored based on lack of pain or swelling after specific activities. Generally, the earliest time for return to unrestricted high impact activity is 1 year.*

16.1 Introduction

Intact articular cartilage surfaces are necessary for smooth motion and pain-free function within the ankle joint. Healthy cartilage surfaces reduce the coefficient of friction, limit peaks of stress, and protect the joint from wear. Damage to the articular cartilage often leads to pain and dysfunction of the joint with limited potential for self-repair [24,

T.T. Antkowiak, MD, MS
Department of Orthopaedic Surgery,
Southern California Orthopedic Institute, University of California, Los Angeles, Van Nuys, CA, USA
e-mail: tom.antkowiak@gmail.com

R.D. Ferkel, MD (✉)
Department of Orthopaedic Surgery, University of California, Los Angeles, Los Angeles, CA, USA

Southern California Orthopedic Institute,
Van Nuys, CA, USA
e-mail: rferkel@scoi.com

M.R. Sullivan, MBBS(Hons), FRACS, FAOrthA
Department of Orthopaedic Surgery, St Vincent's Clinic, Sydney, NSW, Australia
e-mail: drmsullivan@hotmail.com

C.D. Kreulen, MD,MS
Department of Orthopaedic Surgery,
Sutter Auburn Orthopaedics, Sutter Medical Group,
Auburn, CA, USA
e-mail: ckreulen@gmail.com

E. Giza, MD
Department of Orthopaedics, Foot and Ankle Surgery
University of California, Davis, 4860 Y Street,
Suite 3800, Sacramento, CA 95817, USA
e-mail: eric.giza@ucdmc.ucdavis.edu

S.R. Whitlow, MD
Department of Orthopaedics, University of California,
Davis, 4860 Y Street, Suite 3800,
Sacramento, CA 95817, USA

C.N. van Dijk, J.G. Kennedy (eds.), *Talar Osteochondral Defects*,
DOI 10.1007/978-3-642-45097-6_16, © ESSKA 2014

36]. If patients fail conservative management of symptomatic cartilage lesions, several treatment options exist for surgical restoration. There remains controversy regarding what surgical intervention is best. However, the general goals of cartilage restoration techniques are to decrease pain and swelling, maximize function, and prevent further joint degeneration. Effective rehabilitation plays an essential role in the success of any cartilage restoration procedure. In this chapter, we discuss the critical role of rehabilitation for patients undergoing autologous chondrocyte implantation (ACI), matrix-induced autologous chondrocyte implantation (MACI), and juvenile allograft cartilage restoration procedures.

16.2 Rehabilitation After Autologous Chondrocyte Implantation

Autologous chondrocyte implantation is a cell-based technology used for the treatment of chondral defects. ACI has been in clinical use since 1987 and first demonstrated success for focal chondral lesions of the knee [6, 7, 21, 29, 32, 34]. More recently, ACI techniques have been applied for osteochondral lesions of the ankle [4, 12, 23, 33]. Indications for ACI surgery in the ankle include (1) focal contained, unipolar lesions, greater than $1–2$ cm^2 in size; (2) patient age 15–55; (3) pain unresponsive to nonoperative management; (4) persistent pain after previous drilling and/or microfracture; and (5) MRI evidence of a cartilage defect and subchondral irregularity [10, 25]. Significant functional improvements are seen for patients undergoing ACI for osteochondral lesions of the talus (OLT) at 2–5-year follow-up [31]. More recently this same group of patients has been evaluated at a longer follow-up period of 2–10 years [10, 25].

To achieve maximum potential from cartilage restoration procedures, surgeons must ensure appropriate indications, diagnostic workup, technical precision, and adherence to postoperative rehabilitation protocols. The potential benefits of ACI are enhanced when patients are well informed, not only regarding the surgical intervention but also the rehabilitation protocol that will follow. Patients who adhere to a specific rehabilitation

program tend to have improved outcomes [1, 2, 17]. There are two primary goals for an ACI rehabilitation program. The first is local integration and remodeling of the repair. The second is a return to full strength, range of motion, and function of the joint. The challenge is to progressively increase strength and motion while optimizing and protecting integration of the repair site.

Rehabilitation protocols are constructed to take into account the four stages of recovery: (1) healing phase, (2) transitional phase, (3) remodeling phase, and (4) maturation phase [20, 27].

16.2.1 Phase I: The Healing Phase (Weeks 0–6)

The implanted autologous chondrocytes are in the early stages of healing. During this phase, the cells and the overlying patch construct are vulnerable to shear stresses within the joint. However, protection of the construct must be carefully balanced with the known tendency for chondrocytes to atrophy when shielded from joint motion and compressive forces [8]. To achieve this balance, patients are limited to partial weight bearing less than 30 lb in a Cam walker. Range of motion exercises are initiated at 2 weeks postoperatively. Stationary bike activities without resistance are started at 4 weeks. At 6 weeks, patients are placed in a lace-up figure-of-eight brace with tennis shoes, and formal physical therapy is initiated. Physical therapy during phase I focuses on proprioception, motion, and prevention of muscle atrophy (Fig. 16.1). We prescribe isometric exercises for the ankle plantar and dorsiflexors, the toe flexors and extensors, as well as the quadriceps and hamstring muscle groups. In addition to the stationary cycling, we also recommend low-impact activities like swimming or aqua-therapy. Weight bearing is gradually advanced to full weight bearing at 6–8 weeks. The primary goal of phase I is to achieve full range of motion of the ankle by 6 weeks.

16.2.2 Phase II: The Transitional Phase (Weeks 6–12)

The transitional phase is characterized by early maturation of chondrocytes that become less vulnerable

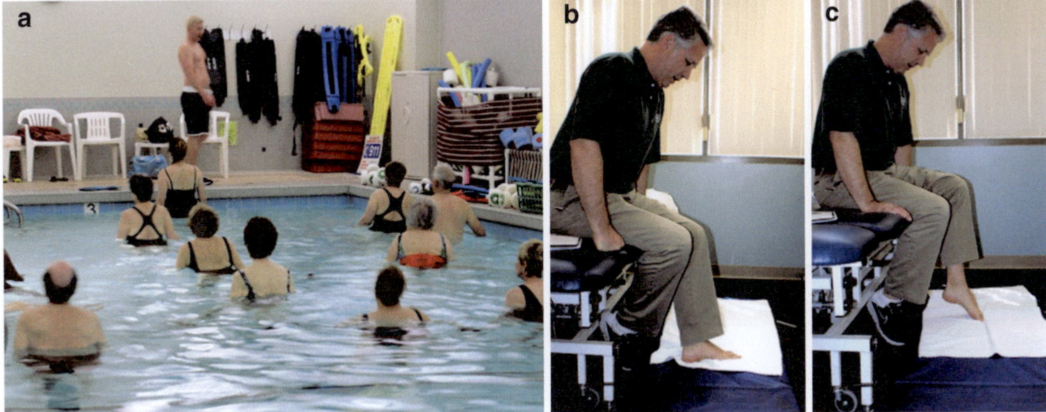

Fig. 16.1 Phase I rehabilitation exercises. Physical therapy during phase I focuses on proprioception, motion, and prevention of muscle atrophy. (**a**) Pool therapy – low-impact activities like swimming or aquatherapy. Range of motion exercises for: (**b**) inversion and eversion (**c**) plantar and dorsiflexion

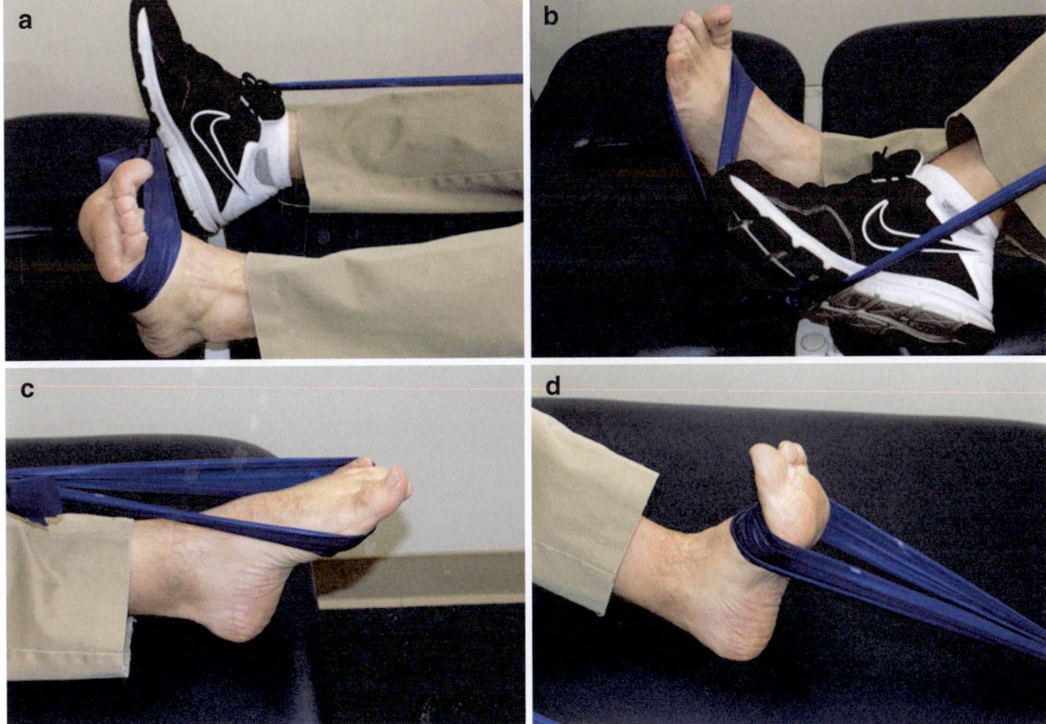

Fig. 16.2 Phase II rehabilitation exercises. Physical therapy during phase II focuses on proprioceptive exercises, isometric and then eccentric strengthening, and closed kinetic chain presses on a progressive basis. Resistive band strengthening for: (**a**) eversion, (**b**) inversion, (**c**) plantar flexion, (**d**) dorsiflexion

to shear forces. At this point, the growing cartilage patch is spongy, and often soft, but durable enough to tolerate increased compressive forces [16]. Physical therapy during phase II should include proprioceptive exercises, isometric and then eccentric strengthening, and closed kinetic chain presses on a progressive basis (Fig. 16.2). The stationary bicycle should be continued with gradually increased resistance. The goal of rehabilitation in phase II is to continue strengthening the periarticular muscles and increasing proprioception in preparation for more high-demand activity in phase III.

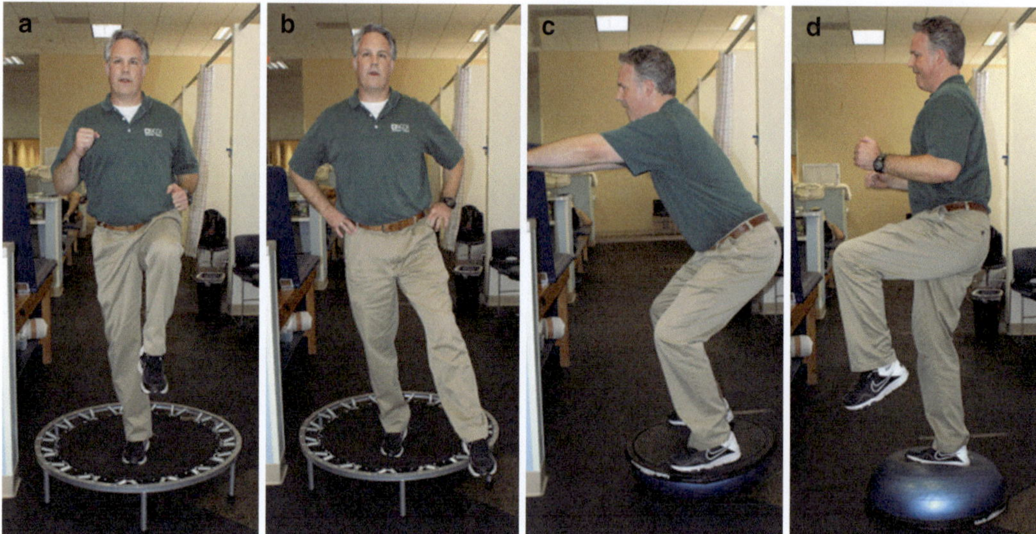

Fig. 16.3 Phase III rehabilitation exercises. Physical therapy during phase III focuses on improving strength and endurance as well as continued progressive proprioception and coordination training especially in weight-bearing positions. Single-leg balance exercise on mini trampoline with (**a**) flexion and extension of the leg and (**b**) abduction/adduction of the leg. (**c**) Progressive balance and proprioception exercises using the flat and (**d**) rounded portions of a wobble board

16.2.3 Phase III: The Remodeling Phase (Weeks 12–32)

At 3 months postoperatively, the graft is becoming firm while it continues to mature. At this point, walking distance and speed can be increased as tolerated by the patient. The goals in this phase are to increase active strengthening and to continue progressive proprioception and coordination training especially in weight-bearing positions (Fig. 16.3). As strength and endurance continue to improve, the patient can gradually return to jogging and running by 6 months. At the end of phase III, patients are assessed for progress in anticipation of possible advancement to light sports-specific activity. To progress to stage IV, patients should demonstrate no pain or swelling after 30 min of weight-bearing exercise as well as full and pain free range of motion.

16.2.4 Phase IV: The Maturation Phase (Weeks 32–54)

Remodeling and maturation of the graft can continue for up to 2 years post operatively [14, 38]. However, by 8 months, the graft is considered stable and mature enough to tolerate sports and higher impact activities. Rehabilitation can now be focused on cross-training and return to sport (Fig. 16.4). Therapists can increase training intensity, load, and volume while maintaining a focus on proper/safe technique. Adequate periods of rest are important as athletes likely remain deconditioned compared to preoperative levels. Progression can continue to occur as long as patients have no pain or swelling after specific activities. Generally, the earliest time for return to unrestricted high-impact activity is 52 weeks.

This four stage protocol and its associated timeline provide the necessary balance between graft protection and return to full strength, range of motion, and function of the joint [31]. The effectiveness of the protocol is further enhanced when it is administered by a knowledgeable physical therapist who is familiar with specific precautions and expectations associated with ACI.

16.3 Rehabilitation After Matrix-Induced Autologous Chondrocyte Implantation

For those patients who fail arthroscopic microfracture of OTL, matrix-induced autologous chondrocyte implantation (MACI) has possibilities with its

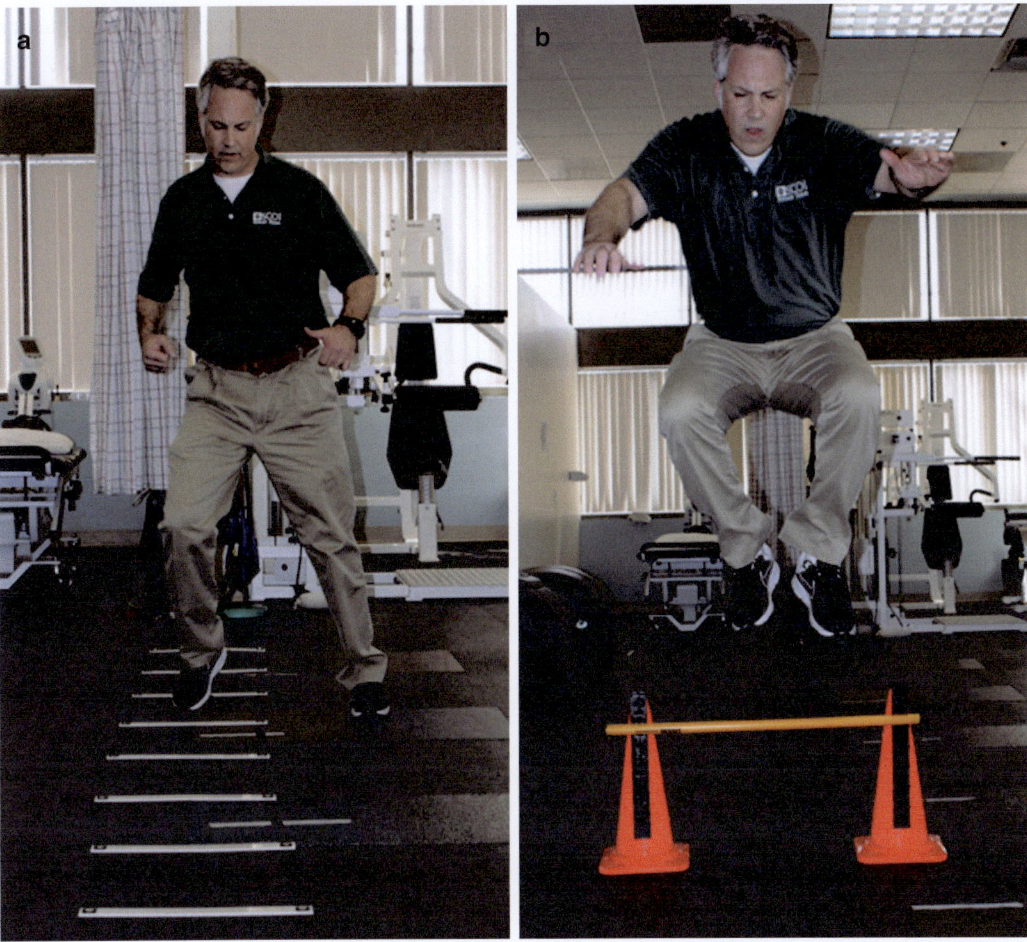

Fig. 16.4 Phase IV rehabilitation exercises. Physical therapy during phase IV focuses on agility, cross-training, and return to sport-specific exercise. (**a**) Lateral motion training on the agility ladder, (**b**) progressive height jump training

potential to generate hyaline-like cartilage [3, 5, 39]. MACI is a second-generation ACI technique used for the treatment of osteochondral defects. Specifically, chondrocytes are harvested from the patient's damaged cartilage [5, 11] during their initial ankle arthroscopy and amplified up to 20–50 times via cell culture. These chondrocytes are then placed onto a 3-dimensional collagen matrix and implanted on the articular defect with fibrin glue [5, 9, 13–15, 19, 26, 30, 35, 37]. This procedure has been performed via an arthrotomy [18, 19]. It can also be performed using an osteotomy of the medial or lateral malleolus. However, osteotomy adds morbidity and can negatively affect patient outcomes [11]. Arthroscopic techniques have also been reported for MACI insertion [14].

Regardless of the technique, postoperative rehabilitation needs to consider the gradual maturation of the repair tissue when designing a postoperative program [16]. As with ACI, the healing tissues associated with MACI must be protected but also stimulated to allow maturation and remodeling. Initial strengthening and range of motion (ROM) exercises are important and should be performed under a controlled environment with gradual progression to limit joint reaction forces and possible shear forces. Joint movement will aid in cartilage growth through the diffusion of the synovial fluid and changes in intra-articular pressure, providing a stimulus for chondrocytes thus promoting healing and maturation [22]. As the healing MACI implant progresses through the stages of healing, the cartilage can accommodate a greater amount of force, tension, and impact. It takes 12–24 months for cartilage tissue to be fully mature [34], which makes the proper rehabilitation very important to a successful long-term outcome.

The short term goals (0–12 weeks) of this protocol work on slowly progressing weight bearing while preventing the deleterious effects of immobilization and rest, including arthrofibrosis, joint adhesions, muscle atrophy, and pain. The long-term goals (>12 weeks) are focused on returning the patient to a normal gait pattern. This includes normal weight-bearing and movement restoration. The important aspects of this protocol are range of motion (ROM) exercises, weight-bearing, strengthening, and the continual progression of these. The goal is to continue to increase the patients' level of function over 12 months and return them to their previous level of pain-free activity.

16.3.1 Phase I: The Healing Phase (Weeks 0–6)

The first 6 weeks is the proliferative stage of healing. During this time, the rehabilitation is focused on decreasing swelling, improving range of motion, preventing adhesions, and conservatively increasing the weight-bearing status. The rehabilitation must begin to create the environment that encourages the cells to proliferate while preventing a certain amount of deconditioning. The goal is to ensure that the implant is strong enough and does not become damaged, disrupted, or displaced by the sheer forces of weight bearing.

At 2 weeks the dressing, splint, and sutures are removed. The patient is placed into a CAM walker boot that is to be worn at all times except during physiotherapy, home exercises, and showering. The patient must maintain strict non-weight bearing (NWB) with crutches at this time. During the 2–4-week post-op period, plantar flexion-dorsiflexion, inversion, and eversion ankle ROM exercises are started under the guidance of a therapist. The therapist also begins manual joint manipulations and gentle scar massage. Strengthening of the intrinsic foot muscles is also initiated.

At the 4–6 week postoperative period, the patient continues to do the same exercises along with hydrotherapy and isometric strengthening of the ankle. From our experience, hydrotherapy provides a great benefit in the rehabilitation process, and we prefer to get the patient in chest high water for all exercises. These exercises include walking forward, backward, sideways, heel raises, cycling in water, and single leg balance. Touchdown weight bearing (TDWB) is started on week 5. Marlovits and coworkers [28] looked at MRI results for MACI in the knee and showed that in 14/16 patients the MACI implant had complete attachment at 34.7 days on the femoral condyle. Thus, on an average of 5–6 weeks, the MACI graft should be completely attached and be able to withstand the forces of weight bearing.

16.3.2 Phase II: The Transitional Phase (Weeks 6–12)

At 6–12 weeks postoperatively, the aim is to increase weight bearing, begin gait reeducation, and restore ROM ankle to normal levels. There is a balance between trying to apply a healthy gradual increase of applied and functional stress to provide a stimulus for the continued healing of the tissue without causing damage to the graft. At week 6, the transition to full weight bearing (FWB) begins and Thera-band strengthening exercises are initiated. Sliding foot-stretching exercises and the exercise bike with no resistance and at low speed are started as well. Joint mobilizations and soft tissue massage should also continue during this time to continue to reduce the amount of swelling. Our experience has shown us that patients will begin to have an increase in pain once they start their weight-bearing transition. Flare-ups occur and the treatment protocol should be adjusted to these on a patient-to-patient basis.

16.3.3 Phase III: The Remodeling Phase (Weeks 12–32)

During weeks 12–6 month postoperatively, remodeling of the graft continues as it further matures. The goals of the rehabilitation protocol at this point are to gradually return to more functional activity, while avoiding high-impact exercise such as running and jumping. Progressive proprioception and strengthening continue and exercises are mainly closed chain. Footwear is also a concern because as patients become more comfortable, they may attempt to wear shoes that are not supportive enough or provide undesired increases in sheer stress or joint force on the graft. Counseling in this area should be a focus throughout the rehabilitation, but especially as the patient begins to ambulate more comfortably.

During the 12–18 week period, the patient is taken out of the boot but is not allowed to have more impact on the joint besides walking. Single leg balance on the floor and transitioning to a pillow are introduced to improve stability and proprioception. More focused stretching and strengthening of the gastrocnemius soleus, including eccentric and concentric calf-raises, are initiated. As the patient continues to improve, a mini trampoline can also be used. The exercise bike is continued for increasing lengths of time and gradual increases in resistance.

The 18–24-week protocol continues to advance the previous activities but still limits high-impact exercises. Wobble board training is started and progression in the time of walking exercises continues. At 6 months the graft will be stable enough to continue to increase balance training and start a gradual increase of impact activities with an aim for full impact activity at 12 months. There have been some MACI rehab protocols of the knee that are more aggressive than this; however, we feel a more conservative approach to this rehab is warranted because of the higher stresses experienced by the talar cartilage.

The MACI procedure previously described has been performed on over 80 patients at our institution (MRS) since 2004. The current protocol was instituted in 2008 and has been used with 26 patients. There were 13 female and 13 male patients in this group. The average age was 38 years old. We have found proper rehabilitation especially important in this group of patients who have often already undergone 2–3 previous surgeries [19]. It is important for patients to have realistic expectations regarding their ankle. We counsel patients that it is unlikely their joint will become completely normal, but it will improve

and they should have little to no pain at the time of full recovery. The protocol may need to be adjusted and individualized to fit particular patients' needs. Overall, we have found our patients to progress well with this rehabilitation protocol, and compliance is generally excellent.

16.4 Rehabilitation After Juvenile Allograft Cartilage Implantation

Ankle arthroscopy is an effective means for the diagnosis and treatment of painful chondral and osteochondral lesions of the talus or tibia. Up to 86 % of patients have been shown to improve with arthroscopic debridement, curettage, and microfracture [38]. The goal of this surgery is to reduce the symptoms of pain and swelling, improve function in the ankle, and aim to prevent secondary osteoarthritis of the ankle. These arthroscopic techniques result in fibrocartilage repair of the defect that has altered biomechanical properties to native articular cartilage [23, 39]. For those patients who fail arthroscopic treatment of these lesions, juvenile allograft NT Natural Tissue Graft (Zimmer Inc., Warsaw, IN) provides possibilities for functional improvement with its potential to generate hyaline-like cartilage.

Juvenile allograft transplantation (DeNovo) is a chondrocyte implantation technique used for the treatment of osteochondral defects. It involves scaffold-free transplantation of particulated juvenile cartilage placed on a bed of prepared bone covered with fibrin glue within the patient's OCD lesion. Each patient will have undergone the necessary work-up and initial conservative treatment prior to ankle arthroscopy. Generally, they have already undergone and failed microfracture and continue to be symptomatic. If the patient has ligamentous laxity, it should be addressed at the time of juvenile allograft transplantation.

16.4.1 Brief Description of Procedure

After induction of general anesthesia, the operative leg is exsanguinated and the remainder of the procedure is performed in a blood-less field under tourniquet. The leg is placed in a holder and an ankle distractor is applied, ideally providing 4–5 mm of distraction. Standard anteromedial and anterolateral portals are made, followed by standard ankle arthroscopy with debridement if necessary. The OCD lesion is identified and debrided to subchondral bone with a circumferentially stable border. This is followed by microfracture to prepare the bed for allograft. The joint is then drained completely, and the portal closest to the lesion is extended. Cotton swabs are used to dry the bed of the defect. A small amount of fibrin glue is placed in the base of the lesion. A 2.9 mm cannula is then inserted through a slightly enlarged portal. Under arthroscopic visualization, the graft is passed down the cannula and deposited onto the lesion until the level of the allograft reaches the height of the surrounding stable border. The graft is then covered with fibrin glue and allowed to cure for at least 4 min. The entire procedure is completed within one surgical setting, as opposed to two for MACI, allowing the healing and rehabilitation process to start immediately. We use a similar rehab protocol for juvenile allograft as we do for MACI, keeping in mind the time course for cartilage maturation and remodeling, which we feel is similar between the two procedures. Using this protocol, we have noted good to excellent AOFAS scores at an average of 16 months follow-up (unpublished data).

16.4.2 Rehabilitation

With this technique, as with others mentioned in this chapter, postoperative rehabilitation is of the utmost importance to optimize a patient's recovery and return the patient to their previous level of activity, while making sure to not damage the graft during the healing process. Rehabilitation needs to consider the gradual maturation of the repair tissue when designing a postoperative program [16]. Healing tissue must be protected but also stimulated to allow maturation and remodeling. A premature overload of the tissue will increase the likelihood of a

failure. Initial strengthening and ROM exercises are important; however, they should be under a controlled environment with gradual progression to limit joint reaction forces and possible shear forces. ROM exercises will aid in cartilage growth through the diffusion of the synovial fluid and changes in intra-articular pressure, providing a stimulus for chondrocyte activity within the matrix to promote healing and maturation [22]. There are three phases observed in the juvenile allograft cartilage healing process: the proliferative phase, the transition or matrix producing phase, and the remodeling and maturation phase. As each phase progresses, the healing cartilage can accommodate a greater amount of force, tension, and impact without sustaining damage. It takes 12–24 months for cartilage tissue to be fully mature [34], which makes the proper rehabilitation very important to a successful long-term outcome. The authors use the same physical therapy protocols for patients receiving MACI grafts and those receiving juvenile allograft.

Conclusions

Effective and safe rehabilitation plays an essential role in the success of cartilage restoration procedures including ACI, MACI, and juvenile allograft. Rehabilitation protocols for cartilage reconstruction must carefully balance protection of the construct with the known tendency for chondrocytes to atrophy when shielded from joint motion and compressive forces. The primary goals of these rehabilitation protocols are to aid in local integration of the repair while optimizing a return to full strength, range of motion, and function of the joint. Patients who adhere to these programs tend to have improved postoperative functional outcomes. It takes 12–24 months for cartilage tissue to be fully mature. Generally, the earliest time for return to unrestricted high-impact activity is 1 year.

Conflict of Interest The author has no current conflict of interests with the products presented

References

1. Alford JW, Cole BJ. Cartilage restoration, part 1: basic science, historical perspective, patient evaluation, and treatment options. Am J Sports Med. 2005;33:295–306.

2. Alford JW, Cole BJ. Cartilage restoration, part 2: techniques, outcomes, and future directions. Am J Sports Med. 2005;33:443–60.

3. Aurich M, Bedi HS, Smith PJ, Rolauffs B, Muckley T, Clayton J, Blackney M. Arthroscopic treatment of osteochondral lesions of the ankle with matrix-associated chondrocyte implantation: early clinical and magnetic resonance imaging results. Am J Sports Med. 2011;39(2):311–9.

4. Bazaz R, Ferkel RD. Treatment of osteochondral lesions of the talus with autologous chondrocyte implantation. Tech Foot Ankle Surg. 2004;3(1): 45–52.

5. Biosurgery G. Carticel Package Insert. Edited June 2007. Genzyme Biosurgery, A division of Genzyme Corporation. http://www.carticel.com. Cambridge, MA.

6. Breinan H, Minas T, Hsu HP, Nehrer S, Sledge CB, Spector M. Effect of cultured autologous chondrocytes on repair of chondral defects in a canine model. J Bone Joint Surg Am. 1997;79:1439–51.

7. Brittberg M, Lindahl A, Nilsson A, Ohlsson C, Isaksson O, Peterson L. Treatment of deep cartilage defects in the knee with autologous chondrocyte transplantation. N Engl J Med. 1994;331:889–95.

8. Brittberg M, Peterson L, Sjogren-Jansson E, Tallheden T, Lindahl A. Articular cartilage engineering with autologous chondrocyte transplantation: a review of recent developments. J Bone Joint Surg Am. 2003;85 Suppl 3:109–15.

9. Cherubino P, Grassi FA, Bulgheroni P, Ronga M. Autologous chondrocyte implantation using a bilayer collagen membrane: a preliminary report. J Orthop Surg (Hong Kong). 2003;11(1):10–5.

10. Chin TY, Mussett S, Ferkel R, Glazebrook M, Tak-Choy Lau J. Osteochondral lesions of the talar dome: autologous chondrocyte implantation. In: Johnson DH, Amendola A, Field LD, Richmond JC, Sgaglione NA, editors. Operative arthroscopy. 4th ed. Philadelphia: Lippincott Williams & Wilkins; 2013. p. 1024–34.

11. Dixon S, Harvey L, Baddour E, Janes G, Hardisty G. Functional outcome of matrix-associated autologous chondrocyte implantation in the ankle. Foot Ankle Int. 2011;32(4):368–74.

12. Giannini S, Buda R, Grigolo B, Vannini F. Autologous chondrocytes transplantation in osteochondral lesions of the ankle joint. Foot Ankle Int. 2001;22:513–7.

13. Giannini S, Buda R, Grigolo B, Vannini F, De Franceschi L, Facchini A. The detached osteochondral fragment as a source of cells for autologous chondrocyte implantation (ACI) in the ankle joint. Osteoarthritis Cartilage. 2005;13(7):601–7.

14. Giannini S, Buda R, Vannini F, Di Caprio F, Grigolo B. Arthroscopic autologous chondrocyte implantation in osteochondral lesions of the talus: surgical technique and results. Am J Sports Med. 2008;36(5): 873–80.

15. Gibson AJ, McDonnell SM, Price AJ. Matrix-induced autologous chondrocyte implantation. Oper Tech Orthop. 2006;16(4):262–5.

16. Gillogly SD, Myers TH. Treatment of full-thickness chondral defects with autologous chondrocyte implantation. Orthop Clin North Am. 2005;36(4): 433–46.

17. Gillogly SD, Voight M, Blackburn T. Treatment of articular cartilage defects of the knee with autologous chondrocyte implantation. J Orthop Sports Phys Ther. 1998;28:241–51.

18. Giza E, Nathe R, Kim J. Talus osteochondritis dissecans: treatment with matrix-based autologous chondrocyte implantation. Tech Orthop. 2010;25(4): 231–6.

19. Giza E, Sullivan M, Ocel D, et al. Matrix-induced autologous chondrocyte implantation of talus articular defects. Foot Ankle Int. 2010;31(9):747–53.

20. Hambly K, Bobic V, Wondrasch B, Van Assche D, Marlovits S. Autologous chondrocyte implantation postoperative care and rehabilitation. Am J Sports Med. 2006;34:1020–38.

21. Horas U, Pelinkovic D, Herr G, Aigner T, Schnettler R. Autologous chondrocyte implantation and osteochondral cylinder transplantation in cartilage repair of the knee joint: a prospective, comparative trial. J Bone Joint Surg Am. 2003;85:185–92.

22. Ikenoue T, Trindade MC, Lee MS, Lin EY, Schurman DJ, Goodman SB, Smith RL. Mechanoregulation of human articular chondrocyte aggrecan and type II collagen expression by intermittent hydrostatic pressure in vitro. J Orthop Res. 2003;21(1):110–6.

23. Koulalis D, Schultz W, Heyden M. Autologous chondrocyte transplantation for osteochondritis dissecans of the talus. Clin Orthop Relat Res. 2002;395: 186–92.

24. Krishnan SP, Skinner JA, Carrington RW, Flanagan AM, Briggs TW, Bentley G. Collagen-covered autologous chondrocyte implantation for osteochondritis dissecans of the knee: two- to seven-year results. J Bone Joint Surg Br. 2006;88:203–5.

25. Kwak S, Ferkel RD. Autologous chondrocyte implantation of the ankle: 2 to 10 year follow-up. AAOS annual meeting podium presentation, San Diego; 2011. Submitted for publication.

26. Lynn AK, Brooks RA, Bonfield W, Rushton N. Repair of defects in articular joints. Prospects for material-based solutions in tissue engineering. J Bone Joint Surg Br. 2004;86(8):1093–9.

27. Mandelbaum BR, Gerhardt MB, Peterson L. Autologous chondrocyte implantation of the talus. Arthroscopy. 2003;19 Suppl 1:129–37.

28. Marlovits S, Striessnig G, Kutscha-Lissberg F, Resinger C, Aldrian SM, Vecsei V, Trattnig S. Early postopera-

tive adherence of matrix-induced autologous chondrocyte implantation for the treatment of full-thickness cartilage defects of the femoral condyle. Knee Surg Sports Traumatol Arthrosc. 2005;13(6):451–7.

29. Minas T, Peterson L. Chondrocyte transplantation. Oper Tech Orthop. 1997;4:323–33.

30. Mitchell ME, Giza E, Sullivan MR. Cartilage transplantation techniques for talar cartilage lesions. J Am Acad Orthop Surg. 2009;17(7):407–14.

31. Nam E, Ferkel R, Applegate G. Autologous chondrocyte implantation of the ankle. A 2- to 5-year follow-up. Am J Sports Med. 2009;37(2):274–84.

32. Peterson L, Brittberg M, Kiviranta I, Akerlund EL, Lindahl A. Autologous chondrocytes transplantation: biomechanics and long-term durability. Am J Sports Med. 2002;30:2–12.

33. Peterson L, Brittberg M, Lindahl A. Autologous chondrocyte trans-plantation of the ankle. Foot Ankle Clin. 2003;8:291–303.

34. Peterson L, Minas T, Brittberg M, Nilsson A, Sjogren-Jansson E, Lindahl A. Two- to 9-year outcome after autologous chondrocyte transplantation of the knee. Clin Orthop Relat Res. 2000;374:212–34.

35. Ronga M, Grassi FA, Montoli C, Bulgheroni P, Genovese E, Cherubino P. Treatment of deep cartilage defects of the ankle with matrix-induced autologous chondrocyte implantation (MACI). Foot Ankle Surg. 2005;11(1):29–33.

36. Salter RB, Simmonds DF, Malcolm BW, Rumble EJ, MacMichael D, Clements ND. The biological effect of continuous passive motion on the healing of full-thickness defects in articular cartilage: an experimental investigation in the rabbit. J Bone Joint Surg Am. 1980;62:1232–51.

37. Schneider TE, Karaikudi S. Matrix-Induced Autologous Chondrocyte Implantation (MACI) grafting for osteochondral lesions of the talus. Foot Ankle Int. 2009;30(9):810–4.

38. Schuman L, Struijs PA, van Dijk CN. Arthroscopic treatment for osteochondral defects of the talus. Results at follow-up at 2 to 11 years. J Bone Joint Surg Br. 2002;84(3):364–8.

39. Zheng MH, King E, Kirilak Y, Huang L, Papadimitriou JM, Wood DJ, Xu J. Molecular characterisation of chondrocytes in autologous chondrocyte implantation. Int J Mol Med. 2004;13(5):623–8.

Mikel L. Reilingh and C. Niek van Dijk

Take-Home Points

- *A new metallic implantation technique for secondary osteochondral defects of the medial talar dome appears to be a promising treatment option.*
- *The surface of the prosthetic device should be placed slightly recessed relative to the surrounding surface of the talar cartilage.*
- *Clinical and radiological short-term follow-up are encouraging; however, more patients and longer follow-up are clearly needed to draw any firm conclusions.*

17.1 Introduction

In 62 % of osteochondral defects of the talus (OCDs), the defect is located on the medial talar dome [6]. These medial defects are generally deep and cup-shaped [4]. An OCD may sometimes heal and stabilize but often progresses to a cystic lesion causing deep ankle pain on weight bearing, prolonged swelling, diminished range of motion, and synovitis [15, 25].

Arthroscopic debridement and bone marrow stimulation is considered the primary treatment and yields 85 % success [29]. In case of failure of the primary treatment, current secondary treatment options include osteochondral autograft transfer, autogenous bone graft, and autologous chondrocyte implantation [3, 8, 9, 20]. However, these techniques are sometimes associated with donor site morbidity, involve two-stage surgery, or poor graft integration [2, 12–14].

For treatment of large lesions of the medial talar dome or after failed primary treatment, a contoured articular inlay implant (HemiCAP®, Arthrosurface Inc., Franklin, MA, USA) with a fixed diameter of 15 mm has been developed [24]. Its goals are to offer relief of pain, return to activity, and prevent degeneration/further cyst formation. There are two components: a Cobalt-Chromium articular component and a Titanium screw. Fifteen articular component offset sizes are available, based on the surface geometry of the medial talar dome. The offset sizes have been found appropriate for a variety of talar specimens in a cadaveric study [24]. Since October 2007, this implant has been used in our institution in patients with persistent complaints more than 1 year after primary surgical treatment of a large osteochondral defect of the medial talar dome

M.L. Reilingh, MD, PhD (✉)
Orthopaedic Research Centre Amsterdam,
Department of Orthopaedic Surgery, Academic
Medical Center, University of Amsterdam,
Amsterdam, The Netherlands
e-mail: m.l.reilingh@amc.uva.nl

C.N. van Dijk, MD, PhD
Department of Orthopaedic Surgery and
Traumatology, Academic Medical Center, University
of Amsterdam, Amsterdam, The Netherlands
e-mail: c.n.vandijk@amc.uva.nl

C.N. van Dijk, J.G. Kennedy (eds.), *Talar Osteochondral Defects*,
DOI 10.1007/978-3-642-45097-6_17, © ESSKA 2014

(anterior-posterior or medial-lateral diameter >12 mm on CT) [21]. Contraindications of this procedure are age <18 years, OCD size >20 mm, ankle osteoarthritis grade II or III [26], concomitant ankle pathology (tibial OCD, instability, fracture <6 months old, tendonitis), diabetes mellitus, advanced osteoporosis, infection, and a known allergy to the implant material. However, these indications/contraindications are not strict because the HemiCap is still in the experimental stage.

17.2   Surgical Technique

The procedure is carried out under general or spinal anesthesia. The patient is placed in the supine position with a tourniquet applied around the upper leg and a rolled-up apron underneath the lateral malleolus to facilitate eversion of the foot and improve exposure of the talus. A curved skin incision of approximately 7 cm is made over the medial malleolus. The anterior skin is mobilized using a scalpel and forceps, and a skin retractor is placed to retract the skin. A Hohmann retractor is placed over the distal tibia. A small anterior arthrotomy exposes the anteromedial talar dome. The level of this anterior superior border of the talar dome will later in the procedure act as a guide to identify the level of the posterior ankle joint. Next, the sheath of the posterior tibial tendon is incised and another Hohmann retractor is placed posterior to the medial malleolus and anterior to the posterior tibial tendon. The posterior capsule of the ankle joint can be visualized now and incised. The posterior intersection between the medial malleolus and tibial plafond is identified using an arthroscopic probe. The surgeon carefully inserts the 5-mm tip of the probe in the posteromedial joint space by sliding along the posterior aspect of the distal tibia at the intersection with the medial malleolus and gently pulls in an oblique craniomedial direction [22]. This maneuver identifies the posterior part of the intersection between the tibial plafond and medial malleolus. The periosteum at the level of the intended osteotomy is marked with a surgical knife, sterile marker pen, or osteotome. Next, the probe is placed in the anteromedial tibial notch

and pulled in an oblique craniomedial direction, identifying the anterior part of the intersection. The anterior intersection is marked, and this is connected to the posterior intersection as a reference guide to the osteotomy. Before creating the osteotomy, two screw holes are predrilled and tapped in the medial malleolus, using a cannulated drill. An oscillating saw is placed on the incised periosteum and directed at the marked intersection of the tibial plafond and medial malleolus. The osteotomy is created up to approximately 2 mm above the articular cartilage, while two Hohmann retractors protect the adjacent soft tissue. The optimal angle for the osteotomy has determined to be at a mean angle of 30° relative to the long tibial axis [23]. The osteotomy is completed with the use of an osteotome. This way, the surgeon controls the osteotomy of the articular surface and minimizes the risk of damaging the talar cartilage. After the osteotomy has been completed, the surgeon manually retracts and everts the medial malleolus using gauze. Optionally, the distal part is temporarily transfixed by drilling a large diameter K-wire into the talus through one of the predrilled holes (Fig. 17.1). Exposure of the talar dome is improved by forced eversion of the heel. The fibula is hereby used as a fulcrum (take care not to use too much force) and the talus is tilted.

The necrotic fragment of the defect can now be identified and debrided. Utilizing a drill guide, a guide pin is placed into the center of the defect, perpendicular to the curvature of the medial talar dome. The guide pin ensures that a perpendicular direction is maintained throughout the procedure. The titanium screw of the metal implant is inserted after drilling a pilot hole. A contact probe is used to determine the radius of curvature in the sagittal and coronal planes to allow for a precise fit of the articular component to the existing articular surface. A matching reamer prepares the site for placement of the articular component. The reamer is a cannulated instrument used over the guide pin with a diameter of 15 mm. A sizing trial with corresponding offsets allows for final verification of proper fit. The selected articular component is oriented into the correct planes and is placed on the screw. It is impacted with a gentle hammer-stroke on an

Fig. 17.1 The osteochondral defect (*arrow*) is exposed through an oblique medial malleolar osteotomy. A K-wire can be inserted into the talus through one of the predrilled holes to hold the medial malleolus in place

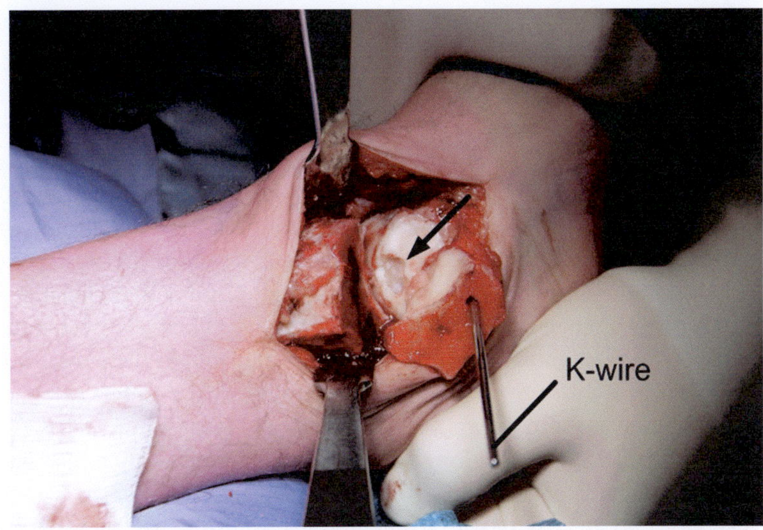

Fig. 17.2 Final view after the articular component (*arrow*) is oriented into the correct planes and is placed on the screw. Note that the edges of the implant are slightly recessed (approximately 0.5 mm) compared to the adjacent cartilage level

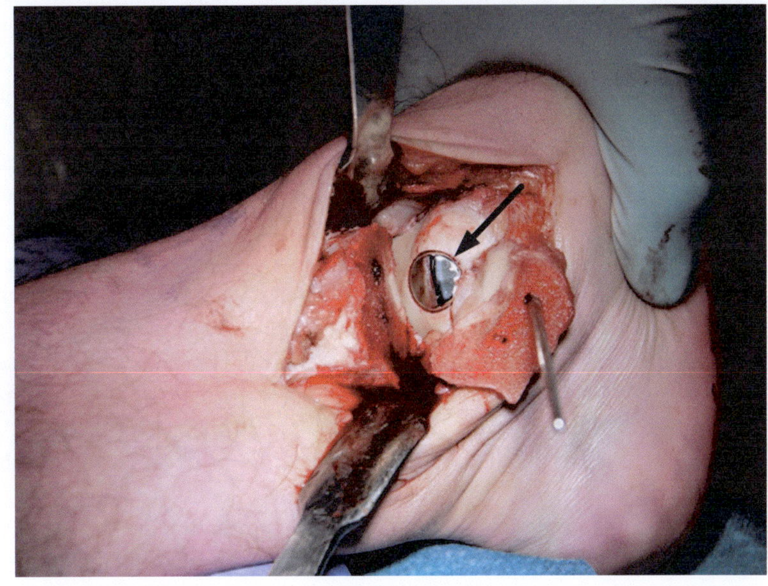

instrument with a plastic tip, thereby engaging the taper interlock (Fig. 17.2). After the confirmation of slightly recessed implant edges, the osteotomy is reduced. Initially, large diameter K-wires are placed through the predrilled screw holes to confirm correct alignment. A Weber bone clamp can be placed for initial compression. Placement of the proximal leg of the Weber clamp is facilitated by creating a small hole in the distal tibial cortex proximal to the osteotomy using a 2.5-mm drill. We routinely use two 3.5-mm cancellous lag screws with a length of 40 or 45 mm. The posterior tibial tendon sheath is not repaired and the wound is closed with Ethilon 3.0 sutures using a vertical mattress (Donati) technique.

17.3 Rehabilitation

The postoperative management consists of a plaster cast for 1 week. A functional non-weight-bearing brace (Walker) or a detachable plaster cast can be applied for another 5 weeks. During this period, non-weight-bearing sagittal range of motion exercises are allowed, i.e., 15 min twice daily. After these 6 weeks, radiographs of the operated ankle are obtained to confirm consolidation of the malleolar osteotomy. Subsequently, physical therapy is prescribed to assist in functional recovery and facilitate the return to full weight bearing over approximately 1 month. Return to normal weight bearing and walking should thus be accomplished 10 weeks after surgery. Impact activities, such as running, are allowed when no signs of prosthetic loosening and migration are seen after 6 months of follow-up. Non-contact sports are allowed after 9 months of follow-up and contact sports 1 year after surgery. However, the risk of periprosthetic fracture during contact sports should be discussed with the patient. We reported the first clinical case report of the talus implant in which the patient was able to play korfball (contact sports) at the preinjury level after 1 year and continued to play at this level at 2 years follow-up [21].

17.4 Discussion

Treatment of osteochondral lesions or osteonecrosis by means of metal resurfacing implants is relatively new, and the literature is scarce. Promising clinical results have been reported for the treatment of the femoral [27] and humeral head [18], as well as the first metatarsal [10] and patellar surface [5]. Two biomechanical cadaveric studies provided foundations for use of the talus implant in the ankle joint [1, 24]. We performed a prospective case series of 15 patients with a clinical follow-up of 1 year [16]. All patients had failed prior surgical treatment of a large defect of the medial talar dome. Failed prior surgical treatments were debridement and bone marrow stimulation, cancellous bone grafting of the defect, and screw fixation. Various outcome measures were recorded prospectively, including numeric rating scales (NRS) of pain at rest, climbing stairs, and running, American Orthopaedic Foot & Ankle Society (AOFAS) Ankle and Hindfoot clinical rating System, Foot and Ankle Outcome Score (FAOS), and

Short Form 36 (SF-36). After 1 year follow-up, there was significant improvement in the NRS, AOFAS, four of five subscales of the FAOS, and the SF-36 physical component scale. There were four minor complications that resolved within the study period. Three patients reported an area of numbness about the scar, which resolved within the postoperative year. Another patient had a superficial wound infection, which was effectively treated by oral antibiotics. On radiographs there were no signs of prosthetic loosening, cyst formation, or degenerative changes at 1 year follow-up (Fig. 17.3). The medial malleolar osteotomy healed in all cases.

Alternative current treatment methods for large or secondary lesions are osteochondral autograft transfer system (OATS), cancellous bone grafting, an osteochondral allograft, ankle arthrodesis, or ankle arthroplasty. Although excellent results of OATS have been published [17], the risk of donor site morbidity in the knee is worrisome [19]. An additional disadvantage of osteochondral autografts is difficulty in matching the talar surface geometry and poor graft integration [12]. Limited availability and donor site pain are also disadvantages of cancellous bone grafting [2]. Osteochondral allografts can be used for massive defects but are not recommended for localized OCDs, based upon the gradual deterioration of the hyaline part of such grafts in the knee and resorption and fragmentation of the graft [20]. Ankle arthrodesis and prosthesis are definite solutions for a recurrent OCD but are not preferable in young patients. Should the metal implant fail in the long term, it can be removed and the ankle joint fused.

The surgical approach is an important part of the implantation technique because the accuracy of implantation of this device strongly depends on the approach and quality of exposure. If the osteotomy is created too medially, i.e., in the articular facet of the malleolus, exposure of the talar dome may be insufficient for adequate treatment. Furthermore, a small distal fragment may be prone to fracture when fixed at the end of the procedure. Conversely, if the osteotomy is created too laterally, it will exit in the tibial plafond. This is undesirable because the medial

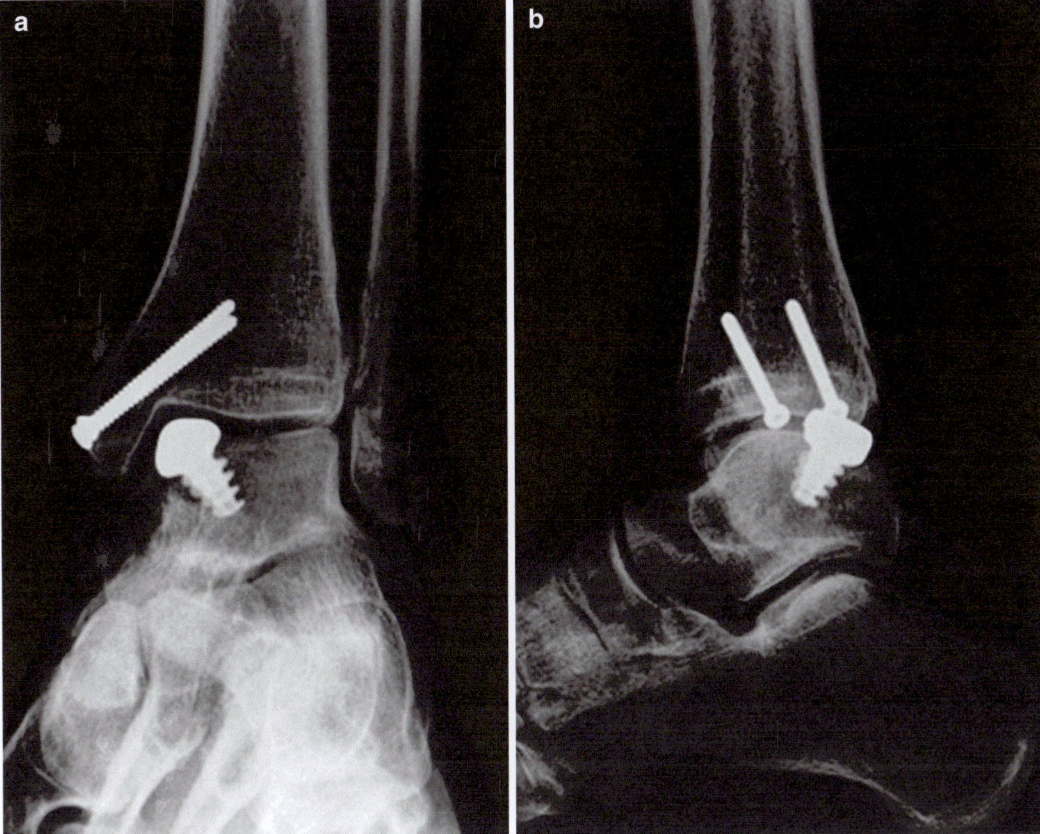

Fig. 17.3 Mortise (**a**) view and lateral (**b**) weight-bearing radiographs of a left ankle 1 year postoperatively showing correct positioning of the implant

tibial plafond directly articulates with the medial talar dome [11, 24], and damage to this weight-bearing area might lead to secondary osteoarthritis [7]. We therefore routinely use a probe to determine the intersection of the tibial plafond and the articular facet of the medial malleolus when performing the osteotomy [22].

The surface of the prosthetic device should be placed slightly recessed relative to the surrounding surface of the talar cartilage because talar cartilage deforms during weight bearing while the implant does not. Wan et al. measured a peak cartilage deformation of 34.5 % ± 7.3 % under full body weight in persons with a medial talar dome cartilage thickness of 1.42 ± 0.31 mm [28]. We therefore aim at an implantation level of 0.5 mm below the adjacent cartilage. This implantation level was found appropriate in a previous cadaveric study [24]. When the prosthetic device is correctly implanted, excessive contact pressures of the implant on the tibial plafond are avoided [24].

Conclusion

In summary, the metallic implantation technique appears to be a new promising treatment option for osteochondral defects of the medial talar dome after failed primary treatment. Although the clinical and radiological results with 1 year follow-up are encouraging, more patients and longer follow-up are clearly needed to draw any firm conclusions and determine if the results continue with time.

Conflict of Interest The author has no current conflict of interests with the products presented

References

1. Anderson DD, Tochigi Y, Rudert MJ, Vaseenon T, Brown TD, Amendola A. Effect of implantation accuracy on ankle contact mechanics with a metallic focal resurfacing implant. J Bone Joint Surg Am. 2010;92:1490–500.

2. Arrington ED, Smith WJ, Chambers HG, Bucknell AL, Davino NA. Complications of iliac crest bone graft harvesting. Clin Orthop Relat Res. 1996;329:300–9.

3. Baums MH, Heidrich G, Schultz W, Steckel H, Kahl E, Klinger HM. Autologous chondrocyte transplantation for treating cartilage defects of the talus. J Bone Joint Surg Am. 2006;88:303–8.

4. Canale ST, Belding RH. Osteochondral lesions of the talus. J Bone Joint Surg Am. 1980;62:97–102.

5. Davidson PA, Rivenburgh D. Focal anatomic patellofemoral inlay resurfacing: theoretic basis, surgical technique, and case reports. Orthop Clin North Am. 2008;39:337–46.

6. Elias I, Zoga AC, Morrison WB, Besser MP, Schweitzer ME, Raikin SM. Osteochondral lesions of the talus: localization and morphologic data from 424 patients using a novel anatomical grid scheme. Foot Ankle Int. 2007;28:154–61.

7. Gaulrapp H, Hagena FW, Wasmer G. Postoperative evaluation of osteochondrosis dissecans of the talus with special reference to medial malleolar osteotomy. Z Orthop Ihre Grenzgeb. 1996;134:346–53.

8. Gautier E, Kolker D, Jakob RP. Treatment of cartilage defects of the talus by autologous osteochondral grafts. J Bone Joint Surg Br. 2002;84:237–44.

9. Hangody L, Kish G, Modis L, Szerb I, Gaspar L, Dioszegi Z, et al. Mosaicplasty for the treatment of osteochondritis dissecans of the talus: two to seven year results in 36 patients. Foot Ankle Int. 2001;22:552–8.

10. Hasselman C, Shields N. Resurfacing of the first metatarsal head in the treatment of hallux rigidus. Tech Foot Ankle Surg. 2008;7:31–40.

11. Millington S, Grabner M, Wozelka R, Hurwitz S, Crandall J. A stereophotographic study of ankle joint contact area. J Orthop Res. 2007;25:1465–73.

12. Nosewicz TL, Reilingh ML, Wolny M, van Dijk CN, Duda GN, Schell H. Influence of basal support and early loading on bone cartilage healing in press-fitted osteochondral autografts. Knee Surg Sports Traumatol Arthrosc. 2013. [Epub ahead of print].

13. Paul J, Sagstetter A, Kriner M, Imhoff AB, Spang J, Hinterwimmer S. Donor-site morbidity after osteochondral autologous transplantation for lesions of the talus. J Bone Joint Surg Am. 2009;91:1683–8.

14. Reddy S, Pedowitz DI, Parekh SG, Sennett BJ, Okereke E. The morbidity associated with osteochondral harvest from asymptomatic knees for the treatment of osteochondral lesions of the talus. Am J Sports Med. 2007;35:80–5.

15. Reilingh ML, van Bergen CJ, van Dijk CN. Diagnosis and treatment of osteochondral defects of the ankle. S Afr Orthop J. 2009;8:44–50.

16. Reilingh ML, van Bergen CJ, van Dijk CN. Novel metal implantation technique for osteochondral defects of the medial talar dome. Tech Foot Ankle Surg. 2012;11:45–9.

17. Scranton Jr PE, Frey CC, Feder KS. Outcome of osteochondral autograft transplantation for type-V cystic osteochondral lesions of the talus. J Bone Joint Surg Br. 2006;88:614–9.

18. Uribe JW, Botto-van Bemden A. Partial humeral head resurfacing for osteonecrosis. J Shoulder Elbow Surg. 2009;18:711–6.

19. Valderrabano V, Leumann A, Rasch H, Egelhof T, Hintermann B, Pagenstert G. Knee-to-ankle mosaicplasty for the treatment of osteochondral lesions of the ankle joint. Am J Sports Med. 2009;37:105S–11.

20. van Bergen CJ, de Leeuw PA, van Dijk CN. Treatment of osteochondral defects of the talus. Rev Chir Orthop Reparatrice Appar Mot. 2008;94:398–408.

21. van Bergen CJ, Reilingh ML, van Dijk CN. Tertiary osteochondral defect of the talus treated by a novel contoured metal implant. Knee Surg Sports Traumatol Arthrosc. 2011;19:999–1003.

22. van Bergen CJ, Tuijthof GJ, Reilingh ML, van Dijk CN. Clinical tip: aiming probe for a precise medial malleolar osteotomy. Foot Ankle Int. 2012;33:764–6.

23. van Bergen CJ, Tuijthof GJ, Sierevelt IN, van Dijk CN. Direction of the oblique medial malleolar osteotomy for exposure of the talus. Arch Orthop Trauma Surg. 2011;131:893–901.

24. van Bergen CJ, Zengerink M, Blankevoort L, van Sterkenburg MN, van Oldenrijk J, van Dijk CN. Novel metallic implantation technique for osteochondral defects of the medial talar dome. A cadaver study. Acta Orthop. 2010;81:495–502.

25. van Dijk CN, Reilingh ML, Zengerink M, van Bergen CJ. Osteochondral defects in the ankle: why painful? Knee Surg Sports Traumatol Arthrosc. 2010;18:570–80.

26. van Dijk CN, Verhagen RA, Tol JL. Arthroscopy for problems after ankle fracture. J Bone Joint Surg Br. 1997;79:280–4.

27. Van Stralen RA, Haverkamp D, van Bergen CJ, Eijer H. Partial resurfacing with varus osteotomy for an osteochondral defect of the femoral head. Hip Int. 2009;19:67–70.

28. Wan L, de Asla RJ, Rubash HE, Li G. In vivo cartilage contact deformation of human ankle joints under full body weight. J Orthop Res. 2008;26:1081–9.

29. Zengerink M, Struijs PA, Tol JL, van Dijk CN. Treatment of osteochondral lesions of the talus: a systematic review. Knee Surg Sports Traumatol Arthrosc. 2010;18:238–46.

Index

A

American College of Radiology (ACR), 41
The American Orthopaedic Foot and Ankle Society
    (AOFAS), 98–99
AOFAS. *See* The American Orthopaedic Foot and Ankle
    Society (AOFAS)
Arthroscopy after ankle fracture
    abnormal motion at tibiofibular joint, 14
    acute osteochondral fragment, 14
    articular cartilage injury
        incidence at time, 10–11
        treatment at operative treatment of ankle
            fracture, 11–12
    bimalleolar ankle fracture with soft tissue
        injury, 16
    distal fibula fracture, medial mortise widening, 15
    distal tibiofibular joint, 14
    indications, 9
    intra-articular injuries, 9–10
    intraoperative photographs, 16–17
    minimally invasive arthroscopic-assisted internal
        fixation, 15
    "nick and spread" technique, 13
    provisional fixation, 17
    residual pain
        articular cartilage damage, 13
        chondral lesions, talus/tibia, 12
        malunion, articular surfaces, 12
    syndesmotic injury, diagnosis, 13
    three-portal technique, 18
    torn fibers, 14
Arthroscopy, OCDs
    characteristics, 48, 49
    chondral lesions, talus, 43
    classification
        ICRS, 44, 45
        imaging studies, 44
        stage D and F medial talar dome lesion, 44
    ICRS grade 4 unconstrained shoulder defect, 48
    vs. imaging (*see* Imaging *vs.* arthroscopy)
    indications, 46
    large superficial flap and fissures, 47
    morbidity with surgical approaches, 43

    notch of Harty, 47
    roughened surface and ICRS grade 2 changes, 47
    with small superficial flap and fissure, 48
    talar dome with no chondral defect, 47
    twenty-one-point ankle arthroscopic
        examination, 46
    zone classification I, II and III, 48, 49
Arthrotomy
    medial talar dome, OCLs, 69
    posterolateral talar dome, OLTs, 58
Articular cartilage injury
    incidence at ankle fracture
        AO-Danis-Weber classification, 10
        articular cartilage lesions, 10
        "cartilaginous injury", 10
    treatment at operative treatment of ankle fracture
        acute osteochondral fractures, 11
        Kirschner wires, advantages, 12
        talar dome, acute osteochondral lesions, 12
Autologous chondrocyte implantation (ACI)
    description, 87
    and MACI (*see* Matrix-induced autologous
        chondrocyte implantation (MACI))
    and OATS, 84
    and OLT, 136
    phase I and II, 136–137
    phase III and IV, 138
    preoperative planning, OCDs, 53–54
    protocols, 136
    regeneration, tissue, 87
    treatment, 90

B

Balanced steady-state free precession (bSSFP), 23
Beam hardening, 33
BMS. *See* Bone marrow stimulation (BMS)
Bone marrow stimulation (BMS)
    drilling/microfracturing, 83
    excision and curettage, 86–87
    and OATS, 89
    preoperative planning, OCDs, 52
    rehabilitation (*see* Rehabilitation)

C.N. van Dijk, J.G. Kennedy (eds.), *Talar Osteochondral Defects*,
DOI 10.1007/978-3-642-45097-6, © ESSKA 2014

C

Cartilage reconstruction
  ACI and MACI, 136
  articular damage, 135
  Juvenile allograft implantation, 141–142
Chondral injury, diagnosis after supination trauma
  ankle arthroscopy, 5–6
  arthroscopic examination, 6
  dGEMRIC technique, 5
  evaluation, 2
  hindfoot valgus and "flatfoot type", 1
  radiological examination
    ankle sprain, 4
    chondral flake medial talus, 5
    CT, 2–4
    radiography, 2
    T2 mapping, 5
    3 T MRI, 4
  sharp deep pain, 2
Computed tomography (CT)
  advantages
    additional bony pathologies, 35
    fast and submillimeter resolution, 35
    operative approach decision, 35
    scanning both ankles at the same time, 35
    weight-bearing cone beam CT, 35
  arthrography
    late-phase SPECT-CT coronal and sagittal
      images, 36–38
    upper ankle joint space, 36
  artifacts, 33
  beam hardening, 33
  disadvantages, 40
  helical, 106
  "kernels", 32
  kissing osteochondral defect, 39–40
  and OCD
    cystic changes, tibial plafond, 34
    field of view (FOV), 33
    fragmentation and detachment, 33
    multicystic osteochondral defect, 34
  partial volume averaging, 33
  pathologies, 107
  plain radiography, 31–32
  postoperative analysis, OCD, 39
  quality of image, 32
  right ankle, 106, 107
  staging systems
    kissing osteochondral defect, 40
    multicystic defect, located medial in talar dome, 39
    medial talar dome, 39
    prognosis and therapeutic planning, 38
Coronal fat-saturated DESS sequence, 26
CT. *See* Computed tomography (CT)

D

Danis-Weber B injuries, 10
Danis-Weber C injuries, 10
Delayed gadolinium-enhanced magnetic resonance
    imaging of cartilage (dGEM-RIC) technique, 5

Dual echo steady state (DESS). *See* Sagittal fat-saturated
    DESS sequence; *See* Coronal fat-saturated
    DESS sequence
dGEMRIC. *See* Delayed gadolinium-enhanced magnetic
    resonance imaging of cartilage (dGEMRIC)
    technique

F

FAAM. *See* Foot and ankle ability measure (FAAM)
FAOS. *See* Foot and ankle outcome score (FAOS)
Fat-suppressed fast spoiled gradient echo (FSPGR), 108
Femoral condyle/tibial plateau
  phase I and II, 121–122
  phase III and IV, 122
  proposed scheme
    phase I and II, 123
    phase III and IV, 123–124
Foot and ankle ability measure (FAAM), 99–100
Foot and ankle outcome score (FAOS), 99, 148
FSPGR. *See* Fat-suppressed fast spoiled gradient echo
    (FSPGR)

G

Gadolinium diethylenetriamine pentaacetic acid
    (Gd-DTPA^{2-}), 5

H

The Hannover ankle score, 99

I

ICRS. *See* The International Cartilage
    Repair Society (ICRS)
Imaging *vs.* arthroscopy
  ankle instability, 46
  MRI, 45
  physical examination and baseline radiographs, 44
  sensitivity and specificity, OCDs, 45
The International Cartilage Repair Society (ICRS), 108

J

Juvenile allograft cartilage implantation
  description, 141–142
  rehabilitation, 142

K

Kissing defect, 39–40

M

MACI. *See* Matrix-induced autologous chondrocyte
    implantation (MACI)
Magnetic resonance imaging (MRI)
  accuracy, OCLs, 26
  ACI, 107
  ankle

bSSFP, 23
chimney coils, 22
clinical sequences and parameters,
    ankle imaging, 23
3D fast spin-echo sequences, 22
fat-saturated intermediate-weighted fast spin-echo
    sequences, 22
MENSA, 23
spinecho sequences, 22
STIR sequences, 23
arthroscopic visual scoring, 107
cartilage repair
    management options, 28
    MOCART scoring system, 28–29
    multidetector helical CT, preoperative planning, 29
    procedures, 28
classification, 24
collagen orientation, 107, 108
coronal fat-saturated
    DESS sequence, 26
    intermediate weighted fast spin echo sequence, 24
    and sagittal weighted fast spin echo sequence, 25,
        27
DESS sequence, 24
FSPGR, 108
maturation, cartilage, 109
MOCART, 107
modified Outerbridge and Noyes classifications, 25
noninvasive follow-up imaging, 109
OATS/mosaicplasty, 28
OCD, 21
sagittal fat-saturated
    fluid sensitive and gadolinium-enhanced spin echo
        sequences, 28
    intermediate weighted and T1-weighted fast spin
        echo sequences, 25–27
signal morphology, repair tissue, 107
stress-related changes, bone marrow, 27
Magnetic resonance observation of cartilage repair tissue
    (MOCART), 28
Matrix-induced autologous chondrocyte implantation
    (MACI)
    description, 138–139
    immobilization, 140
    phase I and II, 140
    phase III, 140–141
    postoperative rehabilitation, 139
    and ROM, 139
Medial talar dome, OCLs
    arthroscopic access
        arthrotomy/osteotomy, 68
        microfracture, 68
        patient, prone and supine position, 68–69
        surgery, ankles, 67–68
    Chevron cut, 70
    extensile exposures, 69–71
    non-arthroscopic access
        arthrotomy, 69
        autograft/allograft transplantation, 69
    osteotomy cut, 70, 71
    techniques and comparison, 69, 70

MENSA. *See* Multiecho in steady-state acquisition
    (MENSA)
Meta-analysis therapy
    ACI, 87, 90
    antegrade drilling, 87
    BMS, excision and curettage, 86–87
    bone graft, curettage and excision, 87
    data extraction and sources, 84
    description, 83
    excision and curettage, 86
    fixation, 88
    nonoperative treatment
        cast immobilization, 86
        NSAIDs, 85–86
        symptoms, 86
    OATS, 87
    OCL, 83
    population characteristics, 85, 86
    quality assessment, 85, 88
    RCT, 90
    retrograde drilling, 87–88
    selection, inclusion and exclusion, 84
    TMD and ACI, 83
    transmalleolar drilling, 89
    treatments, 90
MOCART. *See* Magnetic resonance observation of
    cartilage repair tissue (MOCART)
Mosaicplasty. *See* Osteochondral autograft transfer
    system (OATS)
MRI. *See* Magnetic resonance imaging (MRI)
Multiecho in steady-state acquisition (MENSA), 23

N
Newcastle–Ottawa scale (NOS), 91
"Nick and spread" technique, 13
Nonsteroidal anti-inflammatory drugs (NSAIDs), 85
NRS. *See* Numeric rating scales (NRSs)
NSAIDs. *See* Nonsteroidal anti-inflammatory drugs
    (NSAIDs)
Numeric rating scales (NRSs), 101, 148

O
OATS. *See* Osteochondral autograft transfer system (OATS)
OCDs. *See* Osteochondral defects (OCDs)
OCLs. *See* Osteochondral lesions (OCLs)
Orthopedic procedures, outcome assessment
    ankle joint, radiographic and MRI, 95, 97–98
    clinical and functional scores
        AOFAS, 98–99
        FAAM, 99–100
        FAOS, 99
        foot and ankle, 95–96
        Hannover ankle score, 99
        Ogilvie-Harris and Berndt and Harty scores, 100
    CT, 101–102
    description, 95
    MRI, 102
    pain (*see* Pain assessment)
    radiography, 101

Osteochondral autograft transfer system (OATS)
    metal implant, 53
    secondary treatment options, 51
    and transplantation techniques (*see* Osteochondral
        transplantation techniques)
    treatment methods, 148
Osteochondral defects (OCDs)
    description, 51
    OATS, HemiCAP and ACI, 51
    preoperative planning
        ACI, 53–54
        BMS, 52
        CT and MRI, 52
        fixation, 52
        HemiCAP, OATS and allograft, 53
        operative talar treatment, 52, 53
        retrograde drilling, 54
        sliding calcaneal osteotomy, 53
        soft tissue distraction, 52
    treatment types, 51–52
Osteochondral lesions (OCLs)
    ankle
        cartilage assessment efficacy, 105
        CT, 106–107
        imaging methods, 105
        MRI, 107–109
        OCLs, 105
        second-look arthroscopy, 109–110
        X-ray, 106
    description, 67
    medial talar dome (*see* Medial talar dome, OCLs)
Osteochondral lesions of the distal tibial plafond (OLTP).
        See Tibial plafond
Osteochondral lesions of the talus (OLTs)
    lateral talar dome, 55
    posterolateral talar dome
        arthroscopic access, 56–57
        non-arthroscopic access, 57–61
    resurfacing techniques, 61–62
    retrograde drilling, 57
    surgical management, 55–56
    types, 56
Osteochondral transplantation techniques
    and ACI, 84
    allografts, 87
    application, 129
    cartilage resurfacing procedures, 130
    femoral condyles and patellotrochlear
        surfaces, 129
    medial malleolar fractures, 131
    mosaicplasty, 130
    rehabilitation protocol
        cylindrical autograft and allograft transplantation,
            131–132
        donor knee, 132
        fibular and Chaput osteotomies, 132
        fresh talar osteochondral allografts, 132
        graft integration, 132
        large-volume cystic lesions, 133

    tissue regeneration, 130
    transplants, 87
    treatment, 90
Osteochondritis dissecans (OCD), 21

P
Pain assessment
    NRS, 101
    VAS, 100–101
    VRS, 101
Posterolateral talar dome, OLTs
    arthroscopic access, patients
        prone position, 57
        supine position, 56–57
    non-arthroscopic access
        ACI, 60
        anterior tibial wedge osteotomy, 58–59
        arthrotomy, 58
        cadaveric model, 59
        description, 57
        exposure after ATFL release and oblique fibular
            osteotomy, 59, 60
        microsagittal saw excision, talus, 61
        resurfacing procedures, 57
        sagittal plane exposure, anterolateral
            arthrotomy, 59
        structural allograft reconstruction, 60
        talus extraction, 61

R
Range of motion (ROM)
    ankle, 140
    exercises, 139
    protocol, 140
Rehabilitation
    after arthroscopic BMS
        ankle, 120–121
        tissue healing, 119–120
    cartilage reconstruction (*see* Cartilage reconstruction)
    CPM and BMS, 119
    description, 119
    femoral condyle/tibial plateau, 121–124
    knee microfracture, 121
Retrograde drilling
    OLTs, 57
    preoperative planning, OCDs, 54
Return to sports
    ACI, 115
    activity level, 113
    allograft implant, 114–115
    bone marrow stimulation, 114
    fixation, 115
    HemiCAP, 115
    OATS, 114
    OCD, 113
    retrograde drilling, 115
    return to activity, 114

sliding calcaneal osteotomy, 115
  timeline, activity levels, 115, 116
ROM. *See* Range of motion (ROM)

S
Sagittal fat-saturated DESS sequence, 24
Second-look arthroscopy, 109–110
Short-tau inversion recovery (STIR), 23
Single-photon emission computed tomography
        (SPECT-CT)
  advantages
    implanted hardware, 41
    osteoblast-specific tracers, 41
  disadvantages
    false-positive findings, 41
    infrastructure, 41
  interobserver correlation, 41
  osteoblast-specific tracers, 41
  planar technetium-labeled skeletal scintigraphy, 40
  therapeutic planning, 41
Sliding calcaneal osteotomy, 53
SPECT-CT. *See* Single-photon emission computed
        tomography (SPECT-CT)
Standard radiography (X-Ray), 3, 106
STIR. *See* Short-tau inversion recovery (STIR)
Syndesmotic injury. *See* Arthroscopy after ankle fracture

T
Talar dome resurfacing
  arthroscopic debridement, 145
  bone marrow stimulation, 145
  HemiCap, 146

  metallic implantation technique, 149
  OATS, 148
  osteochondral allografts, 148
  osteonecrosis, 148
  rehabilitation, 147–148
  surgical technique, 146–147
Three-portal technique, 18
Tibial plafond
  ankle instability, 76
  anteroposterior radiograph, 76, 77
  bleeding, microfracture pick, 79, 80
  description, 75
  etiological factors, 75
  intraoperative image intensification
    antegrade packing, bone graft, 79
    curette debriding, 78, 79
    drilling into cyst, 78, 79
    placement, guide pin, 78, 79
  microfracture pick, 79, 80
  nonoperative treatment, 76–77
  OLTP
    arthroscopic view, 78
    post debridement, 78
  osteochondral plugs, 81
  postoperative management, 80
  sagittal cut CT scan, 76, 78
  surgical treatment, 80–81
  "switch stick", 81
Transmalleolar drilling (TMD), 83

V
Verbal rating scale (VRS), 101
Visual analog scale (VAS), 100–101